Treatments That Work With Children

Treatments That Work With Children

*Empirically Supported Strategies
for Managing Childhood Problems*

Edward R. Christophersen and Susan L. Mortweet

American Psychological Association
Washington, DC

Second Printing, June 2002

Published by
American Psychological Association
750 First Street, NE
Washington, DC 20002
www.apa.org

To order
APA Order Department
P.O. Box 92984
Washington, DC 20090-2984
Tel: (800) 374-2721, Direct: (202) 336-5510
Fax: (202) 336-5502, TDD/TTY: (202) 336-6123
Online: www.apa.org/books/
Email: order@apa.org

In the U.K., Europe, Africa, and the Middle East, copies may be ordered from
American Psychological Association
3 Henrietta Street
Covent Garden, London
WC2E 8LU England

Typeset in Goudy by Monotype Composition, Baltimore, MD

Printer: Sheridan Books, Ann Arbor, MI
Cover Designer: NiDesign, Baltimore, MD
Technical/Production Editor: Jennifer L. Macomber

The opinions and statements published are the responsibility of the authors, and such opinions and statements do not necessarily represent the policies of the American Psychological Association.

Library of Congress Cataloging-in-Publication Data

Christophersen, Edward R.
  Treatments that work with children : empirically supported strategies for managing childhood problems / Edward R. Christophersen, Susan L. Mortweet.
    p. cm.
  Includes bibliographical references and index.
  ISBN 1-55798-759-9 (alk. paper)
  1. Child psychiatry.   2. Pediatrics—Psychosomatic aspects.   I. Mortweet, Susan L. II. Title.

RJ499.C492 2001
618.92'891—dc21   00-048526

British Library Cataloguing-in-Publication Data
A CIP record is available from the British Library.

Printed in the United States of America

CONTENTS

List of Exhibits, Tables, and Figures vii

Acknowledgments xi

Introduction 3

Chapter 1.   Diagnosis and Management of Disruptive
Behavior Disorders 11

Chapter 2.   Diagnosis and Management of Anxiety Disorders 49

Chapter 3.   Diagnosis and Management of Habit Disorders 79

Chapter 4.   Diagnosis and Management of Sleep Problems 99

Chapter 5.   Diagnosis and Management of Encopresis 123

Chapter 6.   Diagnosis and Management of Nocturnal
Enuresis 145

Chapter 7.   Assessment and Management of Pain 159

Chapter 8.   Management of Adherence to Pediatric
Medical Regimens 201

Appendix A: The Home Chip System: A Treatment
Manual 223

Appendix B: Progressive Muscle Relaxation Exercises 241

References 245

Author Index 285

Subject Index 297

About the Authors 309

EXHIBITS, TABLES, AND FIGURES

EXHIBITS

Exhibit 1.1 *DSM–IV* Criteria for Oppositional Defiant
Disorder, 313.81 12

Exhibit 1.2 *DSM–IV* Criteria for Conduct Disorder, 312.90 14

Exhibit 1.3 *DSM–IV* Criteria for Attention Deficit Hyperactivity
Disorder, 314.01, 314.00 15

Exhibit 1.4 Time-In 31

Exhibit 1.5 Teaching Your Child to Follow Instructions 32

Exhibit 1.6 Problem-Solving Skills-Training Steps 37

Exhibit 1.7 Barkley Side Effects Questionnaire 43

Exhibit 1.8 Summary of Parent Training Program for Children With
Attention Deficit Hyperactivity Disorder 44

Exhibit 1.9 Therapy Checklist 46

Exhibit 2.1 *DSM–IV* Criteria for Four Common Anxiety Disorders
in Children 51

Exhibit 2.2 Anxiety Disorder Differential 54

Exhibit 2.3 AACAP Components of Anxiety Assessment
for Children 59

Exhibit 3.1 *DSM–IV* Diagnostic Criteria for Tic Disorders and
Tourette's Disorder 80

Exhibit 3.2 *DSM–IV* Diagnostic Criteria for Stereotypic
Movement Disorders and Trichotillomania 81

Exhibit 3.3 Thumb-Sucking Handout 90

Exhibit 3.4 Habit Reversal Training for Reducing Children's Tics .. 93

Exhibit 4.1 *DSM–IV* Criteria for Primary Insomnia and Primary
Hypersomnia 102

Exhibit 4.2 *DSM–IV* Criteria for Nightmare Disorder, Sleep Terrors,
and Sleepwalking Disorder 103
Exhibit 4.3 Intake Form for Children With Sleep Problems 108
Exhibit 4.4 Sleep Diary 109
Exhibit 4.5 Teaching Your Baby to Sleep Through the Night 111
Exhibit 4.6 Day Correction of Bedtime Problems 118

Exhibit 5.1 *DSM–IV* Criteria for Encopresis 124
Exhibit 5.2 Bowel Problem Intake Form 129
Exhibit 5.3 Teaching Muscle Relaxation and Tightening for
Better Bowel Movement 140
Exhibit 5.4 Bowel Symptom Rating Sheet 141

Exhibit 6.1 *DSM–IV* Criteria for Enuresis 146
Exhibit 6.2 Enuresis Intake Form 148
Exhibit 6.3 Practical Tips for Successful Use of an Enuresis Alarm .. 152
Exhibit 6.4 Dry-Bed Training Procedures 153
Exhibit 6.5 Positive Practice for Toileting Accidents 156

Exhibit 7.1 *DSM–IV* Diagnostic Criteria for Pain Disorders and
Somatization Disorder 161
Exhibit 7.2 Types of Pain Experienced by Children With
Chronic Disease 163
Exhibit 7.3 Possible Reasons for the Inadequate Management of
Pain in Children 164
Exhibit 7.4 Examples of Clinical Assessment Measures for
Child Pain and Distress 169
Exhibit 7.5 Poker Chip Tool 174
Exhibit 7.6 Pain Diary 178
Exhibit 7.7 Suggested Elements to Include in Guided Images 186

Exhibit 8.1 Factors That Influence Adherence to Medical
Regimens 203
Exhibit 8.2 Strategies for Providing Effective Patient Education 207
Exhibit 8.3 Pill-Swallowing Handout for Parents 210
Exhibit 8.4 Design Strategies for Developing Low-Literacy
Materials 211
Exhibit 8.5 Examples of Contract Components to Enhance Adherence
to a Medication Regimen 213
Exhibit 8.6 Possible Solutions for Dealing With Problematic
Mealtimes for Children With Diabetes 220

TABLES

Table 1.1   Diagnostic Criteria for Disruptive Behavior Disorders ... 17

Table 1.2   Behavior Rating Scales: Ages and Forms 25

Table 2.1   Five Self-Report Measures for Assessing Anxiety
in Children 62

Table 2.2   Summary of Kendall's CBT Sessions 70

Table 3.1   Differential Diagnosis of Tic Disorders 83

Table 3.2   Pharmacological Treatments for Habit Disorders and Tics   88

Table 3.3   A Comparison of Behavioral Treatments for Habit
Disorders and Tics 95

Table 4.1   The *DSM–IV* Differential Criteria for Primary Insomnia,
Primary Hypersomnia, Nightmare Disorder, Sleep Terror
Disorder, and Sleepwalking 104

Table 5.1   Symptoms of Encopresis and Hirschsprung Disease 131

Table 5.2   *DSM–IV* Diagnostic Criteria for Toileting Problems
in Children 132

Table 5.3   Dietary Fiber Content of Selected Foods 138

Table 6.1   Some Alarm Devices for the Treatment of
Primary Enuresis 155

Table 7.1   Pain Experience History for Acute Pain Management ... 170

Table 7.2   Pain as Impairment-Recommended Self-Report
Measures in Children 172

Table 7.3   Interventions for Addressing Procedure-Related
Pain and Anxiety 184

Table 7.4   Example of Group Cognitive–Behavioral Therapy for
Treating Recurrent Abdominal Pain 193

FIGURES

Figure 5.1   Schematic representation of a normal colon
and a megacolon 135

Figure 7.1   Example of a pain affect facial scale 175

Figure 7.2   Example of a pain thermometer 176

Figure 8.1   Asthma inhaler instruction sheet 209

Figure 8.2   Visual motivation chart for rotating insulin
injection sites 215

ACKNOWLEDGMENTS

We are very grateful to the many people who made this book a reality. First, we are grateful to the researchers and clinicians who are engaging in the endless pursuit of effective interventions to improve the lives of children in need. Your dedication and willingness to share your findings is the foundation of the future of psychology, as well as the reason a book like this can exist. We also gratefully acknowledge the American Psychological Association for providing us the opportunity to create this book and share it with our profession and the public.

I (ERC) would like to thank Nathan Azrin, then at Anna State Hospital in southern Illinois, for the most intense training of my life. He instilled in me a profound appreciation for the scientific method. Later, when Gerald Patterson organized the annual Social Learning in the Family conferences, I was able to use the skills I learned from Azrin.

We are also grateful to the many colleagues who supported our efforts. These include Jane Christophersen, Pat Friman, Michael Luxem, Rita Moser, Ann Palmer, Patricia Purvis, Michael Rapoff, Tammy Watson, Joel Wagaman, Misty Skaff, and Kevin Turner. Of course, the most heartfelt thank you is extended to our respective families and friends, who sacrificed their time and needs as well to support us in our endeavor. Finally, thank you to all of the children who have taught us more than we ever thought we could learn.

Treatments That Work With Children

INTRODUCTION

Parents' concerns about their children's behavioral and emotional development are quite common. Many studies are available that have investigated the prevalence of these concerns in the general population. One in 7 mothers of preschool children report a problem in growth or development, and 1 in 10 mothers report a difficulty in behavior or discipline (Starfield, 1982). More specifically, Starfield stated that 15% of children ages 5–14 years are reported to have a behavioral or discipline problem, with another 10% reported to have problems in social relationships. Temper tantrums and other difficult-to-control behaviors are also common and often persistent in children. Although many children with common emotional and behavior problems may never come to the attention of a pediatrician or a mental health professional, there are a significant number of children[1] in need of psychological intervention to manage issues that are interfering with their development and daily functioning.

Despite the prevalence of such problems in children, there has been relatively little research on therapy with children. In the area of psychotherapy research, few of the published works have addressed the efficacy of interventions with children. A survey of over 3,000 studies revealed a mere 218 (7.3% of those surveyed) on outcomes of child interventions

---

[1]Throughout this book, the terms *child* and *children* are used to refer to both children and adolescents.

(Kazdin, Bass, Ayers, & Rodgers, 1990). Similarly, J. S. Allen, Tarnowski, Simonian, Elliott, and Drabman (1991) examined more than 15,000 studies to locate 904 treatment outcomes (around 6% of those surveyed) that focused on children. The dearth of intervention studies in clinical child psychology only adds to the burden of clinicians who are responsible for the treatment of children. In response to this shortcoming in the field of psychology, an interest in evaluating and developing empirically supported treatments for children has emerged.

EMPIRICALLY SUPPORTED TREATMENTS FOR CHILDREN

Over the past 30 years, there has been a movement, beginning in Canada with the Canadian Task Force on Periodic Health Examination (1979), that has called for an improvement in the "quality of evidence" in studies that purport to benefit children, adolescents, and adults. Within the field of medicine, the term *evidence-based medicine* has been used to stress the importance of the examination of evidence from clinical research (Evidence-Based Working Group, 1992). In clinical psychology, this movement has focused on the need for evidence that procedures are treatments that "work" or treatments that are "empirically supported." In the sense addressed by the American Psychological Association (APA) Task Force on Empirically Supported Treatments, the term *empirically supported treatments* refers to treatments that have been subjected to rigorous scientific investigation (Chambless et al., 1996). That is, the treatments have been studied in more than one setting, using prospective random assignment to alternative treatments, using multiple measures, and using a carefully selected and well-defined participant population.

The APA Task Force identified several procedures that were either "well-established" or "probably efficacious" for the treatment of children. These included the following: behavior modification for enuresis and encopresis, cognitive–behavioral therapy for pain, cognitive–behavioral therapy for generalized anxiety disorder, parent training programs for children with oppositional behavior, token economy programs, and habit reversal and control techniques for habit disorders and tics. Kazdin and Weisz (1998), in a thorough review of the literature on treatment outcome, also identified several promising examples of treatments for problems experienced by children. The example for externalizing problems included cognitive problem-solving skills training and parent management training for oppositional and aggressive children. We review such interventions in the chapters that follow.

The advantages of empirically supported treatments include much greater acceptability of psychological interventions by our colleagues in medicine, better replication of procedures by clinicians in other settings, and greater specificity for trainees at all levels. The main disadvantage of placing such a premium on empirically supported treatments is that procedures that are very effective but that have not been studied scientifically will be much more difficult to get accepted into mainstream clinical psychology. And, much of the research that was done in the past, before these newly agreed-on criteria, may have the appearance of "falling short" of the new criteria.

As either a part of, or in addition to, the increased importance attributed to empirically supported treatments, three major issues have been discussed and argued: manualized treatments, the impact of comorbidity on assessment and treatment outcome, and the impact of cultural and ethnic diversity on assessment and treatment of child problems. These issues are discussed briefly below, followed by a description of the purpose of this book.

Treatment Manuals

Treatment manuals are used to describe the precise treatment procedures that were used in an outcome study, both during the actual conduct of the study and when the treatment is described in the written report of the study. Typically, treatment manuals have been used in large research projects that evaluate treatment outcomes. Often, researchers measure the degree to which the therapists in the study have followed the treatment manual. Doing so provides a level of specificity that would otherwise not be possible and provides for the measurement of treatment integrity.

The development of treatment manuals represents an effort to operationalize treatments and facilitate the standardization of treatments across participants, settings, and therapists (Hibbs et al., 1997). Manuals that are more detailed and scripted tend to offer greater reproducibility across different studies, therapists, and settings; that is, interventions will more likely be delivered in the same way every time. The manuals increase confidence that only active treatment elements account for observed effects, rather than unique characteristics of the therapist or setting (Hibbs et al., 1997). If treatment manuals can be developed that enable a properly trained psychologist to know when and how to implement an intervention strategy that alleviates even one aspect of human suffering, deficiency, or excess, the field of psychology will experience a growth and standing unparalleled in psychology's history.

Despite the potential contribution of treatment manuals, there are some concerns reported in the literature about "manualization." Hibbs et al. (1997) stated the concern that clinical treatment is an interactive, very personal process that cannot be adequately described in manual form. When blindly adhered to, treatment can become far too direct, rigid, and less adaptable to unique client issues. There is also a concern that the manualization of therapy used in outcome research does not adequately or validly represent the psychotherapy that is conventionally practiced.

It is interesting to note that one of the major concerns regarding "manualized treatment"—that the needs of individual clients would not be taken into consideration—has not been realized. In fact, in a review of the published research on treatment manuals, Eifert, Schulte, Zvolensky, Lejuez, and Lau (1997) concluded just the opposite. They stated that tailoring treatment to target an individual's particular problem beyond the level of clinical diagnosis does not seem to improve overall treatment outcome. Moreover, many studies involved a more flexible application of standardized treatment manuals than was intended or anticipated. That is, although there has been a fear expressed that manualized treatment will remove or at least deemphasize the importance of the clinician's own skills when implementing treatments, this fear has not been supported in the published literature.

Iwamasa and Orsillo (1997) emphasized that graduate students must, at a minimum, be exposed to manualized treatment to foster a comprehensive understanding of behavioral and cognitive–behavioral theory. Being exposed to manualized treatments clearly does not mean that the trainee must mechanically implement the procedures described in the manuals. Rather, the treatments described in the manuals provide the details that the authors of the respective studies thought were important. Such details may also contribute to the evolution of treatment procedures as other researchers and clinicians are able to investigate the effectiveness of intervention modifications. One example of the evolution of treatment procedures is the *habit reversal* procedures, originally described by Azrin and Foxx (1974) and later empirically shortened by Miltenberger, Finney, and their colleagues (Miltenberger, Fuqua, & McKinley, 1985; Finney, Rapoff, Hall, & Christophersen, 1983). Beginning with the 13 treatment components described by Azrin and Foxx, both Miltenberger and Finney have shortened the habit reversal procedures to include only 4 components. These procedures are discussed in detail in chapter 3 on the diagnosis and management of habit disorders. As we discuss the treatment of common child problems throughout this book, we will note when treatment manuals are available.

Comorbidity

50%

One limitation of the current state of empirically supported treatments is their representativeness of the true picture of mental health problems for children. For example, Hufford (2000) made the case that the disparity between the single diagnoses seen in the treatment literature and the complexity of cases seen in actual practice cannot be ignored. *Comorbidity*, which refers to the co-occurrence of a least two different disorders in the same individual, happens with great frequency in child, adolescent, and adult populations. In fact, epidemiological studies show that half of all people with mental disorders have more than one diagnosable disorder, and comorbidity rates are even higher in clinical samples (Clark, Watson, &

Reynolds, 1995). The exclusionary criteria used by some of the most important and widely cited psychotherapy outcome trials reveal that the full spectrum of psychopathology is not adequately represented.

Throughout this book, unless otherwise stated, the research that is reviewed and the interventions that are discussed have been hampered by the fact that they address specific problems as though they have occurred in isolation, when in fact they are almost always complicated by comorbidity. One notable exception is found in some research on anxiety done by Kendall et al. (1997), who explored the effects of comorbid disorders such as depression on the effectiveness of a cognitive–behavioral treatment for anxiety. In subsequent editions of this book, we hope that we will be able to review many more studies that address the issue of comorbidity in much greater depth.

Cultural Diversity

Although numerous discussion articles have highlighted the importance of the issue of cultural diversity, there are virtually no published research studies that have compared the outcomes of two or more ethnic groups that were exposed to identical treatments. When clients in different countries have presented with the same problems, similar treatments have reportedly produced comparable results. For example, when children with encopresis, enuresis, or habit disorders have been treated using empirically supported or probably efficacious procedures, the outcomes have been essentially similar. The lack of empirical data on cultural diversity makes it impossible to estimate when and where cultural differences are important. But, as ethnic minorities make up an increasingly greater percentage of the population of the United States, cultural diversity takes on more and more importance as a possible variable to consider in developing effective assessment and treatment tools for children.

As Hall (1997) pointed out,

> with the changing demographics occurring in the United States, psychology must make substantive revisions in its curriculum training, research, and practice. Without these revisions, psychology will risk professional, ethical, and economic problems because psychology will no longer be a viable professional resource to the majority of the U.S. population. (p. 642)

In support of her position, Hall (1997) stated that by the year 2050, approximately one half of the U.S. population will be people of color, with many U.S. cities currently at or near this percentage. The vast majority of published research in psychology has excluded diverse populations from the participant pool. Although the reasons for this exclusion are many, the reality is that when a clinician prepares to assess a child or to provide treatment services for a child and his or her family, the research on which the assessment and treatments are based was, in all likelihood, on White families.

There can be no argument that Hall (1997) is correct in her call for more cultural diversity in psychology. Without a practical awareness of cultural norms, even a definition of "deviant," "abnormal," or "unusual" is difficult to defend. In spite of the differences that have surfaced about the need, or lack thereof, for empirically supported treatments, the call for procedures that meet the needs of the population that they serve cannot readily be argued. For example, in the chapter on sleep disorders (chapter 4), the point is made that in some countries children are encouraged to sleep with either their parents or their siblings, whereas in other countries sleeping with a parent is not only unacceptable but is often the reason why parents seek clinical services. Similar issues may be found for both externalizing and internalizing behavior problems. A child's level of "hyperactivity" or "depressed mood" must be considered in the cultural context of the family, even when such behaviors are disruptive to the standards of the majority culture. Cultural expectations may also influence how a child responds to pain. Thus, the clinician who is not aware of prevailing cultural norms is at a decided disadvantage. Similar to the issue of comorbidity, we hope that future research addresses cultural considerations to improve the representativeness of the true child population that we serve as clinicians. Our next volume would then most likely include entire sections in each chapter that would guide readers in the implications of cultural factors in the effective treatment of children.

PURPOSE OF THIS BOOK

The purpose of this book is to provide a comprehensive review of therapies that work with common childhood behavioral problems. Our goal was to provide the reader with the current state of empirically based interventions for children in the framework of "empirically validated" treatments offered by the APA Task Force. The present volume, based on our review of the treatment literature for children, includes the problems that are most common and that have procedures that have been evaluated in formal outcome studies. For example, as two recent literature reviews showed, the areas of encopresis (M. L. McGrath, Mellon, & Murphy, 2000) and enuresis (Mellon & McGrath, 2000) have a number of published outcome studies.

The reader must bear in mind that the guidelines for what constitutes empirical support have only recently been agreed on. Given the large number of recent studies that have met the criteria for "empirically supported," it is obviously only a matter of time, now that the criteria have been agreed on, before many more studies appear in the literature. Fortunately, the studies that are now appearing in the published literature certainly do not contradict the results published previously. Rather, they have been a direct outgrowth of previous work.

The chapters in this book address the most commonly encountered problems in childhood that may come to the attention of the clinician. They include disruptive behavior disorders, anxiety disorders, habit disorders and tics, sleep disorders, encopresis, enuresis, pain management, and adherence to medical regimens. The two notable omissions are depression and obsessive-compulsive disorders. We felt that these areas were quite adequately covered in other texts, particularly in Hibbs and Jensen's (1996) edited book, *Psychosocial Treatments for Child and Adolescent Disorders*, which had four chapters on depression and one chapter on obsessive–compulsive disorder.

The chapters are organized to include a definition of the problem area, diagnostic symptoms based on the *Diagnostic and Statistical Manual of Mental Disorders* (4th ed., *DSM–IV*; American Psychiatric Association, 1994), a discussion of the prevalence and causes of the problem, and a review of the pharmacological and nonpharmacological treatments. The decision to use the *DSM–IV* was predicated on the fact that the majority of training programs, in both psychology and pediatrics, use formal diagnostic codes and that third-party payers require a formal diagnosis. The descriptions assume, unless otherwise specified, that the assessment and treatment take place in an outpatient setting.

This volume can be used as a reference book, a training tool, and a resource to share with other mental health practitioners and primary care providers. As a reference book, it reviews most of the common problems encountered in delivering mental health services to children and adolescents. For the reader who is interested in pursuing any of the topics at greater length, there is an extensive list of references at the end of this book. In this age of computer and online literature searches, the references are current to the summer of 2000.

For trainees at the doctoral level, internship level, and postdoctoral level, this book acquaints them with what empirically supported treatments are available and provides examples of these treatments. The clinical child psychology trainee, as well as the pediatric resident and fellow who is familiar with the conditions, assessment tools, and intervention strategies reviewed herein, will become well acquainted with the current state of empirically supported treatments as well. The *DSM–IV* diagnostic codes were intentionally included to acquaint the trainee and the practitioner with not only the major diagnostic categories but also the actual symptoms on which these categories are based. There are diagnostic forms included in most chapters that can literally be used as an aid in the differential diagnosis of common childhood problems.

Finally, this book may provide a comprehensive resource for primary care providers, who are often the major providers of mental and behavioral health services in the United States (Pace, Chaney, Mullins, & Olson,

1995). Magill and Garrett (1988) reported that 60% of all health care visits related to mental health are to primary care physicians. Thus, primary care providers have long been faced with the dual purpose of needing to stay current with the literature on primary care while also needing to be well acquainted with the services that are available from subspecialists, such as mental health providers.

REFERRALS FROM PRIMARY CARE PHYSICIANS

Mental health professionals depend on referrals from primary care physicians. Children, regardless of whether they present with disruptive behaviors, sleep problems, toileting problems, or anxiety-related issues, will typically be seen first by the primary care professional, then referred to the mental health professional. Thus, referral of appropriate patients is essential if the child or pediatric psychologist is to be able to provide services for them.

Schroeder (1999) and Perrin (1999) recommended that psychological services be physically available in the primary care office. Yet the current system for delivering medical care to children depends almost entirely on referrals from the primary care provider to the specialist. Referral of mental health concerns can be greatly facilitated if psychologists are involved in the training of pediatricians (Perrin, 1999), and if the psychologist and the pediatrician practice out of the same office. In the absence of such a close physical arrangement, the psychologist can encourage referral of mental health concerns by routine communication with primary care physicians. This can be in the form of the traditional timely written feedback on each patient who is referred, but also by aligning him or herself more closely with the primary care physician by becoming involved in local discussion groups and continuing education offerings (Christophersen, Cataldo, Russo, & Varni, 1984).

Pace et al. (1995) attributed the good working relationship between primary care providers, such as pediatricians, and psychologists to the fact that psychologists often provide some of the training to pediatricians during their residency, which serves to introduce the pediatrician to the services that are offered by psychologists. Pace et al. stated that psychologists may not be consulted, however, because the pediatrician lacks confidence in the process of psychological intervention, seeing it as less quantifiable than biological variables and physicians as lacking information about consulting psychologists' roles and areas of expertise vis-à-vis other mental health, behavioral science, and medical professionals. With *Treatments That Work With Children*, they will be able to make decisions about referring children on the basis of whether or not empirically supported treatments exist for the presenting problem. Thus, this book serves to educate, inform, and possibly further establish the important relationship between clinicians and primary care providers who seek to meet the mental health needs of the children in their care.

1

DIAGNOSIS AND MANAGEMENT OF DISRUPTIVE BEHAVIOR DISORDERS

Disruptive behavior is often brought to the attention of the clinician because such behavior is distressing to others and often does not conform to social norms that rule appropriate social interactions. Even when identified and treated early, disruptive behavior disorders are often associated with, but not always predictive of, more serious disruptive behavior and psychiatric diagnoses in later phases of development (C. G. Baum, 1989; Robins, 1966). The three classifications of disruptive behavior disorders that are included in this chapter are oppositional defiant disorder, conduct disorder, and attention deficit hyperactivity disorder. Definitions of these disorders are provided along with some information about differential diagnoses, as these conditions frequently coexist (Shaffer, 1989). Information on the prevalence of these disorders, causes and correlates, and assessment and intervention strategies is also provided. There are probably more office visits with mental health professionals for disruptive behavior disorders than for any other condition. For example, in our clinical practices, approximately 55% of all office appointments are for disruptive behavior disorders.

OPPOSITIONAL DEFIANT DISORDER

Oppositional defiant disorder (ODD) "consists of an enduring pattern of uncooperative, defiant, and hostile behavior toward authority figures that does not involve major antisocial violations, is not accounted for by the child's developmental stage, and results in significant functional impairment" (Vitiello & Jensen, 1995, p. 2317). It should be considered a disorder only when the behaviors are more frequent and intense than in unaffected peers and when they cause dysfunction in social, academic, or work-related situations. Children with ODD have problems controlling their temper, often appear to be angry and easily annoyed, and may be described by other children as being bullies or mean. Furthermore, their defiance is often expressed through temper tantrums, arguing, and stubbornness (Cantwell, 1989b). Oppositional behavior is often setting-specific, occurring more often with parents and other familiar adults, such as teachers or sitters, with whom the child has frequent contact (Cantwell, 1989b). Exhibit 1.1 lists the diagnostic criteria for ODD from the *Diagnostic and Statistical Manual of Mental Disorders* (4th ed., *DSM–IV*; American Psychiatric Association, 1994).

Problem behaviors of ODD are greater than the normal oppositional behavior often displayed throughout the developmental period, including the opposition of children from 18 to 36 months of age and some types of adoles-

---

EXHIBIT 1.1
DSM–IV Criteria for Oppositional Defiant Disorder, 313.81

Oppositional Defiant Disorder

A. A pattern of negativistic, hostile, and defiant behavior lasting at least 6 months, during which four (or more) of the following are present:
   1. often loses temper
   2. often argues with adults
   3. often actively defies or refuses to comply with adults' requests or rules
   4. often deliberately annoys people
   5. often blames others for his or her mistakes or misbehavior
   6. is often touchy or easily annoyed by others
   7. is often angry and resentful
   8. is often spiteful or vindictive.

Note: Consider a criterion met only if the behavior occurs more frequently than is typically observed in individuals of comparable age and developmental level.

B. The disturbance in behavior causes significant impairment in social, academic, or occupational functioning.

C. The behaviors do not occur exclusively during the course of a psychotic or mood disorder.

D. Criteria are not met for conduct disorder and, if individual is age 18 or older, criteria are not met for antisocial personality disorder.

Note. Information from *Diagnostic and Statistical Manual of Mental Disorders* (4th ed.), by the American Psychiatric Association, 1994, Washington, DC: Author. Copyright 1994 by the American Psychiatric Association. Reprinted with permission.

cent rebellion. In a detailed comparison of children with ODD and conduct disorder, Schachar and Wachsmuth (1990) found that most of the children in the study who were diagnosed with conduct disorder also met diagnostic criteria for ODD. Thus, they concluded that ODD, rather than being a variant of normality or being a distinct disorder, is more accurately viewed as a variant of conduct disorder, perhaps at the milder end of the spectrum.

CONDUCT DISORDER

Conduct disorder (CD) describes a persistent pattern of behavior that is not socially acceptable and may violate the rights of others. The behaviors that are characteristic of CD are more serious than oppositional behavior. In young children, CD may include disobedience, defiance, bullying, or aggressive attacks on other children and cruelty toward animals. If the disorder begins later in childhood, established patterns of behavior may include repeated lying; stealing; truancy; aggression toward others, including parents and teachers; destruction of property; staying out late or running away; substance abuse; and precocious sexual behavior. The diagnosis of CD should be made only if antisocial behavior is persistent, repetitive, and associated with functional impairment (Cantwell, 1989a). The *DSM–IV* criteria for CD are found in Exhibit 1.2.

Current clinical uses of this diagnosis are usually based on the repetitive, aggressive patterns of violating others' rights and violating social norms or rules. Many children have conduct-problem behaviors. A smaller number will have a time-limited clinical problem at some point in their lives that can be diagnosed but that is not persistent. An even smaller number of children will have a distinct CD that has persisted over time (Cantwell, 1989a). CD can have onset in childhood or adolescence, and it can occur in a mild, moderate, or severe form (Vitiello & Jensen, 1995). The lack of specific subtyping or exclusion criteria may result in CD being an overinclusive disorder, often associated with other diagnoses such as attention deficit hyperactivity disorder, substance use disorders, psychotic disorders, and mood disorders.

The various *DSM–IV* diagnostic criteria do not carry equal weight and significance. In fact, only 3% of adolescents self-reported having engaged in a robbery or a car theft, compared with 37% who reported having initiated a physical fight and 82% having skipped school (Vitiello & Jensen, 1995). In general, the *DSM–IV* criteria have good positive but poor negative predictive value; that is, the presence of a criterion strongly predicts CD in that child, but its absence does not exclude it. That attests to the heterogeneity of the disorder and to the existence of subtypes. Thus, on the basis of the symptoms' severity, CD is also divided into mild, moderate, and severe types. The severity of the aggressive behavior has an important clinical and

EXHIBIT 1.2
DSM–IV Criteria for Conduct Disorder, 312.90

Conduct Disorder

A. A repetitive and persistent pattern of behavior in which the basic rights of others or major age-appropriate societal norms or rules are violated, as manifested by the presence of three (or more) of the following criteria in the past 12 months, with at least one criterion present in the past 6 months.

Aggression to people and animals
1. often bullies, threatens, or intimidates others
2. often initiates physical fights
3. has used a weapon that can cause serious physical harm to others (e.g., a bat, brick, broken bottle, knife, gun)
4. has been physically cruel to people
5. has been physically cruel to animals
6. has stolen while confronting a victim (e.g., mugging, purse snatching, extortion, armed robbery)
7. has forced someone into sexual activity

Destruction of property
8. has deliberately engaged in fire setting with the intention of causing serious damage
9. has deliberately destroyed others' property (other than by fire setting)

Deceitfulness or theft
10. has broken into someone else's house, building, or car
11. often lies to obtain goods or favors or to avoid obligations (i.e., "cons" others)
12. has stolen items of nontrivial value without confronting a victim (e.g., shoplifting, but without breaking and entering; forgery)

Serious violations of rules
13. often stays out at night despite parental prohibitions, beginning before age 13 years
14. has run away from home overnight at least twice while living in parental or parental surrogate home (or once without returning for a lengthy period)
15. often truant from school, beginning before age 13 years

B. The disturbance in behavior causes clinically significant impairment in social, academic, or occupational functioning.

C. If the individual is age 18 years or older, criteria are not met for Antisocial Personality Disorder.

Note. Information from *Diagnostic and Statistical Manual of Mental Disorders* (4th ed.), by the American Psychiatric Association, 1994, Washington, DC: Author. Copyright 1994 by the American Psychiatric Association. Reprinted with permission.

prognostic value, because a high level of aggressiveness is predictive of criminal offences in adulthood (Vitiello & Jensen, 1995).

ATTENTION DEFICIT HYPERACTIVITY DISORDER

Attention deficit hyperactivity disorder (ADHD) is a chronic and pervasive condition characterized by developmentally inappropriate levels of attention, impulsivity, hyperactivity, or some combination of these traits

(Anastopoulos, Barkley, & Shelton, 1996). The clinical features of ADHD are difficulty paying attention to tasks such as academic work, poor impulse control (e.g., calling out in class, not waiting turn), and motor restlessness. These behaviors are often most disruptive at school, given the requirement that the child pay attention and limit motor activity for extended periods of time. The *DSM–IV* provides diagnostic criteria to differentiate between three subtypes of ADHD, which are listed in Exhibit 1.3.

EXHIBIT 1.3
DSM–IV Criteria for Attention Deficit Hyperactivity Disorder, 314.01, 314.00

Attention Deficit Hyperactivity Disorder

A. Either (1) or (2):
   1. six (or more) of the following symptoms of inattention have persisted for at least 6 months to a degree that is maladaptive and inconsistent with developmental level:

Inattention
   a. often fails to give close attention to details or makes careless mistakes in schoolwork, work, or other activities
   b. often has difficulty sustaining attention in tasks or play activities
   c. often does not seem to listen when spoken to directly
   d. often does not follow through on instructions and fails to finish schoolwork, chores, or duties in the workplace (not due to oppositional behavior or failure to understand instructions)
   e. often has difficulty organizing tasks and activities
   f. often avoids, dislikes, or is reluctant to engage in tasks that require sustained mental effort (such as schoolwork or homework)
   g. often loses things necessary for tasks or activities (e.g., toys, school assignments, pencils, books, or tools)
   h. is often easily distracted by extraneous stimuli
   i. is often forgetful in daily activities

   2. six (or more) of the following symptoms of hyperactivity–impulsivity have persisted for at least 6 months to a degree that is maladaptive and inconsistent with developmental level:

Hyperactivity
   a. often fidgets with hands or feet or squirms in seat
   b. often leaves seat in classroom or in other situations in which remaining seated is expected
   c. often runs about or climbs excessively in situations in which it is inappropriate (in adolescents or adults, may be limited to subjective feelings of restlessness)
   d. often has difficulty playing or engaging in leisure activities quietly
   e. is often "on the go" or often acts as if "driven by a motor"
   f. often talks excessively

Impulsivity
   g. often blurts out answers before questions have been completed
   h. often has difficulty awaiting turn
   i. often interrupts or intrudes on others (e.g., butts into conversations or games)

(continued)

EXHIBIT 1.3 *(continued)*

B. Some hyperactive–impulsive or inattentive symptoms that caused impairment were present before age 7 years.

C. Some impairment from the symptoms is present in two or more settings (e.g., at school [or work] and at home).

D. There must be clear evidence of clinically significant impairment in social, academic, or occupational functioning.

E. The symptoms do not occur exclusively during the course of a Pervasive Developmental Disorder, Schizophrenia, or other Psychotic Disorder and are not better accounted for by another mental disorder (e.g., Mood Disorder, Anxiety Disorder, Dissociative Disorder, or a Personality Disorder).

Code based on type:

   314.01 Attention-Deficit/Hyperactivity Disorder, Combined Type: if both Criteria A1 and A2 are met for the past 6 months

   314.00 Attention-Deficit/Hyperactivity Disorder, Predominantly Inattentive Type: if Criterion A1 is met but Criterion A2 is not met for the past 6 months

   314.01 Attention-Deficit/Hyperactivity Disorder, Predominantly Hyperactive–Impulsive Type: if Criterion A2 is met but Criterion A1 is not met for the past 6 months

---

Note. Information from *Diagnostic and Statistical Manual of Mental Disorders* (4th ed.), by the American Psychiatric Association, 1994, Washington, DC: Author. Copyright 1994 by the American Psychiatric Association. Reprinted with permission.

ADHD is one of the most significant disorders of our time because it is a prevalent and persistent problem that may change its manifestation with development from preschool through adult life, and it interferes with many areas of normal development and functioning in a child's life (Cantwell, 1996). Generally, diagnostic criteria for ADHD are based on extensive empirical research and, if applied appropriately, lead to the diagnosis of a syndrome with high interrater reliability, good face validity, and high predictability of course and medication responsiveness (Goldman, Genel, Bezman, & Slanetz, 1998). In a large-scale study on the identification of attention and hyperactivity problems in primary care, Wasserman et al. (1999) reported that clinicians do not appear to overdiagnose attention problems, nor are they predisposed to label children from disadvantaged backgrounds as having attention problems.

DIFFERENTIAL DIAGNOSIS

Many behaviors defined under each of the disruptive behavior disorders described above seem to be present in most children and overlap with each other, often varying only by intensity or frequency. Thus, the differential diagnosis of these disorders usually involves discriminating between normal behavior and behavior that is outside of the normal range, and further discriminating between each disorder alone or in combination. For example, it is always important to distinguish ODD from normal oppositional behavior. Normal oppositional behavior should not cause substantial and persistent dysfunction, whereas ODD results in significant functional impairment. To illustrate, Vitiello and Jensen (1995) reported that in a community sample of children and adolescents, the prevalence of ODD-type symptoms was as high as 20% on the basis of criteria of the *DSM–III* (American Psychiatric Association, 1987). Once the additional criterion of functional impairment was applied, however, the rate dropped to approximately 10%. To facilitate the differential diagnosis of ODD, CD, and ADHD, Table 1.1 presents the *DSM–IV* diagnostic criteria for each of the disruptive behavior disorders. This format is offered as a means of structuring the diagnostic interview with the child and parents to include comprehensive and systematic questioning about the child's presenting symptoms.

TABLE 1.1
Differential Diagnosis Criteria

Diagnostic Criteria for Disruptive Behavior Disorders

ADHD 314.01 Hyper-Impulsive Type	ADHD 314.00 Inattentive Type	ODD 313.81 Oppositional	CD 312.90 Conduct Disorder
❏ Fidgets, squirms	❏ Lacks attention to detail	❏ Often loses temper	❏ Bullies
❏ Leaves seat	❏ Lacks sustained attention	❏ Argues with adults	❏ Initiates fights
❏ Runs and climbs	❏ Not listening	❏ Actively defiant	❏ Used a weapon
❏ Difficulty with leisure	❏ Lacks follow-through	❏ Deliberately annoys	❏ Cruel to people
❏ Always on the go	❏ Not organized	❏ Blames others	❏ Cruel to animals
❏ Talks excessively	❏ Avoids mental effort	❏ Touchy	❏ Stolen with confrontation
❏ Blurts out answers	❏ Loses things	❏ Angry and resentful	❏ Forced sex
❏ Difficulty waiting turn	❏ Easily distracted	❏ Spiteful, vindictive	❏ Fire setting
❏ Often interrupts	❏ Forgetful		❏ Destroyed property
			❏ Broken into house
			❏ Often lies
			❏ Stolen without confrontation
			❏ Stays out late
			❏ Has run away
			❏ Often truant
__ of 9 (6+ = dx)	__ of 9 (6+ = dx)	__ of 8 (4+ = dx)	__ of 15 (3+ = dx)

Note. Information from *Diagnostic and Statistical Manual of Mental Disorders* (4th ed.), by the American Psychiatric Association, 1994, Washington, DC: Author. Copyright 1994 by the American Psychiatric Association. Reprinted with permission.

PREVALENCE

Most parents, at one time or another, have to deal with their children's behavior problems. As universal as they are, these problems are often dealt with by parents without any professional intervention. When such problems exceed the parents' knowledge or capabilities, and when the problems begin to interfere with the normal growth and development of the child, however, professional intervention is often sought.

The majority of the common behavior problems that parents encounter come under the category of oppositional behaviors. In fact, childhood behavior problems are the most frequently occurring disorder in both clinic-referred and general populations (Quay, 1986). Richman, Stevenson, and Graham (1982b), in a study of non-clinic-referred, 3-year-old children, showed that temper tantrums were present in approximately 5% of the children, equally distributed between boys and girls. Nearly 11% of the population was described as difficult to control, with boys slightly more represented than girls. Richman et al. reported that, according to maternal reports, the problems persisted in 63% of the children at age 4 and 62% at age 8. Teacher ratings also indicated more persistent problems at age 8 among the children rated as problematic in preschool. Furthermore, the problems were more likely to persist in boys than in girls, with 73% of the boys reported to be having difficulties at age 8, compared with 48% of the girls. Similar prevalence rates have been reported in both referred and nonreferred Dutch preschool children (Koot & Verhulst, 1991). Campbell (1995) reviewed a number of follow-up studies of preschool children identified as having potentially significant problems and also showed that the problems persisted over time. Although predictions were not diagnosis-specific, given the overlap in symptoms of attention and discipline problems noted in young children, Campbell concluded that early problems appear to be associated with a range of negative outcomes that include externalizing problems, academic difficulties, or both.

A significant number of children who exhibit CD at early ages continue to exhibit these same behaviors as adolescents. For example, in prepubertal children, the incidence rate of CD is 1.9–8% in boys and 0–1.9% in girls. Among adolescents, the incidence is 3.4–10.4% in boys and 0.8–8% in girls (Vitiello & Jensen, 1995). The continuity of CD demonstrates the importance of programs that focus on prevention and early treatment of conduct problems. These programs may be especially important for boys through adolescence, who generally have greater estimates of CD (6–16%) than do girls (2–9%) throughout childhood (Vitiello & Jensen, 1995).

Prevalence estimates for ADHD vary widely, depending on the diagnostic criteria used, but reasonable estimates suggest that 3–5% of children nationwide are affected (Hibbs & Jensen, 1996). More specifically, children with ADHD, predominantly the inattentive type, constitute approximately one third of the total number of youths diagnosed with ADHD (Cantwell,

1996). Wasserman et al. (1999) conducted a prospective cohort study of over 22,000 consecutive children ages 4–15 seen for acute, chronic, and health supervision visits. They reported that clinicians did not appear to overdiagnose attention and hyperactivity problems, although boys were more likely than girls to be identified as having attention and hyperactivity problems.

COMORBID DISORDERS

Disruptive behavior disorders often occur in the presence of other mental health problems, such as anxiety disorders, obsessive–compulsive disorder, major depressive disorder, and communication disorders. Although a diagnosis of CD supersedes a diagnosis of ODD, as many as 90% of children with CD of early onset also meet criteria for ODD (Vitiello & Jensen, 1995). CD, with peak of onset at age 9, is quite often preceded by ODD, which peaks earlier, at about age 6.5. Most cases of ODD, however, do not result in CD (Vitiello & Jensen, 1995).

Children with CD are at risk for comorbid mood disorders such as anxiety and depression (Kazdin, 1996). According to Vitiello and Jensen (1995), the association of CD with mood disorders, especially major depressive disorder and dysthymic disorder, tends to be higher than expected by chance, reaching 50% in some studies. In adolescents, CD can be a major precursor of depressive disorders. Adolescents with depression can display antisocial behaviors, but it is often not clear whether they meet the full criteria for CD. The association between CD and anxiety disorders is less consistent. Children with CD are also more likely to show academic deficiencies, as reflected in achievement level, grades, retention, early termination from school, and deficiencies in specific skill areas such as reading (Kazdin, 1996).

Children with ADHD present unique challenges in terms of both assessment and intervention. This challenge is due, in large part, to the fact that the majority of children with ADHD (both the hyperactive/impulsive type and the combined type) have comorbid ODD or CD. Children with ADHD of predominantly inattentive type, in contrast, are more likely to have comorbid anxiety problems. Lalonde, Turgay, and Hudson (1998) showed that, of the three subtypes of ADHD, children with the inattentive type showed lower rates of comorbid ODD than those with the combined type or the hyperactive/impulsive type. Youths diagnosed with the hyperactive/impulsive type showed much higher rates of CD than those with either the inattentive type or the combined type.

In general, diagnoses involving CD, ODD, or ADHD often coexist. In studies of community and clinic samples, a large percentage of youths with CD or ADHD (45–70%) also meet criteria for the other disorder (Kazdin, 1996). Among clinic-referred youths who meet criteria for CD, 84–96% also meet concurrent diagnostic criteria for ODD. Biederman et al. (1996)

conducted a study to evaluate the overlap among ADHD, ODD, and CD. They recruited 260 children, ages 6–17, 140 of whom had been diagnosed with ADHD and 120 of whom did not meet the diagnostic criteria for any of the disruptive behavior disorders. Their results showed that, of the children with ADHD, 65% had comorbid ODD and 22% had comorbid CD. Of those with ADHD and ODD, 32% also met the criteria for CD. With all but 1 child with ADHD and CD, the ODD preceded the onset of the CD by several years. Biederman et al. concluded that children diagnosed with ODD followed by CD had more comorbid psychiatric disorders, lower Global Assessment of Functioning scores, and more abnormal behavior rating scale scores when compared with ADHD children without these disorders. In addition, ODD without CD at baseline assessment in childhood did not increase the risk for CD at the 4-year follow-up, by the time the child has reached mid-adolescence. Thus, the outlook for children with ODD is more optimistic with respect to symptom improvement than it is for children with CD, both in the short and the long term.

CAUSES AND CORRELATES

Many biological, individual, and family factors have been associated with behavioral problems in children and adolescents (Quay, 1986), and all may play a role in the etiology of disruptive behavior disorders. Although these correlates have been identified in a number of studies, additional evidence of their contribution to the etiology of disruptive behavior disorders is needed. Three such factors—gender, age, and family functioning—that have been studied more extensively are discussed below.

Gender

Several studies have examined gender differences in reports of young children's problem behaviors in community samples. Whereas some studies report that externalizing problems such as tantrums, overactivity, fighting, and disobedience are higher in boys, other studies have revealed relatively trivial gender differences (Campbell, 1995). Gender differences have not been found to be remarkable in preschoolers, whereas school-age boys have been found to demonstrate higher rates of externalizing behaviors than school-age girls (Campbell, 1995). Campbell also reported a shift toward more internalizing problems in girls by early adolescence.

Age

Major parental concerns about their child's aberrant behavior vary with age or developmental level of the child. Parental concerns about toddlers are related to eating, sleeping, and toileting problems, whereas their concerns about discipline peak at about age 3 (e.g., Jenkins, Bax, & Hart, 1980). In general, parents' and teachers' reports of problems with discipline and peer relationships tend to increase from about age 2–3 (Crowther, Bond, & Rolf, 1981). Between ages 3 and 5, tantrums, overactivity, attention problems, and fighting with peers seem to decrease in nonclinical samples (Coleman, Wolkind, & Ashley, 1977; Crowther et al., 1981). Overall, cross-sectional studies suggest that problems around management, self-control, and aggression decrease in meaningful and predictable ways with development (Campbell, 1995).

Disruptive behavior disorders generally begin in the early to middle grade school years and will have developed by early adolescence. The onset of each disorder is, however, variable within this age range. Early onset conduct problems (i.e., high rates of oppositional defiant, aggressive, and noncompliant behaviors in the preschool years) are fairly stable and predict not only problems in school but also serious health and behavioral problems in adolescence, such as drug abuse, depression, juvenile delinquency, and school dropout (Webster-Stratton, 1998). One of the first major studies to address the longitudinal aspects of children with behavior problems was Richman et al. (1982a). They studied a representative sample of 3-year-olds in an inner London borough who were identified as "hard to manage." They reported that behavior problems persisted in 63% of the group at age 4 and 62% at age 8, according to maternal reports. Teacher ratings also indicated more persistent problems at age 8 among the children rated as problematic in preschool. Furthermore, problems were more likely to persist in boys than in girls; 73% of problem boys were still reported to be having difficulties at age 8 in contrast to 48% of girls (Campbell, 1995).

The Cambridge Study in Delinquent Development (Farrington, 1991) provided a longitudinal study of 411 male participants who displayed high rates of antisocial behavior at age 8. There was evidence of continuing aggressive behavior from ages 8 to 32. Children who were rated as aggressive by their teachers at ages 8 to 10 were significantly more likely to be rated as aggressive on the basis of self-reports at age 32 and to have been convicted of a violent crime before age 32 (Oxford & Bennett, 1994). Thus, although some acting-out behaviors in toddlers and preschoolers may be attributed to either a developmental "stage" or to the fact that a child is "all boy," many of the more aberrant behaviors have been demonstrated to persist, in the absence of any intervention, into the school years and adolescence.

Family Functioning

Research suggests that certain family characteristics put children at particular risk for developing conduct problems, namely, low income, low education, teenage pregnancy, isolation, high levels of stress, and high levels of marital discord and depression (Webster-Stratton, 1998). Children whose parents are inconsistent in their discipline, physically abusive, or highly critical and hostile are also at greater risk for conduct disorder, as are children whose parents are disengaged from their children's school experiences and provide little cognitive stimulation. Moreover, the risk of a child developing conduct problems seems to increase exponentially with the child's exposure to each additional risk factor (Webster-Stratton, 1998).

The most influential developmental model for describing the family dynamics that may underlie early antisocial behavior is Patterson's (1982) theory of the "coercive process." In this process, children learn to escape or avoid parental criticism by escalating their negative behaviors, which in turn leads to increasingly more aversive parental interactions. These negative parental behaviors, in turn, directly reinforce the child's deviant behaviors. Such mutual training in aversive responding intensifies both the child's aggressive behavior and the parents' hostile, nonresponsive behavior. Parents are inadvertently teaching their children noncompliance and aggression by modeling and reinforcing those behaviors in their daily interactions with their children.

Coercive Process (handwritten margin note)

ASSESSMENT

Behavioral assessment for a child and family includes several overlapping functions (Mash & Terdal, 1988):

- determining the problem behaviors for which services are being sought
- determining the child's and family's history of relevant problems, if any
- formulating a treatment plan based on the assessment and presenting problems
- evaluating the effectiveness of treatment and reformulating the plan when less-than-optimal progress is achieved
- evaluating the long-term outcomes of treatment.

Assessment should have clinical utility (Ollendick & King, 1998). That is, the most useful assessments provide an accurate estimate of the type and extent of "problems" or "areas of concern" prior to any intervention and give direction to effective treatment options. Thus, when considering assessment tools for any childhood disorder, including the disruptive behavior disorders discussed in this chapter, clinicians must use assessment tools that are helpful in selecting an appropriate treatment modality.

The accurate diagnosis of disruptive behavior disorders most often requires multimethod assessment, which involves considering the conclusions reached by at least two qualitatively different assessment methods (Eyberg,

1985). For example, results from a parent rating scale of child behavior can be compared with interview data, direct observations, and teacher rating scale scores. The American Academy of Child and Adolescent Psychiatry (1997a) provides practice guidelines for ADHD that also support multi-method assessment. They recommend including parent and child interviews, standardized rating scales from parents and teachers, school performance information from current and past teachers, and a physical examination of the child. It is also important to consider using more traditional standardized intelligence, achievement, and personality tests to identify other possibly relevant problems and to help formulate a diagnosis. The American Academy of Pediatrics, in their published *Clinical Practice Guidelines for ADHD* (2000), also recommend multimethod assessment, with multiple informants. They state that assessment of the child with ADHD should include assessment for coexisting conditions, such as ODD, CD, mood disorders, anxiety, and learning disabilities. However, they did not recommend other diagnostic tests such as blood lead levels, thyroid hormone levels, brain imaging studies and EEGs, or continuous performance tests.

Such multimethod assessment can incorporate the advantages of empirically based assessment and the *DSM–IV* diagnostic criteria (Achenbach & McConaughy, 1996). Empirically based assessment has the advantage that the various clinical syndromes actually reflect patterns of co-occurring problems that are reported for particular samples of children. The parent and teacher rating scales that are discussed below do not require the rater to choose between the presence or absence of each symptom. Rather, the rater is instructed to quantify the degree to which a child exhibits each symptom using terms such as "absent," "mild or infrequent," and "severe or frequent." The sets of co-occurring problems are then viewed as "syndromes" in the sense that they occur together. Achenbach and McConaughy made the case that the disruptive behavior disorders of ODD, CD, and ADHD from the *DSM–IV* manual were quite similar to the empirically based syndromes.

Several useful assessment tools for diagnosing disruptive behavior disorders and other childhood problems are described below.

Interviewing

Interviews may be conducted with the parent or child alone, possibly followed by an interview of the family together. La Greca (1983) suggested taking a thorough family history, which may include the following:

- questions about disruptive behavior problems in both biological families
- descriptive information from both the parent and the child about situations in which the current behavioral problems are manifested

- apparent antecedents for episodes of problem behavior
- child and parent characteristics that might be important contributors to the problem
- likely consequences that may be maintaining or exacerbating
problem behaviors.

For children with disruptive behavior disorders, the clinician may be able to identify parental child-rearing practices that may be contributing to the problem (Kazdin, 1985; Snyder & Patterson, 1986). Although inter-viewing as an exclusive assessment method will not provide all of the needed information, it is the beginning of an assessment process designed to identify child, parent, and family characteristics that contribute to prob-lematic behavior (Patterson, 1982).

One standardized interview format that is available for children ages 9–17 is the Diagnostic Interview Schedule for Children (Shaffer, Fisher, Lucas, Dulcan, & Schwab-Stone, 2000). A similar interview, the Children's Interview for Psychiatric Syndromes (Weller, Weller, Fristad, Rooney, & Schecter, 2000), is under development for interviewing children ages 6–18. Although both of these formats are fairly lengthy (estimated time of 20–30 minutes to complete), when studies have been done to correlate their use with empirically based assessments, they are potentially useful to the clinician.

Behavior Rating Scales

In addition to the data and impressions that can be obtained from the clinical interview, behavior rating scales provide the clinician with input from multiple informants (e.g., the parents and one or more of the child's teachers). Data from multiple informants can be valuable for detecting con-sistencies and inconsistencies in how a child is viewed (Achenbach & McConaughy, 1996). Several studies have demonstrated significant associa-tions between DSM diagnoses of children and the scores that they obtained on the corresponding empirically based syndrome derived from parent, teacher, and self-reports (e.g., Biederman, Faraone, et al., 1993; Weinstein, Noam, Grimes, Stone, & Schwab-Stone, 1990). These findings suggest that the DSM criteria, in conjunction with parent and child interviews and be-havior ratings scales, are useful in the differential diagnosis of disruptive behavior disorders. In fact, according to Barkley (1981), "no other area of child psychopathology has spawned more rating scales than that of conduct problem or hyperactive children" (p. 104).

Three of the most widely used parent rating scales are the Conners Parent Rating Scale (Goyette, Conners, & Ulrich, 1978), the Child Behav-ior Checklist (Achenbach, 1991), and the Behavior Assessment System for Children (Reynolds & Kamphaus, 1998). Table 1.2 summarizes the different

TABLE 1.2
Behavior Rating Scales: Ages and Forms

Scale Ages in Years (Norms)	Teacher Form (Computer form)	Parent Form (Computer form)	Youth Form (Computer form)
Conners			
2–3	No	Yes	Yes
4–16	Yes	Yes	Yes
CBCL			
2–3	No	Yes	Yes
4–16	Yes	Yes	Yes
12–16	Yes	Yes	Yes
BASC			
2–3	No	Yes	Yes
4–16	Yes	Yes	Yes
12–18	Yes	Yes	Yes

Note. Conners = Conners Parent Rating Scale; CBCL = Child Behavior Checklist; BASC = Behavior Assessment System for Children.

forms of these rating scales. On each of these rating forms, the parents, teachers, and child (older than age 11) are asked to rate the extent to which the child is experiencing a number of different problems such as "can't sit still," "mean to other children," and "argues with adults."

- *Conners Rating Scale.* The CRS was originally constructed to assess hyperactivity from the perspective of the child's parents and teacher. The CRS consists of 48 items, rated on a 4-point scale, and has been shown to discriminate hyperactive from normal children (Conners, 1969). Separate scales are available for children from ages 2 to 17 (Goyette et al., 1978). The manual version of the CRS takes a fair amount of time to score; however, the Quick Scoring Form that uses NCR (no carbon required) paper is much quicker to score.

- *Child Behavior Checklist.* The CBCL was developed so that the answers from the parent, teacher, and youth forms are sorted into scores on subscales, including social withdrawal, attention problems, and aggression, normed according to the child's age and sex (Achenbach, 1991). The 118-item scale, rated on a 3-point scale, has norms for children from ages 2 to 17. Separate norms are provided for boys and girls at each of four age levels, and Achenbach has provided evidence that the CBCL can discriminate effectively between clinic-referred and normal children (Achenbach, 1991). The manual scoring versions of the CBCL require a good deal of time to score; the computerized scoring form is much faster. Also, the printout from the computerized scoring includes the scores on each of the subscales, as well as *t* scores, and offers a much more efficient means of scoring.

- *Behavior Assessment System for Children.* The BASC is available in Teacher Rating Scales, Parent Rating Scales, and Self-Report of Personality for children ranging from ages 4 to 18 (Reynolds & Kamphaus, 1998). Each form of the BASC can be scored using a computer-scoring program available from the publisher (American Guidance Service). The computer printout, like the CBCL, includes the scores on each of the subscales as well as *t* scores.

These behavioral checklists provide a current description of parents' perceptions of their children's conduct and other behavioral problems. Checklists also provide a means for repeated assessment during and after treatment. Behavioral checklists do not, however, provide specific and detailed information on dimensions of problem behaviors that may be necessary for developing a treatment formulation. For this information, clinicians often turn to direct observation of the child's behavior and, in some situations, self-monitoring by the child.

The diagnostic utility of both the BASC and the CBCL rating scales for differentiating students with ADHD from those without and for discriminating between the predominantly inattentive-type and combined-type of ADHD has been documented by Ostrander, Weinfurt, Yarnold, and August (1998). The BASC was more accurate than the CBCL for distinguishing students with ADHD from those without. In another comparison of the BASC and the CBCL parent and teacher rating scales, Vaughn, Riccio, Hynd, and Hall (1997) reported that there was no strong advantage of either measure in differentiating children with ADHD from those without. The one exception was the BASC Teacher Rating Scale, which had better predictive validity for children who did not meet ADHD criteria. These studies indicate that, for subtypes of ADHD, and specifically the ADHD inattentive type, the best results are obtained with the BASC over the CBCL (Ostrander et al., 1998). The fact that there are no empirical data to suggest that one behavior rating scale is superior to another suggests that the clinician may use either.

Clinic-Based Diagnostic Procedures

Several diagnostic tests that can be administered in the clinician's office have been used to assess for disruptive behavior disorders. Most of the work in this area has been done to assist in the diagnosis of ADHD. For example, DuPaul, Anastopoulos, Shelton, Guevremont, and Metevia (1992) examined the utility of two clinic-based tests: the Matching Figures Test

(MFT; Kagan, 1966) and one version of the Continuous Performance Task (CPT; Gordon, 1983). They reported that scores on the MFT and the CPT were found to share little variance with parent and teacher reports on several behavior rating scales used to evaluate ADHD. Furthermore, they reported that clinic test scores, either alone or in combination, resulted in classification decisions that frequently disagreed with a diagnosis of ADHD based on parent interviews and behavior rating scales completed by parents and teachers. In fact, Baren and Swanson (1996) made the point that none of the three available continuous performance tasks (Conners' Continuous Performance Test, Conners, 1995; Gordon Diagnostic System, Gordon, 1983; and Tests of Variables of Attention, Forbes, 1998) are really useful either for screening or for clinical diagnosis of ADHD. There are simply too many times when the results from a CPT conflict with the other screening and diagnostic tools that are available in the form of parent and teacher rating scales.

Barkley and Grodzinsky (1994) compared the performance of four groups of children, ages 6–12, with the different subtypes of ADHD on a variety of tests designed to measure frontal lobe functions, including the following tests:

- Gordon Continuous Performance Test (Gordon, 1983)
- Controlled Word Association Test (Benton & Hamsher, 1978)
- Hand Movements Scale (Kaufman & Kaufman, 1983)
- Porteus Mazes (Porteus, 1965)
- Rey–Osterrieth Complex Figure (Lezak, 1983)
- Stroop Color–Word Association Test (Stroop, 1935)
- Trail Making Test (Reitan & Wolfson, 1985)
- Wisconsin Card Sorting Test (Heaton, 1981)
- Grooved Pegboard Test (Reitan & Wolfson, 1985).

Barkley and Grodzinsky (1994) concluded that these neuropsychological tests, with the exception of the CPT, were not particularly helpful for clinical diagnostic purposes with ADHD children at this time. "Abnormal scores on the CPT may be predictive of ADD, though not of which subtype, while normal scores are not indicative of an absence of ADD and should go uninterpreted" (p. 121).

The data published by Barkley and Grodzinsky (1994) were not especially encouraging regarding the inclusion of neuropsychological tests of presumed frontal lobe functions in children as part of a clinical diagnostic battery for the diagnosis of ADHD. Most tests did not perform much above base-rate levels of positive predictive power for the hyperactive/impulsive subtype of ADHD and rarely exceeded that which could be achieved with a coin toss. They cautioned that because a "normal score" on these same tests was not especially helpful at ruling out ADHD, the score should probably be disregarded for purposes of clinical diagnostic interpretation.

Although there is a tremendous need for objective measurement to determine the presence and extent of attention problems, the use of clinic-based diagnostic tests and continuous performance tests has yet to be perfected to the point at which the tests are useful in the diagnosis of children with attention deficit problems. This may be a temporary condition that will be remedied by further research and demonstration.

INTERVENTIONS

Although disruptive behavior disorders have been the topic of literally hundreds of research publications, only recently have there been many well-controlled intervention studies. The interventions that have been developed for disruptive behavior disorders do, however, represent some of the best intervention studies in all of clinical child psychology. Most of the interventions can be described as pharmacological or behavioral in nature.

Oppositional Defiant Disorder

Pharmacological Interventions

Currently, there is limited support for using pharmaceutical treatment to manage ODD. Cantwell (1989b) stated that pharmacotherapy generally has not been found to be effective for children with ODD or for children with ODD combined with or resulting from an underlying behavior disorder. Children with ADHD and ODD may, however, benefit from some types of psychopharmacological intervention, including stimulants or tricyclic antidepressants. Cantwell (1989a) also cautioned that pharmacotherapy should never be used as the sole treatment for a child or adolescent with ODD or ODD combined with or resulting from an underlying behavior disorder. When a drug is prescribed, it should be prescribed only in conjunction with psychological interventions. In the case of children and most adolescents, psychological interventions almost always include parent training as well.

Behavioral Interventions

Two major research findings lend significant support to the concept of intervening with young children who are hard to manage. Campbell and Ewing (1990) reported on the long-term follow-up of children who were seen as hard to manage at age 3. In the absence of intervention, 67% of these children still met the diagnostic criteria for an externalizing disorder at age 9 on the basis of maternal and teacher interviews and behavior rating scales. A comparison group of children who were identified as problem-free at age 3 continued, for the most part, to be well adjusted at age 9. Similarly,

Long, Forehand, Wierson, and Morgan (1994) reported on the long-term follow-up of 26 late adolescents and young adults who had participated in parent training with their mothers when they were young, ranging in age from 2 to 7. At the follow-up, which was approximately 14 years posttreatment, the individuals who had been treated earlier were compared with a matched community sample on various measures of delinquency, emotional adjustment, academic progress, and relationship with their parents. No differences were noted between the two groups, leading Long et al. to conclude that noncompliant children who participated during their early years in parent training functioned as well as nonclinical individuals. Thus, it appears that effective early intervention for children with noncompliant or more severe behavior problems may be beneficial for remediating behavior problems in children and that, in the absence of any intervention, behavior problems will probably continue.

Parent training. Teaching parents improved behavior management techniques is a mainstay of behavior therapy for oppositional children (Patterson, 1982). In his early studies, Patterson used what by today's standards would be called "treatment manuals," such as *Families* (Patterson, 1971) and *Living With Children* (Patterson & Gullion, 1968). Parents were instructed to read parts of these manuals as their homework, and therapists used the manuals as a blueprint for conducting the interventions. Patterson and his colleagues were able to empirically validate their parent training and social learning interventions as effective methods of decreasing deviant behavior in males (Fleischman, 1981; Patterson, 1974). More recently, Kazdin (1995) commented about the effectiveness of parent training, stating that perhaps no other technique has been as carefully documented and empirically supported as parent management training in treating the conduct problems of children.

Recent evidence of the effectiveness of parent training has been provided by Forehand and colleagues (e.g., Long et al., 1994). The parent training intervention consisted of 8 to 10 clinic sessions in which a parent was initially taught to pay attention to and reward appropriate behavior and to ignore minor inappropriate behavior. The parents were then taught how to issue commands and to use reinforcement for compliance and time-out for noncompliance. Didactic instruction, modeling, role play, interaction with the child in the clinic, and structured times to practice skills in the home were used as teaching procedures. At follow-up, the children who were treated, when compared with a nonclinic community control group, were not different in functioning across multiple areas, including delinquency, emotional adjustment, academic performance, and relationship with parents.

More recently, Forehand and Long (1996) published a similar stepwise set of recommendations for teaching parents how to change the manner in which they were interacting with their noncompliant children. The major elements included the following:

- using differential attention
- using rewards
- ignoring inappropriate behavior
- giving effective directions
- using time-out to decrease undesirable behaviors
- integrating these newly learned skills into a comprehensive plan for dealing with their children.

With young children, parent training often focuses on differential attention for compliance and other desirable behaviors, ignoring problem behaviors when possible, and time-out for misbehaviors such as noncompliance and tantrums (see Christophersen, 1994, 1998b). One way we teach parents in our clinic to provide differential attention to their children is to describe and model "time-in." *Time-in* is defined as frequent and consistent physical contact with the child when he or she is not engaged in inappropriate behavior. For example, a mother might pat her child on the head while he plays independently with his blocks or rub her child's arm for sitting quietly while she talks on the telephone. An example of our information for parents that describes time-in is found in Exhibit 1.4.

The time-in handout was developed to address an important point made by Solnick, Rincover, and Peterson (1977), that time-out is a much more effective procedure when parents provide their children with "enriched" time-in. Conversely, when time-in is "impoverished," time-out is a much less effective procedure. Forehand and Long's (1996) discussion of differential attention is one way of making time-in more enriched. So is the rewarding of appropriate behavior, discussed by Patterson, Reid, Jones, and Conger (1975).

In addition to providing structured learning opportunities for techniques of differential attention, parent behaviors that serve as antecedents, such as the vague or nagging ways that parents give instructions to their children, are also important to address in the clinic (Forehand & McMahon, 1981). Exhibit 1.5 describes effective instruction-giving techniques that facilitate compliance. Other programs use "token economy" systems (see below) to help structure the parents' use of reinforcement to reward appropriate behaviors and response-cost procedures to change their children's problem behaviors (Christophersen, 1994). The use of a token economy often provides parents with the structure that is necessary to encourage them to use differential attention, response cost, and practicing in order to assist their child to develop more appropriate behavioral repertories.

Token economy. The term *token economy* refers to an organized exchange system in which conditioned reinforcers are earned and lost contingent on the individual engaging in or refraining from specific and clearly defined behaviors. *Conditioned reinforcers* are items or activities that alone may not be reinforcing but when paired with the availability of a known reinforcer take on reinforcing properties.

EXHIBIT 1.4
Time-In

By their very dependent nature, newborns and young infants require a lot of physical contact from their parents. As they get older and their demand characteristics change, parents usually touch their children much less. By the time children are four years old, they are usually toilet trained, can get dressed and undressed themselves, can feed themselves, and can bathe themselves. Thus, if parents don't conscientiously put forth an effort to maintain a great deal of physical contact with their child, he or she will be touched much less than at earlier ages. There are several things that parents can do to help offset these natural changes.

1. Physical proximity. During the boring or distracting activities, place your child close to you where it is easy to reach him. At dinner, in the car, in a restaurant, when you have company, or when you are in a shopping mall, keep your child near you so that physical contact requires little, if any, additional effort on your part.

2. Physical contact. Frequent and brief (one or two seconds) nonverbal physical contact will do more to teach your child that you love him than anything else that you can do. Discipline yourself to touch your child at least 50 times each day for one or two seconds—touch him anytime that he is not doing something wrong or something that you disapprove of.

3. Verbal reprimands. Children don't have the verbal skills that adults do. Adults often send messages that are misunderstood by children, who may interpret verbal reprimands, nagging, and pleading as signs that their parents do not like them. Always keep in mind the old expression, "If you don't have anything nice to say, don't say anything at all."

4. Nonverbal contact. Try to make most of your physical contact with children nonverbal. With young children, physical contact usually has a calming effect, whereas verbal praise, questioning, or general comments may only interrupt what your child was doing.

5. Independent play. Children need to have time to themselves—time when they can play, put things into their mouths, or stare into space. Generally, children don't do nearly as well when their parents carry them around much of the time and constantly try to entertain them. Keep in mind that although your baby may fuss when frustrated, he or she will never learn to deal with frustration if you are always there to help him or her out. Give children enough freedom to explore the environment on their own, and they will learn skills that they can use the rest of their lives.

Remember:
Children need lots of brief, nonverbal physical contact. If you don't have anything nice to say, don't say anything at all.

Note. From *Beyond Discipline: Parenting That Lasts A Lifetime* (pp. 131–132), by Edward R. Christophersen, 1990, Kansas City, MO: Westport Publishers. Copyright 1990 by Edward R. Christophersen. Reprinted with permission.

The token economy was originally developed to add flexibility to the use of tangible rewards with children and adolescents. For example, when a child has completed a required task, whether a homework assignment, a chore, or a social interaction, he or she is presented with a token that can be exchanged later for any of a wide variety of rewards. Tokens can also be used to reward children for practicing skills that they are working to acquire. If a child is working to learn anger management skills by using procedures

EXHIBIT 1.5
Teaching Your Child to Follow Instructions

Parents frequently have problems getting their children to follow instructions. Your child's compliance can improve if you follow the suggestions given below.

GIVING INSTRUCTIONS OR COMMANDS

Step 1. Get your child's attention when giving a direction: Say the child's name and request that he look at you (for example, "Bob, look at me").

Step 2. Thank the child when she has complied by looking at you.

Step 3. Give the child a simple, clear command, like, "Please shut the door."

THINGS TO REMEMBER

1. Be realistic. Give your child instructions that you know he is *physically* and *developmentally* capable of following.

2. Be direct. Say things like, "Joey, please put your shoes in the closet" and "Open the door." Avoid questions that imply choice when there really is no choice, like, "Won't you go to your room?" or "Don't you want to go downstairs?"

3. Give one instruction at a time, and allow your child 5 seconds to begin to obey. Do not repeat the same instruction a second time.

4. Avoid giving a second command while the child is working on the first command.

5. *Avoid giving your child a command unless you are prepared to use time-out for not minding.*

WHEN YOUR CHILD OBEYS

Step 1. When your child begins to comply, praise and encourage her so that she will continue the desired behavior.

Step 2. Thank the child immediately for following the direction by saying something like, "Thank you for putting your bear in the toy box, Joey."

Step 3. Kids love hugs and pats, so be sure to touch your child as well as praise his behavior.

WHAT TO DO IF YOUR CHILD DOES NOT BEGIN
TO OBEY WITHIN 5 SECONDS

Step 1. Put her in time-out immediately.

Step 2. Be careful not to unintentionally give your child attention for not obeying or for behaving unacceptably.

Step 3. After time-out, require your child to complete the requested task. This will give her a chance to receive attention when she obeys and will teach her that you are serious when you give a command.

Note. From *Pediatric Compliance: A Guide for the Primary Care Physician* (pp. 63–64), by Edward R. Christophersen, 1994, New York: Plenum. Copyright 1992 by Edward R. Christophersen. Reprinted with permission.

like progressive muscle relaxation, he or she can be rewarded with tokens each time the child practices his or her skills. Thus, although a child may be willing to clean his room or practice her anger management skills in exchange for the opportunity to play a video game, play with friends, or accumulate additional money, these rewards are unlikely to be available immediately on completion of the required task. The use of a token, which can take the form of a chip or an earned point on a point card, serves to bridge the time delay between the time that the child completes the activity and the time that the child is able to "consume" or use the reward.

Child populations served by token economies have ranged from children with mental retardation to children who are gifted, as well as to those with a wide variety of behavioral and medical problems. Kazdin (1977, 1982) provided an excellent review of early and extensive therapeutic applications of token economies. Two of the largest projects to use token economies have been the work with juvenile delinquents using the Achievement Place Teaching Family Model (M. M. Wolf, Kirigan, Fixsen, Blasé, & Braukmann, 1995) and the Follow Through Head Start Program (Bushell, 1978). The present discussion is limited to the use of a token economy as it is implemented by parents in the home or clinicians in the office as part of an intervention to improve the behavior of the child. For that reason, token economies that have been implemented in institutional settings, including schools, are only referenced as they relate to children's behavior in the home. Information on how token economies can be used to address behavior problems related to medical issues can be found in the chapter on adherence issues (see chapter 8).

Token economies have been successfully implemented to decrease common childhood behavior problems at home (e.g., Christophersen, Arnold, Hill, & Quilitch, 1972) and in public (e.g., Barnard, Christophersen, & Wolf, 1977). A treatment manual for the Home Chip System for children ages 3–7, based on Christophersen, Barnard, and Barnard (1981), is included in Appendix A. This manual provides detailed instructions on the implementation of a token economy by parents in the natural home. Barkley (1981) included a copy of this manual in his book on ADHD. Other examples of token systems and their uses can be found by Barkley and Benton (1998), Barkley, Guevremont, Anastopoulos, and Fletcher, (1992), and Kazdin, Siegel, and Bass (1992), who included the use of token reinforcement as a method of improving the child's cooperation during therapy sessions.

Although Kazdin (1977) reported that a number of problems had been encountered when using token economies in institutional settings, many of these are avoided when using the tokens in the natural home. For example, Kazdin mentioned that the token economy procedures used in a therapeutic treatment setting did not necessarily generalize to the child's natural home. When the token economy is originally implemented in the natural home, however, problems with generalization have not been reported.

Structural Family Therapy

One comprehensive comparison of behavior management training, problem-solving and communication training, and structural family therapy

(Barkley et al., 1992) concluded that all three treatments resulted in significant reductions in negative communications, conflicts, and anger during conflicts, as well as improved ratings of school adjustment, reduced internalizing and externalizing symptoms, and decreased maternal depressive symptoms. The structural family therapy procedures used is this study were based on the principles set forth in Minuchin (1974) as described by Aponte and Van Deusen (1981) for helping families to identify and alter maladaptive family systems or interactional processes.

Szapocznik et al. (1989) compared the effectiveness of structural family therapy with psychodynamic child therapy for boys who presented with behavioral and emotional problems. Their results showed that both therapy groups were significantly more effective than a control condition consisting of recreational activities, such as doing arts and crafts, learning songs, and learning to play musical instruments. By the follow-up, all three groups maintained the improvement shown at posttest on the behavioral, self-report, and psychodynamic measures but did not differ significantly among themselves. Szapocznik et al. reported a dramatic effect on the family functioning measure, with the family therapy condition improving, the child therapy condition deteriorating, and the control group remaining the same.

The structural family therapy demonstrated improved family functioning and greater safety in that it protected the integrity of the family. The "integrity of the family" was measured by the direct observation of the family interacting during three types of tasks: planning a menu that everyone would enjoy, describing things that others do in the family that please or displease each family member, and discussing a previous family argument. The comparison of structural family therapy with psychodynamic child therapy, including random assignment of children and their families to alternative treatments and a control condition, represents a significant advancement in the quest to identify effective intervention strategies for children with behavior disorders. In time, such rigorous evaluation strategies will certainly help to identify the therapies that work with children. Clearly, the short- and long-term follow-up data from the structural family therapy treatment would argue for subsequent comparison of structural family therapy treatment with both the cognitive–behavioral therapy and the parent management training. It is only through such comparisons that accurate recommendations about intervention can be made.

Conduct Disorder

Pharmacological Intervention

Only a few controlled studies are available on the use of medication with CD. Three drugs that have been investigated for their effectiveness with CD children are clonidine, lithium, and risperidone. Clonidine was tested in 17 outpatients ranging in age from 5 to 15 years with severe, treatment-resistant, aggressive behavior (Kemph, DeVane, Levin, Jarecke, & Miller, 1993). Fifteen of the 17 patients showed a significant decrease in aggressive behavior during treatment with clonidine. Although these results are promising, data were collected for only about 2 weeks, and Kemph et al. did not report the use of a control condition (placebo, alternative treatment, or wait list). Clonidine alone or in combination with methylphenidate has also been studied for reducing the aggressive symptoms of CD and ODD (Connor, Barkley, & Davis, 2000). Connor et al. reported significant improvements in all three groups (methylphenidate alone, clonidine alone, and both methylphenidate and clonidine), with only a few measures showing differences between the three treatments. This study also showed similar improvements for children with ADHD, which is often comorbid with CD. In fact, both methylphenidate (Ritalin) and d-amphetamine (Dexedrine) have proved effective in decreasing aggression and other disruptive behaviors in children with comorbid CD and ADHD (Vitiello & Jensen, 1995), but virtually all of the studies were with older children.

Vitiello and Jensen (1995) stated that lithium carbonate has proven antiaggressive properties in children with explosive aggression that are as good as haloperidol but with fewer side effects, but they cautioned that it has not been studied in nonhospitalized patients. Information on Eskalith (lithium carbonate) in the *Physician's Desk Reference* (1999) does not recommend use in children younger than 12 because of the lack of any controlled studies. Although there is widespread use of clonidine for the aggressive and impulsive components of CD, there have been few studies investigating this drug.

Risperidone has been shown to be superior to a placebo in the treatment of the aggressive behavior of CD patients ages 5–15. Unfortunately, the brevity of the study (10 weeks), combined with the high dropout rate (40%) and problems with side effects, dramatically reduces the applicability of these results (Findling et al., 2000).

Similar to the medical treatment of ODD, Cantwell (1989a) stated that although pharmacological interventions have not been sufficiently demonstrated to be effective with CD, they have been effective for the ADHD component in children who have both CD and ADHD. (Pharmocotherapy for ADHD is discussed in the following section on ADHD.)

The lack of outcome studies with children with CD must be contrasted with the recent reports on the tremendous increase in the use of psychotropic medications with children (Zito et al., 2000). The increase in the use of such medications in the absence of proof of their effectiveness has been viewed by the medical community with alarm (see Coyle, 2000). In fact, Coyle stated,

> It appears that behaviorally disturbed children are now increasingly subjected to quick and inexpensive pharmacological fixes as opposed to informed, multimodal therapy associated with optimal outcomes. These

disturbing prescription practices suggest a growing crisis in mental health services to children and demand more thorough investigation. (p. 1060)

Further discussion of this phenomenon can be found in the section on ADHD.

Behavioral Interventions

The programs that have been effective in dealing with CD have been characterized by both their breadth and their intensity. Most require a large number of sessions, often in excess of 20 sessions, to achieve treatment gains. And in an effort to provide more cost-effective interventions for children with CD, numerous clinicians have resorted to group interventions. The interventions discussed here include cognitive–behavioral therapy and a combination of cognitive–behavioral therapy and parent management training.

Cognitive–behavioral therapy. Kazdin and his colleagues have provided several empirical demonstrations of the effectiveness of cognitive–behavioral therapy on reducing severe conduct problems in children. For example, Kazdin, Bass, Siegel, and Thomas (1989) evaluated alternative treatments for 112 children (ages 7–13) who exhibited severe antisocial behavior. Children were randomly assigned to one of three treatment groups: problem-solving skills training (PSST); problem-solving skills training with in vivo practice (PSST-P), which included therapeutically planned activities to extend training to settings outside treatment; or client-centered relationship therapy (RT). The PSST training emphasized interpersonal situations in everyday life, using structured games and stories. The training combined cognitive and behavioral techniques to teach a step-by-step approach to managing interpersonal situations with parents, teachers, siblings, peers, and others. Within the sessions, practice, modeling, role playing, corrective feedback, and social and token reinforcement were used to develop their problem-solving skills. Exhibit 1.6 summarizes the problem-solving steps included in the program.

PSST and PSST-P children showed significantly greater reductions in antisocial behavior and overall behavior problems, as well as greater increases in prosocial behavior than RT children. These effects were evident on measures obtained immediately after treatment, at 1-year follow-up, and on measures of child performance at home and at school. Despite the significant improvements, however, comparisons with nonclinic (normative) samples revealed that the majority of youths were still not within the normal range of deviant behavior.

Parent management training (PMT) draws on the procedures described by Patterson et al. (1975), including how to

- observe and define behavior
- use reinforcement to encourage appropriate behaviors

EXHIBIT 1.6
Problem-Solving Skills-Training Steps

1. What am I supposed to do?
   This step requires that the child identify and define the problem.
2. I have to look at all my possibilities.
   This step asks the child to delineate or specify alternative solutions to one problem.
3. I had better concentrate and focus in.
   This step instructs the child to concentrate and evaluate the solutions that he or she has generated
4. I need to make a choice.
   During this step, the child chooses the answer that he or she thinks is correct.
5. I did a good job, or Oh, I made a mistake.
   This step entails checking to verify the solution: whether it was the best among those available, whether the problem-solving process was followed correctly, or whether a mistake or less-than-desirable solution was selected (in which case the process should begin anew).

Note: These steps are used by the child to develop an approach toward responding to interpersonal situations. The steps, as presented here, provide the initial set of statements. Over the course of treatment, use of the steps change in separate ways, for example, Steps 2 and 3 merge to form a separate question ("What could I do and what would happen?), which is then answered as the child generates multiple ways of responding and the likely consequences of each. Also, the steps move from overt (aloud) to covert (silent, internal) statements.

- use shaping to teach new behaviors
- use negotiating and behavioral contracting
- use time-out to discourage inappropriate behavior
- reduce or eliminate the use of verbal reprimands.

In a large prospective study with random assignment to treatment groups, Kazdin et al. (1992) compared the effectiveness of PMT with PSST. Each group improved over the course of treatment, with further improvements at 1-year follow-up on parental measures of overall child dysfunction, prosocial competence, and aggressive, antisocial, and delinquent behavior. The best results were obtained in the combined group, with the PMT training alone showing the fewest changes.

Finally, one of the largest prospective studies on the treatment of children with CD was published by Kazdin and Wassell (2000). They analyzed the outcomes of 250 children (ages 2–14) whose families were treated using cognitive PSST, PMT, or both. Their main findings were as follows:

- Child, parent, and family functioning improved over the course of treatment.

- The effects were evident across multiple measures of child symptoms, parent symptoms and stress, and family relations, functioning, and support.
- The magnitude of these changes indicated large effects for child outcome measures and smaller effects for parent and family outcome measures.
- Changes in children, parents, and family measures were significantly and moderately correlated.
- Socioeconomic disadvantage, child severity of dysfunction, and perceived barriers to participation in treatment predicted therapeutic change, but the patterns of predictors varied among child, parent, and family outcome.

The Kazdin model has produced some of the most promising results to date and has been subjected to rigorous scientific evaluation.

Parenting groups for children with CD. Webster-Stratton and her colleagues have conducted a number of studies using group designs with multiple measures, random assignment to treatment groups, and long-term follow-up. Webster-Stratton (1996) described her parent training model, based primarily on Patterson's (1982) coercion hypothesis, as using videotaped vignettes depicting children in a variety of situations and settings (e.g., at home with parents, in the classroom, and on the playground). The interested reader is referred to *The Parents and Children Series*, by Webster-Stratton (n.d.), for a comprehensive description of her video-based course for parents, teachers, and other adults who are living or working with children ages 2–8.

Webster-Stratton and Hammond (1997) studied children with CD (ages 4–8). They compared group child therapy (CT) in which only the child received treatment, group parent training (PT) in which only the parents received treatment, a combination of CT + PT in which both the child and the parent received treatment at the same point in time, and a wait list (WL) control. One of the major components in the Webster-Stratton therapy is the use of videotapes to depict such events as children cooperating with time-outs, children using positive self-talk, and parents dealing with a variety of situations. They used the videotapes to show parents' models in natural situations with their children "doing it right" and "doing it wrong" to debunk the notion that there is perfect parenting and to illustrate how parents can learn from their mistakes.

The results showed that the combined CT + PT group had significantly more improvements in child behavior at the 1-year follow-up. Comparisons of the three treatment conditions showed that the CT and the CT + PT children showed significant improvements in their problem-solving skills as well as conflict resolution skills, as measured by observations of their interactions with a best friend. Differences among treatment conditions on these measures consistently favored the CT condition over the PT condition. One-year follow-up assessments indicated that all the significant changes noted immediately after treatment had been maintained over time. Moreover, the children's conduct problems at home had significantly lessened over time. Webster-Stratton (1990) did report 3-year follow-up data on children with CD treated individually and those treated individually and in groups. Her results showed that, although mothers and fathers from all three treatment groups (individual videotapes, group videotapes, and group discussion without videotapes) continued to report fewer total child behavior problems at the 3-year follow-up in comparison with baseline, only the parents treated in groups using videotapes showed stable improvements. The publication of Webster-Stratton's *The Parents and Children Series* (n.d.) represents one of the most systematic attempts to produce and distribute "treatment manuals" for use with children with CD.

Parenting groups for the prevention of conduct problems. In their review of outcome studies for treatment of CD, Offord and Bennett (1994) stated that, because of the heavy burden of suffering CD, there is a compelling argument in favor of an increased emphasis on primary prevention efforts. Webster-Stratton has conducted pioneering work in the area of the "prevention" of conduct problems in children who are at high risk for developing them. For example, Webster-Stratton (1998) conducted research on preventing conduct problems with Head Start mothers and their 4-year-old children. The major intervention component involved teaching positive discipline strategies, effective parenting skills, and ways of strengthening their child's social skills using videotapes. Intervention children showed significantly more improvement than the children in the control group as measured by changes in their conduct problems, compliance, and affect. One year later, most of the improvements had been maintained. Webster-Stratton should be commended for attempting prevention research in natural settings with children at high-risk for development of conduct problems. The appeal of such prevention programs is that they are implemented at a time when the problems are still relatively mild and the intervention is relatively inexpensive. Ultimately, Head Start programs across the United States could be used to disseminate information on parenting to mothers from high-risk groups.

Attention Deficit Hyperactivity Disorder

A wide variety of treatments have been used for ADHD, including but not limited to various psychotropic medications, psychosocial treatment, dietary management, herbal and homeopathic treatments, biofeedback, meditation, and perceptual stimulation. Of these treatment strategies, medications and psychosocial interventions have been the major focus of research. Studies on the efficacy of medication and psychosocial treatments for ADHD have focused primarily on a condition equivalent to *DSM–IV* combined type, meeting criteria for inattention and hyperactivity/impulsivity (National Institutes of Health Task Force, 1998).

Pharmacological Intervention

Psychostimulant medications have been the most extensively studied intervention for ADHD and related disruptive behavior disorders. Anastopoulos, DuPaul, and Barkley (1992) reported that more than 70% of children with ADHD who take these medications exhibit behavioral, academic, and attention improvements according to parent ratings, teacher ratings, direct observations, or a combination of these measures. The Council of Scientific Affairs of the American Medical Association (Goldman et al., 1998) concluded, after an exhaustive literature review, that there is little evidence of widespread overdiagnosis or misdiagnosis of ADHD, or of widespread overprescription of methylphenidate by physicians. For example, in a large-scale study, Jensen et al. (1999) reported that medication treatments were often not used in treating ADHD children identified in the community, and they decided that, on the basis of their data, it cannot be concluded that too many children are being treated with medications.

Several other studies, however, have been more concerned about the increasing use of medications for children with ADHD and other disorders. Rappley et al. (1999) identified 223 children ages 3 and under who were diagnosed with ADHD, with more than half receiving psychotropic medications (57%), whereas less than half of these children were receiving any type of psychological services. L. M. Robinson, Sclar, Skaer, and Galin (1999) reported a 2.3-fold increase in the population-adjusted rate of office-based visits documenting a diagnosis of ADHD, a 2.9-fold increase in the population-adjusted rate of ADHD-patient-prescribed stimulant pharmacotherapy, and a 2.6-fold increase in the population-adjusted rate of ADHD-patient-prescribed methylphenidate.

It is worth noting that there has been a significant increase in the overall use of psychotropic medications with children, particularly with preschoolers. For example, Zito et al. (2000) reported on the prescribing patterns for preschoolers in two states across a 5-year span. The largest increase was in prescriptions for clonidine, which increased 28 times from a low of 0.1% of children in 1991 to 2.3% of children by 1995. During this same time frame, Zito et al. reported a 3-fold increase in the use of stimulant medications and a 2.2-fold increase in the use of antidepressants. The increase in prescription medications for psychotropic drugs for very young children (3 years old or younger) is even more alarming considering the fact that, after polling the physician members of the Editorial Board of the *Journal of Child and Adolescent Psychopharmacology*, Coyle (2000) reported that 80% of them reported either no use or very rare use of prescription medications for children in this age group. Coyle further stated that the lack of clinical research on the long-term consequences of pharmacological treatment of behavior problems in young children was a strong basis of concern for these prescribing practices.

There is one comprehensive study of the efficacy of the use of medication with children with ADHD published by the MTA Cooperative Group (1999). A total of 579 children were randomly assigned to 14 months of medication management, intensive behavioral treatment, both medication and behavioral treatment, and standard community care. Although there were a number of shortcomings to the study (not the least of which was that in the community sample virtually all received medication similar to the children in the medication-alone group), this is the largest scale and longest study to date. The main conclusions of the study were that medication management was superior to behavioral treatment and that the combined (medication plus behavioral treatment) was no better than medication alone, although the combination group may have provided modest advantage for non-ADHD symptoms and for positive functioning outcomes. In fact, parent satisfaction scores for combined treatment and behavioral treatment alone were significantly superior to medication management alone. This suggests that the parent placed a high value on the services received in the behavioral treatment.

The MTA Cooperative Group (1999), the largest and best-designed study published to date, clearly supported the efficacy of the use of stimulant medication with children diagnosed with ADHD. At the time of this writing, the treatment of choice for children and adolescents with ADHD, without any comorbid conditions such as ODD and CD, is stimulant medication. Because there are virtually no outcome studies on the efficacy of medications for the most common comorbid conditions, behavioral interventions remain the treatment of choice for these children. In response to concerns about medicating young children, the White House, upon the recommendation of the American Medical Association, has directed the Food and Drug Administration and the National Institutes of Health to implement a nationwide study on the use of Ritalin in children younger than age 6 (Pear, 2000).

Medication side effects. Barkley and his colleagues (Ahmann et al., 1993; Barkley, McMurray, Edelbrock, & Robbins, 1990) used a questionnaire as an assessment device to estimate the extent and severity of negative side effects that children with ADHD experienced when stimulant medication (Ritalin) was prescribed. The use of the questionnaire, which has been referred to as the Barkley Side Effects Questionnaire (BSEQ), both before any medication was prescribed and at weekly intervals after the medication was prescribed, revealed that the most significant side effects were decreased appetite, insomnia, stomachaches, and headaches. The remaining nine items (prone to crying, tics, drowsiness, talking less, disinterest in other children, euphoria, nightmares, sadness, and staring) did not differ. At higher dosages, children were nearly twice as likely to experience decreased appetite than the same children taking lower dosages. Ahmann et al. reported high baseline rates for both daydreaming and anxiety, suggesting that these are not side effects of Ritalin but, rather, symptoms or behaviors associated with ADHD that are possibly benefited by stimulant therapy.

Ahmann et al. (1993) further reported that, in general, the number of patients reporting side effects was higher, and in some cases substantially higher, during baseline than during the placebo condition. Ahmann et al. suggested that parents may have overreported symptoms in the baseline condition in the hope that their physician would be convinced that treatment was needed. In any event, the use of the BSEQ or a similar instrument, at least during baseline and after each change in medication dosage, provides the clinician with objective estimates of the incidence and severity of side effects to the medication.

Exhibit 1.7 is a Side Effects Questionnaire based on Barkley et al. (1990) that we routinely use before and after administration of stimulant medication. At the appointment during which a medication trial is discussed, we ask the parent or parents to rate their child on each of the BSEQ items. A letter is then prepared for the primary care physician summarizing the results of the evaluation, recommending a trial on stimulant medication, and informing the physician that the parent or parents completed the BSEQ for baseline. If the primary care physician elects to give the child a trial on stimulant medication, the parents are asked to complete the BSEQ again after the dosage of the medication has stabilized.

Medication recommendations. When ADHD evaluations are conducted by psychologists, it is quite common for them to conclude that an individual child might benefit from a trial on stimulant medication. Several states have ruled on the legality of psychologists making recommendations to primary care physicians about medication trials and dosing. The courts have ruled that psychologists who by training and experience are knowledgeable about certain diagnostic conditions and the medications used to treat them can legally make such a recommendation (Clay, 1998). Because the physician is ultimately responsible for writing the prescription, the courts in Missouri, Florida, Maryland, and Massachusetts have ruled that psychologists cannot be prosecuted for practicing medicine without a license. Unfortunately, there have not been any cases in which the issue of competence based on education, training, supervised experience, or appropriate professional experience has been clarified. Until such issues are addressed, it is in the best interest of nonphysicians, and the patients they serve, to err in the direction of too much training or experience rather than too little. Regardless of whether the psychologist actually initiates discussion of the use of stimulant medication, however, familiarity with the possibility of negative side effects of stimulant medication is in the best interest of the child, the psychologist, and the prescribing physician.

EXHIBIT 1.7
Barkley Side Effects Questionnaire

CHECKLIST OF SYMPTOMS SOME CHILDREN EXPERIENCE

NAME: _____ DATE: _____

PERSON FILLING OUT FORM: _____

INSTRUCTIONS: Please rate each behavior from 0 (*absent*) to 9 (*serious*). Circle only one number beside each item. A zero means that you have not seen the behavior in this child during the past week, and a 9 means that you have noticed it and believe it to be either very serious or to occur very frequently.

Behavior	Absent									Serious
Insomnia/trouble sleeping	0	1	2	3	4	5	6	7	8	9
Drowsiness	0	1	2	3	4	5	6	7	8	9
Nightmares	0	1	2	3	4	5	6	7	8	9
Stares a lot or daydreams	0	1	2	3	4	5	6	7	8	9
Bedwetting	0	1	2	3	4	5	6	7	8	9
Talks less with others	0	1	2	3	4	5	6	7	8	9
Uninterested in others	0	1	2	3	4	5	6	7	8	9
Decreased appetite	0	1	2	3	4	5	6	7	8	9
Irritable	0	1	2	3	4	5	6	7	8	9
Hair loss	0	1	2	3	4	5	6	7	8	9
Stomachaches	0	1	2	3	4	5	6	7	8	9
Headaches	0	1	2	3	4	5	6	7	8	9
Nervous movements	0	1	2	3	4	5	6	7	8	9
Muscle cramping	0	1	2	3	4	5	6	7	8	9
Seizures	0	1	2	3	4	5	6	7	8	9
Sad/unhappy	0	1	2	3	4	5	6	7	8	9
Prone to crying	0	1	2	3	4	5	6	7	8	9
Anxious	0	1	2	3	4	5	6	7	8	9
Bites fingernails	0	1	2	3	4	5	6	7	8	9
Euphoric/unusually happy	0	1	2	3	4	5	6	7	8	9
Dizziness	0	1	2	3	4	5	6	7	8	9
Tics	0	1	2	3	4	5	6	7	8	9
Diarrhea	0	1	2	3	4	5	6	7	8	9
Constipation	0	1	2	3	4	5	6	7	8	9

Note. From "Side Effects of Methylphenidate in Children With Attention Deficit Hyperactivity Disorder: A Systemic, Placebo-Controlled Evaluation," by R. A. Barkley, M. B. McMurray, C. S. Edelbrock, & K. Robbins, 1990, *Pediatrics, 86,* pp. 184–192. Copyright 1990 by American Academy of Pediatrics. Adapted with permission.

Behavioral Interventions

Although stimulants can lead to significant behavioral improvements in a large percentage of children with ADHD, behavioral parent training may be necessary when the child experiences undesirable negative side effects, during those times when medication is not taken, and in order to assist the parents in dealing with comorbid ODD (Anastopoulos et al., 1996). An example of an effective parent training program is provided by Anastopoulos and his colleagues. They reported on a 2-year evaluation of behavior parent training (PT) for 36 children who met the diagnostic criteria for ADHD, 14 of whom were also diagnosed with ODD. Exhibit 1.8 summarizes the steps in the PT program. Anastopoulos et al. reported that, compared with the wait list controls, children receiving PT displayed significant changes in several areas of psychosocial functioning immediately after treatment and during a 2-month follow-up period.

The behavioral treatment component of the MTA Cooperative Group (1999) intervention included PT, child-focused treatment, and a school-based intervention organized and integrated within the school year. The parent training was based on the work of Barkley (1987) and Forehand and McMahon (1981). The groups with the behavioral treatment showed greater benefits than community care (which was essentially a medication-alone component) for oppositional/aggressive behaviors, internalizing symp-

EXHIBIT 1.8
Summary of Parent Training Program for Children With
Attention Deficit Hyperactivity Disorder

Session	Therapeutic Content
1	Overview of attention deficit hyperactivity disorder
2	Discussion of four-factor model of parent–child conflict; review of behavioral management principles
3	Using positive attending and ignoring skills during special play time
4	Using positive attending and ignoring skills to promote appropriate independent play and compliance with simple requests; discussion of how to give commands more effectively
5	Setting up a comprehensive, reward-oriented home token/point system
6	Using response cost for minor noncompliance and rule violations
7	Using time out from reinforcement for more serious rule violations
8	Handling child behavior problems in public
9	Handling future problems; working cooperatively with school personnel (e.g., setting up daily report card systems)

Note. From "Family-Based Treatment: Psychosocial Intervention for Children and Adolescents With Attention Deficit Hyperactivity Disorder" (p. 271), by A. D. Anastopoulos, R. A. Barkley, and T. L. Shelton. In E. D. Hibbs & P. S. Jensen (Eds.), *Psychosocial Treatments for Child and Adolescent Disorders: Empirically Based Strategies for Clinical Practice,* 1996, Washington, DC: American Psychological Association. Copyright 1996 by the American Psychological Association. Reprinted with permission.

toms, peer interactions, parent–child relations, and reading achievement. These results have not been previously reported in long-term studies. Perhaps as interesting as the outcome on the behavioral measures was the fact that parents reported significantly higher satisfaction ratings with the combined (medication plus behavioral treatment) and behavioral treatment groups.

Cognitive–Behavioral Therapy

Kendall and Braswell (1985) provided a treatment manual for implementation of their self-control program for impulsive children. Each of the 12 sessions involves the therapist teaching the child to use the self-instructional procedures by means of modeling while working on a variety of impersonal and interpersonal problem-solving tasks. The program includes the use of a token economy during the therapy sessions. Although the children are required to buy one prize at the end of each therapy session, they may choose to bank some of their tokens to purchase a more expensive prize after a future session.

Kendall and Braswell's (1985) 12 sessions include how to teach children to

- use self-statements
- follow directions
- use verbal self-instructions, first to solve arithmetic problems and later to address social and interpersonal tasks
- identify the emotions involved in social interactions
- physically act out what they would do in specific social situations
- handle actual social situations.

Kendall and Braswell (1985) also included a therapy checklist (see Exhibit 1.9) as a reminder of the process and activities that were supposed to be covered within each session and across sessions.

Barriers to Effective Interventions

The most commonly encountered problem in dealing with disruptive behaviors is maintaining parental adherence to the treatment recommendations for their child. As Patterson (1982) pointed out, some parents get into a coercive cycle—their coercive behavior produces coercive behavior on the child's part, which in turn leads to further coercive behavior on the parents' part. Breaking this cycle is sometimes difficult. Also, when dealing with disruptive behaviors, whether the oppositional component is dealt with directly (e.g., with discipline) or less directly (e.g., with ignoring), there is sometimes an escalation in the child's oppositional behavior prior to a decrease (Drabman & Jarvie, 1977). This initial increase is sometimes

EXHIBIT 1.9
Therapy Checklist

1. Begin each session by checking whether the child remembers the self-instructions and has an example of when and how they can be used.

2. Fade from overt to covert speech over the course of the treatment and occasionally during each session.

3. Enact a response-cost when the child
   a. Forgets a self-instruction
   b. Solves the task incorrectly
   c. Goes too fast

4. Label each response-cost. Be specific in the very beginning, but emphasize conceptual labeling in latter sessions.

5. Teach self-evaluation and give bonus chips for accurate self-evaluation.

6. Model the task immediately following a response-cost. Highlight the coping statement when you model a task following a response-cost.

7. Watch for mechanical use of the self-instruction.

8. Banking; reward menu

Note. From *Cognitive–Behavioral Therapy for Impulsive Children* (p. 207), by P. C. Kendall and L. Braswell, 1985, New York: Guilford Press. Copyright 1985 by Guilford Press. Reprinted with permission.

a cause for the parents' concern if they have not been prepared for it in advance.

Patterson and Chamberlain (1994) showed that a similar phenomenon occurs between the parents and the therapist. As the therapist increased efforts to intervene with the parents, there were corresponding increases in the parents' resistance to follow the therapist's recommendations. Patterson and Chamberlain were particularly intrigued with the set of findings demonstrating that the client may be changing the behavior of the therapist while the therapist is changing the behavior of the client. They also presented data suggesting that families with younger children in treatment are more like to stay in treatment and are more likely to benefit from treatment than families with older children.

Eyberg, Edwards, Boggs, and Foote (1998) reviewed the literature on strategies for maintaining treatment effects of parent training. They identified two major strategies for maintenance. First, maintenance strategies used during treatment typically involve "fading," or gradually lengthening the time between treatment sessions, as well as teaching self-management, problem-solving, and communication skills. Second, maintenance strategies used after treatment typically involve the use of brief, periodic contacts between parents and therapists. An important function of posttreatment professional contact is to help parents sustain motivation and behavioral changes needed for long-term success. Eyberg et al. stated that, to their knowledge, no one has actually evaluated the effectiveness of booster sessions on maintaining treatment gains. Although the MTA Cooperative Group (1999) study included some provisions for addressing long-term gains in the behavioral treatment group, the study design did not allow for an analysis of any single component of the treatment. Thus, at this point in time, the issue of maintenance of long-term treatment gains has not been adequately addressed in the literature.

CONCLUSION

The combination of the high incidence as well as the intrusiveness of disruptive behavior disorders makes them particularly troublesome for parents. When parents are unable to manage these behaviors at home, or when the child begins to demonstrate significant struggles with school and social relationships, assistance from mental health providers is often sought.

The assessment of disruptive behavior disorders is aimed at estimating the extent to which a given child or adolescent exhibits these behaviors as well as the degree of impairment in the child's academic or social functioning. The use of multiple informants, including both the parents and the teachers, is preferred. Parent and teacher rating scales are used extensively in the diagnosis of disruptive behavior problems, primarily because they are readily available, inexpensive, and well accepted in the mental health community. Although clinic-based diagnostic tests, such as continuous performance tasks, have a tremendous appeal in that they can be readily administered with little monitoring by office personnel, the information that is gleaned from them is, at least at the present time, of little value in formulating a diagnosis. Although our assessment tools for diagnosing disruptive behavior disorder can be quite convincing, it is important to bear in mind that such a diagnosis can have a significant impact on the child and family, and thus must be made cautiously. In many clinical settings, a child diagnosed as having ADHD may almost immediately be considered for a trial on stimulant medication.

With the exception of ADHD, pharmacological therapies are of limited effectiveness for children's disruptive behavior disorders. With ODD and CD, the literature on pharmacological therapies is characterized by weak experimental designs, the lack of random assignment, and little, if any, long-term data.

There has been much discussion in the literature about the large number and young ages of children diagnosed with ADHD. Although several authors have provided convincing evidence that ADHD is not being overdiagnosed in children and adolescents, there is cause for concern for children ages 5 and younger. Zito et al. (2000) reported increases in prescriptions for very young children, from 220% for antidepressants to up to 2,800% for clonidine. Neither of these increases is actually supported by the literature.

That is, there are no well-designed research studies documenting the efficacy of either antidepressants or clonidine with young children.

In terms of behavioral interventions, there have been major contributions. Parent management training is one of the best-researched therapy techniques for the treatment of oppositional and aggressive youths (Kazdin & Weisz, 1998). The treatment of children with disruptive behavior disorders has been approached from parent training as well as child-focused and group perspectives. The finding that a combination of problem-solving skills treatment and parent management training was superior to either treatment alone is not surprising. These treatment approaches produce significant improvements in children's behavior, but children with disruptive behavior disorders often are rated as having clinical problems after treatment when compared with their nonclinical peers.

Webster-Stratton's (1996) approach, in which the parents are seen in small groups, is potentially more cost-effective, with the research to date demonstrating outcomes at least as efficacious with groups as with individual families. In fact, Webster-Stratton made the point, in her published work, that parents accept the group interventions well, appreciating the discussion and togetherness afforded by the group. Acceptability of the groups, both by the general public and by third-party payers and HMOs, has yet to be addressed.

The clinician treating children with disruptive behavior disorders now has numerous assessment tools that are empirically based and that are economical to administer and to score. With respect to treatment, although there are not any studies that have compared parent training, problem solving, Webster-Stratton's parent training using videotaped vignettes, and structured family therapy, the outcomes of these strategies are such that the clinician can really choose any one of them. The treatment manuals that have been developed for use with each of these strategies are comprehensive and practical. And although they were developed with the goal of evaluating the overall intervention strategy, they do offer numerous empirically based procedures for use by the clinician.

2

DIAGNOSIS AND MANAGEMENT
OF ANXIETY DISORDERS

Most children have various fears and worries throughout their childhood, and such apprehensions are often labeled as *anxiety*. For example, it is developmentally appropriate for an 8-month-old to demonstrate *stranger anxiety* by perhaps crying and clinging to a caregiver when approached by an unknown person. Many children also display some *separation anxiety* from approximately ages 10 months to 18 months as they protest being away from caregivers. As children age, other common anxieties develop, such as fear of the dark, worries about social performance, fear of harm to loved ones, and fear of dying. Anxiety symptoms are, indeed, a common occurrence in childhood. At times, however, these worries or fears can become exacerbated to the point of causing significant impairment in the child's functioning. When both symptoms of anxiety and impairment are present, the child should be evaluated for a possible anxiety disorder.

There are numerous anxiety disorders defined in the *Diagnostic and Statistical Manual of Mental Disorders* (4th ed., *DSM–IV*; American Psychiatric Association, 1994) that characterize the symptoms of worry and fear that afflict children. The disorders that are included in this chapter are those seen most frequently by clinicians and that have empirically supported treatments reported in the literature. They include separation anxiety disorder, generalized anxiety disorder, social phobia, and specific phobia. The anxiety disorders that are not discussed in this chapter include panic disorder, obsessive–compulsive disorder, acute stress disorder, and posttraumatic stress disorder.

Separation anxiety disorder is defined as excessive distress and fearfulness on the part of the child when asked to separate from a major attachment figure. This distress may be manifested as persistent worry about the safety of the person whom they are separated from, refusal to go to school, sleep problems, and somatic complaints. Generalized anxiety disorder, which includes the previous classification of overanxious disorder of childhood, is defined as excessive worry about numerous events and activities that is difficult for the person to control. Common worries may include fear of displaying a poor performance at school, fear of imperfection, and a general fear of catastrophes. More specific fears are included under social and specific phobias. Children with this disorder may suffer from restlessness, fatigue, irritability, or sleep disturbance. Social phobia, which has also been called social anxiety disorder, is the fear of social performance and potential evaluation by others. The child may avoid the social situation and may or may not be aware that his or her distressed response is excessive. Finally, specific phobias are excessive reactions to the presence or anticipated presence of a specific situation or object. The child may react by excessively crying, clinging, or having a tantrum when faced with the feared stimulus. Common specific phobias include fear of animals, occurrences in the natural environment such as storms, fear of injury or blood, and fears related to situations such as flying or being in enclosed places. Exhibit 2.1 lists the DSM–IV criteria for the anxiety disorders described above.

DIFFERENTIAL DIAGNOSES

Definitions of anxiety disorders for children have been modified over the years. These modifications may be a result of the uncertainty surrounding such diagnoses given their significant symptom overlap with each other and with other disorders (Labellarte, Ginsburg, Walkup, & Riddle, 1999). In the DSM–III–R (American Psychiatric Association, 1987), three anxiety diagnoses were listed in the child and adolescent disorders section: separation anxiety disorder, overanxious disorder, and avoidant disorder. Further refinement of these definitions resulted in only separation anxiety disorder remaining in the section on childhood disorders found in the DSM–IV (American Psychiatric Association, 1994). The other two disorders in the DSM–III–R were subsumed under generalized anxiety disorder and social phobia, respectively. To assist the clinician with making a differential diagnosis between the various anxiety disorders, Exhibit 2.2 presents the diagnostic criteria for each disorder in a checklist format that can be used during the diagnostic interview. It is important to remember, however, that many

EXHIBIT 2.1
DSM–IV Criteria for Four Common Anxiety Disorders in Children

Separation Anxiety Disorder	Generalized Anxiety Disorder

Separation Anxiety Disorder

A. Developmentally inappropriate and excessive anxiety concerning separation from home or from those to whom the individual is attached, as evidenced by three (or more) of the following:
  1. recurrent excessive distress when separation from home or major attachment figures occurs or is anticipated
  2. persistent and excessive worry about losing, or about possible harm befalling, major attachment figures
  3. persistent and excessive worry that an untoward event will lead to separation from a major attachment figure (e.g., getting lost or being kidnapped)
  4. persistent reluctance or refusal to go to school or elsewhere because of fear of separation
  5. persistently and excessively fearful or reluctant to be alone or without major attachment figures at home or without significant adults in other settings
  6. persistent reluctance or refusal to go to sleep without being near a major attachment figure or to sleep away from home
  7. repeated nightmares involving the theme of separation
  8. repeated complaints of physical symptoms (such as headaches, stomachaches, nausea, or vomiting) when separation from major attachment figures occurs or is anticipated
B. The duration of the disturbance is at least 4 weeks.
C. The onset is before age 18 years.
D. The disturbance causes clinically significant distress or impairment in social, academic (occupational), or other important areas of functioning.
E. The disturbance does not occur exclusively during the course of

Generalized Anxiety Disorder

A. Excessive anxiety and worry (apprehensive expectation), occurring more days than not for at least 6 months, about a number of events or activities (such as work or school performance).
B. The person finds it difficult to control the worry.
C. The anxiety and worry are associated with three (or more) of the following six symptoms (with at least some symptoms present for more days than not for the past 6 months). Note: Only one item is required in children.
  1. restlessness or feeling keyed up or on edge
  2. being easily fatigued
  3. difficulty concentrating or mind going blank
  4. irritability
  5. muscle tension
  6. sleep disturbance (difficulty falling or staying asleep, or restless unsatisfying sleep)
D. The focus of the anxiety and worry is not confined to features of an Axis I disorder, e.g., the anxiety or worry is not about having a Panic Attack (as in Panic Disorder), being embarrassed in public (as in Social Phobia), being contaminated (as in Obsessive–Compulsive Disorder), being away from home or close relatives (as in Separation Anxiety Disorder), gaining weight (as in Anorexia Nervosa), having multiple physical complaints (as in Somatization Disorder), or having a serious illness (as in Hypochondriasis), and the anxiety and worry do not occur exclusively during Posttraumatic Stress Disorder.
E. The anxiety, worry, or physical symptoms cause clinically significant distress or impairment in social, occupational, or other important areas of functioning.

(continued)

EXHIBIT 2.1 *(continued)*

Separation Anxiety Disorder	Generalized Anxiety Disorder
Pervasive Developmental Disorder, Schizophrenia, or other Psychotic Disorder and, in adolescents and adults, is not better accounted for by Panic Disorder With Agoraphobia.	F. The disturbance is not due to the direct physiological effects of a substance (e.g., a drug of abuse, a medication) or a general medical condition (e.g., hyperthyroidism) and does not occur exclusively during a Mood Disorder, a Psychotic Disorder, or a Pervasive Developmental Disorder.

Social Phobia	Specific Phobia

Social Phobia

A. A marked and persistent fear of one or more social or performance situations in which the person is exposed to unfamiliar people or to possible scrutiny by others. The individual fears that he or she will act in a way (or show anxiety symptoms) that will be humiliating or embarrassing. Note: In children, there must be evidence of the capacity for age-appropriate social relationships with familiar people and the anxiety must occur in peer settings, not just in interactions with adults.

B. Exposure to the feared social situation almost invariably provokes anxiety, which may take the form of a situationally bound or situationally predisposed Panic Attack. Note: In children, the anxiety may be expressed by crying, tantrums, freezing, or shrinking from the social situations with unfamiliar people.

C. The person recognizes that the fear is excessive or unreasonable. Note: In children, this feature may be absent.

D. The feared social or performance situations are avoided or else are endured with intense anxiety or distress.

E. The avoidance, anxious anticipation, or distress in the feared social or performance situation(s) interferes significantly with the person's normal routine, occupational (academic) functioning, or social activities or

Specific Phobia

A. Marked and persistent fear that is excessive or unreasonable, cued by the presence or anticipation of a specific object or situation (e.g., flying, heights, animals, receiving an injection, seeing blood).

B. Exposure to the feared social situation almost invariably provokes an immediate anxiety response, which may take the form of a situationally bound or situationally predisposed Panic Attack. Note: In children, the anxiety may be expressed by crying, tantrums, freezing, or clinging.

C. The person recognizes that the fear is excessive or unreasonable. Note: In children, this feature may be absent.

D. The phobic situation(s) is avoided or else is endured with intense anxiety or distress.

E. The avoidance, anxious anticipation, or distress in the feared situation(s) interferes significantly with the person's normal routine, occupational (or academic) functioning, or social activities or relationships, or there is marked distress about having the phobia.

F. In individuals under age 18 years, the duration is at least 6 months.

G. The anxiety, Panic Attacks, or phobic avoidance associated with the specific object or situation are not better accounted for by another mental disorder, such as

(continued)

EXHIBIT 2.1 *(continued)*

Social Phobia	**Specific Phobia**
relationships, or there is marked distress about having the phobia. F. In individuals under age 18 years, the duration is at least 6 months. G. The fear or avoidance is not due to the direct physiological effects of a substance (e.g., a drug of abuse, a medication) or a general medical condition and is not better accounted for by another mental disorder (e.g., panic disorder with or without agoraphobia, separation anxiety disorder, body dysmorphic disorder, a pervasive developmental disorder, or schizoid personality disorder. H. If a general medical condition or another mental disorder is present, the fear in Criterion A is unrelated to it, e.g., the fear is not of stuttering, trembling in Parkinson's disease, or exhibiting abnormal eating behavior in anorexia nervosa or bulimia nervosa.	Obsessive–Compulsive Disorder (e.g., fear of dirt in someone with an obsession about contamination), Posttraumatic Stress Disorder (e.g., avoidance of stimuli associated with a severe stressor), Separation Anxiety Disorder (e.g., avoidance of school), Social Phobia (e.g., avoidance of social situations because of fear of embarrassment), Panic Disorder With Agoraphobia, or Agoraphobia Without History of Panic Disorder.

Note. Information from *Diagnostic and Statistical Manual of Mental Disorders* (4th ed.), by the American Psychiatric Association, 1994, Washington, DC: Author. Copyright 1994 by the American Psychiatric Association. Reprinted with permission.

children with anxiety disorders often have comorbid anxiety and other disorders. For example, Kendall (1994) found that 60% of the children in his study with overanxious disorder, separation anxiety, or avoidant disorders also had simple phobias. Further discussion of comorbidity is found in the next section.

PREVALENCE

Epidemiological studies and clinical samplings have been conducted to determine the prevalence of anxiety disorders in children and adolescents. Anxiety disorders have been labeled as the most common type of psychopathology in children and adults (Castellanos & Hunter, 1999; E. J. Costello et al., 1996). In a review of epidemiological studies since 1986, E. J. Costello and Angold (1995) reported that anxiety disorders as a group were present in approximately 6% to 18% of the population of children ages 6–17. Information on the prevalence of specific anxiety disorders that

EXHIBIT 2.2
Anxiety Disorder Differential

Separation Anxiety Disorder (309.21)	Generalized Anxiety Disorder (300.02)
❑ Distress when separation from home or attachment figure (AF)	❑ Excessive anxiety and worry about a number of events or activities
❑ Worry about losing or harm befalling AF	❑ Difficult to control the worry
❑ Worry that bad event will lead to separation from AF	❑ One or more: restlessness, fatigue, sleep problems, irritability, tension, or concentration problems
❑ Reluctance to go to school due to fear of separation	❑ Focus of anxiety is not confined to another disorder such as fear of panic attacks (Panic Disorder)
❑ Reluctance/refusal to go to sleep without AF	❑ Duration of at least 6 months
❑ Repeated nightmares with theme of separation	
❑ At least 4 weeks' duration	
❑ Younger than 18	

Social Phobia (300.23)	Simple Phobia (300.29)
❑ Fear of social/performance situations involving unfamiliar people or possible scrutiny	❑ Excessive fear cued by presence/ anticipation of specific situation
❑ Capacity for age-appropriate relationships with familiar people	❑ Exposure to situation provokes anxiety/Panic Attack (child may freeze, cry, tantrum)
❑ Occurs in peer settings	❑ May or may not recognize fear as excessive/unreasonable
❑ Exposure provokes anxiety	❑ Situation is avoided or endured with intense distress
❑ May or may not recognize fear as excessive/unreasonable	❑ Duration of at least 6 months
❑ Situation is avoided or endured with intense distress	❑ R/O other anxiety disorders such as OCD, PTSD, etc.
❑ Duration of at least 6 months	❑ Not physiological due to substances or medical condition

* All disorders must cause significant interference with the child's normal routine, academic functioning, or social activities or relationships.

Note. From *Diagnostic and Statistical Manual of Mental Disorders* (4th ed.), by the American Psychiatric Association, 1994, Washington, DC: Author. Copyright 1994 by the American Psychiatric Association. Reprinted with permission. R/O = rule out; OCD = obsessive–compulsive disorder; PTSD = posttraumatic stress disorder.

present to a mental health clinic is also available. For example, Last, Perrin, Hersen, and Kazdin (1992) found that separation anxiety disorder was the most frequent anxiety disorder seen in a community outpatient clinic. Other common diagnoses were social phobia, simple phobia, and overanxious disorder.

The prevalence of a specific anxiety disorder varies on the basis of the child's age. For example, separation anxiety is more prevalent than the other anxiety disorders for younger children (Last et al., 1992; Westenberg, Siebelink, Warmenhoven, & Treffers, 1999), with average age on onset being 7.5 years (Last et al., 1992). Overanxious disorder is reportedly more prevalent as children age (Castellanos & Hunter, 1999; Westenberg et al., 1999). Adolescents with anxiety disorders are also more at risk for having anxiety disorders as adults. An epidemiological study of adolescents and young adults showed that the presence of an anxiety disorder in adolescence was a strong risk factor for anxiety disorders in adults, especially for simple and social phobias (Pine, Cohen, Gurley, Brook, & Ma, 1998). In a review of epidemiological studies, Costello and Angold (1995) found that 20% to 30% of children diagnosed with an anxiety disorder at a later point in time also had had a diagnosis at an earlier time. These studies demonstrate that anxiety disorders are not only prevalent but also often persist well into adulthood. They also found that such persistence in diagnosis occurred more frequently in girls than in boys.

There are several other disorders that have been found to be comorbid with anxiety disorders. The most common comorbid disorder is another anxiety disorder. For example, Last et al. (1992) found that over 90% of the children in their clinic sample with overanxious disorder and avoidant disorder also had another anxiety disorder. Kendall and his colleagues have also found that children with anxiety disorders frequently have another anxiety disorder, such as a specific phobia (Kendall, 1994; Kendall et al., 1997). The other most common comorbid disorders include depressive disorders and disruptive behavior disorders, such as attention deficit hyperactivity disorder (ADHD) and oppositional defiant disorder (Kendall, 1994; Last et al., 1992; Nilzon & Palmerus, 1998).

CAUSES AND CORRELATIONS

There is very little information reported in the literature about the causes and correlations of anxiety disorders. In fact, the available literature is generally limited to a description of potential "risk factors" for developing an anxiety disorder in childhood. These risk factors can be divided into genetic or individual characteristics of the child and environmental factors, although the contribution of each to anxiety disorders remains unclear (Legrand, McGue, & Iacono, 1999).

Child Factors

Many child factors have been explored as contributors to the etiology of anxiety disorders. Most twin studies of anxiety suggest that a genetic predisposition to anxiety does exist. For example, Legrand et al. (1999) assessed over 500 sets of twins, ages 10–18, and found moderate heritability for anxiety symptoms. As mentioned above, a child's age may also be considered as a risk factor in the development of a specific type of anxiety disorder, such as separation anxiety disorder. Younger children also endorse symptoms of simple phobias more frequently than do older children (Muris, Schmidt, & Merckelbach, 1999).

Less consistent evidence has been found for gender as a contributing factor for the development of anxiety disorders. Although boys are reportedly more at risk for developing any psychiatric disorder, gender differences for the development of anxiety disorders specifically have not been consistently demonstrated (Costello et al., 1996). Spence (1997) found no significant differences in the presenting pattern of anxiety symptoms for school-age boys and girls. Similarly, Last et al. (1992) found no significant differences in gender for the occurrence of the anxiety disorders discussed in this chapter in their clinic sample of school-age children. In contrast, Muris et al. (1999) found that more girls than boys reported a higher frequency of phobia symptoms. The presence of comorbid disorders, however, may have some influence on gender presentations of anxiety. For example, Nilzon and Palmerus (1998) found gender differences and symptoms of fear, worry, and social anxiety for girls with depression when compared with boys with depression. Finally, as mentioned previously, anxiety disorders may be more persistent for girls than for boys (Costello & Angold, 1995). In addition, girls may demonstrate more impairment in functioning once diagnosed with an anxiety disorder. For example, Schwartz, Snidman, and Kagan (1999) found that adolescent girls with generalized social anxiety were more functionally impaired than their male counterparts. Of course, it is difficult to determine if such differences are due to genetic or environmental influences or both. Finally, regardless of gender issues, the presence of other mental health and behavioral disorders may also increase a child's risk for anxiety. For children with recognized anxiety disorders, comorbid problems such as depression, oppositional behaviors, and developmental delays may put them at risk for more impairment than anxious children without these problems (Manassis & Hood, 1998).

Temperament, or more specifically a child's level of behavioral inhibition, has also been studied as a correlate of anxiety. Behavioral inhibition has been characterized as the tendency to withdraw, react negatively, or both to negative stimuli (Prior, Smart, Sanson, & Oberklaid, 2000). Children with behavioral inhibition often demonstrate such behaviors at a very young age and may be labeled as shy, timid, or fearful. Numerous studies have demonstrated that the presence of persistent behavioral inhibition in childhood is a risk factor for the development of anxiety disorders (Biederman et al., 1993; Hirshfeld et al., 1992; Prior et al., 2000; Schwartz et al., 1999). For example, Hirshfeld et al. reported on a longitudinal study that compared the rates of anxiety disorders for children rated as behaviorally inhibited or uninhibited from age 4 years to age 7. They found that children with stable behavioral inhibition had higher rates of anxiety disorders than their uninhibited peers. More specifically, Schwartz et al. found that the majority of children rated as inhibited at 2 years old displayed symptoms of social anxiety at 13 years old. Inhibition, however, was not a predictor of differences in the presence of other anxieties, such as separation anxiety, performance anxiety, or specific fears.

Environmental Factors

Two frequently reported correlates of child anxiety are parental psychopathology and impaired family functioning. Several studies have found that a significant number of children with anxiety disorders have at least one parent with psychopathology. When compared with parents of children without anxiety disorders, parents of children with anxiety disorders suffer more frequently from anxiety disorders, with and without comorbid disorders such as depression (Hirshfeld et al., 1992; Manassis & Hood, 1998; Rosenbaum et al., 1992). In fact, Turner and colleagues reported that children with anxious parents are at least seven times more likely to develop an anxiety disorder than their peers without anxious parents (Turner, Beidel, & Costello, 1987; Turner, Beidel, & Epstein, 1991). Differences in parental psychopathology have also been found for children with subclinical levels of anxiety. For instance, Bell-Dolan, Last, and Strauss (1990) found that when compared with nonanxious children, children with subclinical levels of anxiety came from households with fathers with a psychiatric diagnosis, such as major depression or alcohol dependence. Thus, parental psychopathology may certainly be a contributing factor to the development of anxiety disorders in children. The presence of psychopathology in a parent may also have a negative impact on the severity of their child's anxiety disorder. For example, Manassis and Hood (1998) found that mothers with phobic anxiety contributed to increased impairment in their anxious children. Significant psychopathology is not necessarily needed, however, for parental behavior to have a major impact on their child's level of anxiety. Simple modeling of fearfulness to situations or specific objects may also influence the development of an anxiety disorder in children. Parental modeling, for example, has been implicated as one path of transmission for the development of dog and spider phobias in children (e.g., De Jong, Andrea, & Muris, 1997; N. J. King, Clowes-Hollins, & Ollendick, 1997; Merckelbach & Muris, 1997).

Finally, some characteristics of families and their interactions have been suggested as contributors to increased risk for anxiety disorders in children. For example, Last et al. (1992) found that children diagnosed with separation anxiety disorder were more frequently being raised in single-parent homes when compared with children with other anxiety disorders. Other factors, such as large families that have experienced psychosocial adversities such as divorce, are predictive of increased impairment in children with diagnosed anxiety disorders (Manassis & Hood, 1998). Interactions between anxious parents and their children have also been studied to determine what types of interaction styles may contribute to anxiety in children. Interaction styles in families with children with anxiety disorders have been described as disengaged and rigid for older children (e.g., G. A. Bernstein, Warren, Massie, & Thuras, 1999) and less granting of autonomy and criticizing for younger children (e.g., Whaley, Pinto, & Sigman, 1999). Certainly, these studies are not discussed to implicate single parenthood or divorce as definitive factors for the development of anxiety disorders in children. They are simply presented as an example of the possible impact of environmental factors in the complicated etiology of anxiety.

Thus, although numerous studies have been conducted to determine the etiology and maintenance of anxiety disorders in children, a clear profile of all the contributing factors and their complex interactions has yet to emerge. As with other mental health disorders, the development of anxiety disorders is undoubtedly a complicated interface between genetic and environmental mechanisms. The importance of identifying such causes, of course, is to improve the state of assessment and intervention tools for diagnosing and managing anxiety disorders in children.

ASSESSMENT

The diagnostic assessment for anxiety requires a multimodal approach similar to that described in the previous chapter on disruptive behavior disorders. March and Albano (1998) suggested that an adequate diagnostic process should be able to provide valid and reliable anxiety symptom recognition and discrimination, assess severity, integrate information from multiple informants, and be sensitive to symptom changes on the basis of treatment effects. The American Academy of Child and Adolescent Psychiatry (AACAP; 1997b), in its practice guidelines on anxiety disorders in children and adolescents, suggests the following components for a thorough assessment: parent and child interviews; caregiver and child report measures; recent physical examination of the child to rule out physical conditions or medication reactions that mimic anxiety; screening for comorbid psychiatric diagnoses, including other anxiety disorders; and educational testing if concerns arise about intellect or learning problems. Exhibit 2.3

EXHIBIT 2.3
AACAP Components of Anxiety Assessment for Children

Caregiver Interview	Child Interview

Symptom History
  Onset of symptoms
  Specific, spontaneous, or anticipatory
  Presence of avoidant behavior
  Social reinforcement of symptoms
	Self-report of symptoms and impairment
	Objective signs of anxiety (vigilance, excessive motor activity, separation difficulties)

Developmental History
  Temperament
  Adaptability
  Self-calming skills
  Response to separation
  Fears and worries
	Screen for Psychiatric Disorders
	Consider comorbid disorders, including
	  Mood disorders
	  ADHD
	  Adjustment disorders
	  Substance use
	  Personality disorders

Medical History
  Number of medical visits for symptoms
  Medications that may produce symptoms (antihistamines, anti-asthmatics, steroids, haloperidol, SSRIs, diet pills, cold medicines)
  Medical disorders (hypoglycemia, hyperthyroidism, cardiac arrhythmias, seizure disorders, migraines)
	Eating disorders
	  Somatoform disorders
	  Tics
	  Habit disorders (trichotillomania)
	  Reactive attachment disorder
	  Pervasive developmental disorders
	  Schizophrenia
	*Remember that anxiety disorders are often comorbid with other anxiety disorders.

School History
  Attendance
  Academic, social, behavioral functioning
  Disparity between aptitude and achievement
	Physical Examination
	Consider referral to a physician to rule out physical conditions and medication reactions that may mimic anxiety symptoms (see Medical History in Caregiver Interview)

Family History
  Stressors, resources, coping style
  History of loss, separation
  Exposure to abuse, violence, death
  Psychiatric history (anxiety, mood disorders, attention or learning problems, tic disorders, psychotic disorders, suicidal behavior)
  Parental response to psychotropics
  Medical conditions that may mimic anxiety	

Note. From "Practice Parameters for the Assessment and Treatment of Children and Adolescents With Anxiety Disorders," by the American Academy of Child and Adolescent Psychiatry (AACAP), 1997, *Journal of the American Academy of Child and Adolescent Psychiatry, 36*(Suppl.), 69S–84S. Copyright 1997 by AACAP. Adapted with permission. ADHD = attention deficit hyperactivity disorder; SSRI = selective serotonin reuptake inhibitor.

highlights several important issues to address in the assessment of anxiety in children based on these AACAP recommendations. More extensive information on structured interviews and rating measures available to assist in the assessment of anxiety is then provided.

Structured and Semistructured Interviews

Structured and semistructured interviews have been developed to assist clinicians and researchers in establishing an accurate diagnosis. Such interviews improve diagnostic reliability by quantifying clinical data and reducing the potential for interviewer bias (Eisen & Kearney, 1995). The feasibility of available structured and semistructured interviews for use in the clinical setting is variable. For example, structured interviews can be lengthy to administer and demand exact administration of the questioning format, thus allowing little flexibility for informant- or clinician-driven elaboration or for consideration of cultural influences (March & Albano, 1998). Some semistructured interviews do exist, however, that are more clinically friendly and also demonstrate adequate psychometric properties overall as well as specifically for diagnosing anxiety disorders. Two diagnostic interviews that have been used most frequently in outcome studies for children with anxiety are the Anxiety Disorders Interview Schedule for Children (ADIS-C) and Parents (ADIS-P; Silverman & Nelles, 1988) and the Diagnostic Interview Schedule for Children (DISC; A. J. Costello, Edelbrock, Dulcan, Kalas, & Klaric, 1984). The ADIS-C and ADIS-P are designed to assess the etiology, symptomatology, course, and function of anxiety disorders in children. The ADIS-P asks more detailed questions about symptom history and consequences of anxiety behavior in the child, whereas the ADIS-C focuses on symptomatology and phenomenology. Upon completion of the interview, the clinician is able to make primary and secondary diagnoses, as well as to rate the severity of symptoms and extent of their interference for a wide range of internalizing and externalizing disorders.

The DISC (A. J. Costello et al., 1984) is a more structured interview that does not allow for nonstandard probing or elaboration. The most recent version of this measure, the DISC-IV (Shaffer et al., 2000) was updated from previous versions to accommodate the diagnostic criteria of the *DSM–IV* (American Psychiatric Association, 1994) and the International Classification of Diseases (ICD-10; World Health Organization, 1993). The DISC-IV assesses over 30 psychiatric diagnoses, including nine specific anxiety disorders. There are parallel versions of the interview for parents of children over 6 years old (DISC-P) and for children older than 9 (DISC-Y). Both formats address the nature and range of behaviors in the child, with a change in pronouns to accommodate inquiries about internal states for the child. The DISC-IV also has a Spanish version and a computerized version available from the Division of Child and Adolescent Psychiatry at Columbia University (Shaffer et al., 2000).

One concern often presented about clinical interviews that offer both parent and child data is how to reconcile differing results with respect to diagnoses. Silverman and Nelles (1988) suggested that a child receive a diagnosis of an anxiety disorder if both parent and child reports meet diagnostic criteria, if the child's data alone meet criteria, or if both reports indicate barely meeting criteria but either person rated the interference or severity as high. These criteria, along with the consideration of information gathered from other sources, could increase the likelihood of a reliable diagnosis.

Child's Self-Report of Anxiety

Measures are also available that assess the child's report of his or her own anxiety and behaviors. Such information is important not only for the diagnostic process but also to identify relevant symptomatology and level of severity for the individual child (March & Albano, 1998). The child's data may be especially significant as parents and teachers often underreport anxiety symptoms in children (Bell-Dolan et al., 1990; E. J. Costello & Angold, 1995). Self-report measures are typically administered easily and quickly, leaving time for the clinician to seek additional diagnostic information. Despite the potential importance of self-report data from children, however, some controversy exists over the reliability and validity of many available measures. Many studies of pharmacological and nonpharmacological interventions have relied on self-report measures, such as the Fear Survey Schedule for Children–Revised (FSSC-R; Ollendick, 1983), the Revised Children's Manifest Anxiety Scale (RCMAS; Reynolds & Richmond, 1985), and the State–Trait Anxiety Inventory for Children (STAIC; Spielberger 1973). A summary of the format, factor structure, and psychometric properties of these scales is presented in Table 2.1. All three of these measures have demonstrated adequate internal validity, test–retest reliability, and concurrent validity. Less conclusive evidence has been reported, however, for the discriminant validity of these measures. For example, Perrin and Last (1992) found that the FSSC-R was unable to discriminate between boys with anxiety, ADHD, or boys without previous or current psychiatric illness. A more recent study of the FSSC-R, however, found adequate discriminant validity for simple phobias but not for social phobia (Weems, Silverman, Saavedra, Pina, & Lumpkin, 1999). The RCMAS and a modified version of the STAIC (STAIC-M; Fox & Houston, 1983) were able to adequately discriminate the children with anxiety and ADHD from the non-ill group but not from each other. Such confounding may occur for the RCMAS because of questions that also tap attention and impulsivity problems (March & Albano, 1998). Given the fact that most children experience fears to some extent, as well as the fact that anxiety disorders are often comorbid with other disorders, the ability for self-report measures to reliably differentiate between populations is vital.

These limitations have led to the development of other self-report measures that purport to demonstrate adequate reliability and validity, particularly for discriminating between nonclinical levels of anxiety, multiple anxiety disorders, and other psychiatric diagnoses. Table 2.1 also describes the properties of two such measures: the Multidimensional Anxiety Scale for Children (MASC; March, Parker, Sullivan, Stallings, & Conners, 1997) and the Screen for Child Anxiety Related Emotional Disorders (SCARED; Birmaher et al., 1997, 1999). The MASC (March et al., 1997) was designed to assess common anxiety symptoms for school-age children across many domains, including physical symptomatology, social and separation anxiety, and harm avoidance. The MASC reportedly has adequate internal consistency and test–retest reliability (March et al., 1997; March, Sullivan, & Parker, 1999). It also has adequate convergent validity with other measures of anxiety such as the RCMAS (Reynolds & Richmond, 1985). Evidence of discriminant validity is provided by the scale's ability to differentiate children with anxiety from children with depression and externalizing disorders. A recent study of the MASC also supports its ability to recognize anxiety in

TABLE 2.1
Five Self-Report Measures for Assessing Anxiety in Children

Self-Report Measure	Format	Factor Structure	Sample Items	Psychometric Properties
Fear Survey Schedule for Children (FSSC-R; Ollendick, 1983)	80 items 3 ratings (none, some, a lot)	Fear of failure and criticism Fear of unknown Fear of injury and small animals Fear of danger and death Medical fears	Giving an oral report. Meeting someone for the first time. Bears and wolves. A burglar breaking into our house. Going to the dentist.	Adequate internal and test–retest reliability; adequate convergent validity; poor divergent validity except for simple phobias.
Revised Children's Manifest Anxiety Scale (RCMAS; Reynolds & Richman, 1985)	37 items Yes or No ratings	Worry/Oversensitivity Fear/Concentration Physiological	I worry when I go to bed at night. I have trouble making up my mind. I am afraid of a lot of things. I feel alone even when there are people with me. My hands feel sweaty.	Adequate internal and test–retest reliability; adequate convergent validity; poor divergent validity, especially for ADHD

(continued)

TABLE 2.1 *(continued)*

Self-Report Measure	Format	Factor Structure	Sample Items	Psychometric Properties
State–Trait Anxiety Inventory for Children (STAI-C; Spielberger, 1973)	Two, 20 item inventories (Trait Scale; State Scale)			Adequate test–retest reliability for the Trait scale; poor divergent validity
Multidimensional Anxiety Scale for Children (MASC; March et al., 1997)	39 items 4-point Likert scale ratings	Physical Symptoms -Tense/restless -Somatic/autonomic Social Anxiety -Humiliation/ rejection -Public performance fears Harm Avoidance -Perfectionism -Anxious coping Separation Anxiety	I have pains in my chest. I'm afraid other kids will make fun of me. I keep my eyes open for danger. I check to make sure things are safe. I sleep next to someone in my family.	Adequate internal and test–retest reliability; adequate convergent validity; adequate divergent validity reported for depression and externalizing disorders; and for anxiety disorders in children with ADHD.
Screen for Child Anxiety Related Emotional Disorders (SCARED; Birmaher et al., 1999)	41 items 3 ratings (not true or hardly ever true; sometimes true; true or often true)	Panic/Somatic Generalized Anxiety Separation Anxiety Social Phobia School Phobia	When I feel frightened, I feel like I am going crazy. I am a worrier. I get scared if I sleep away from home. I worry about how well I do things. I am scared to go to school.	Adequate internal and test–retest reliability; adequate convergent validity; adequate divergent validity reported for normals, depression, externalizing disorders, and multiple anxiety disorders

children with ADHD (March, Conners, et al., 1999). Such a finding is important given the prevalence of comorbid disorders for children with anxiety disorders and with ADHD. Because of its recent development, the MASC has not been used extensively in treatment research. This measure has, however, been chosen as the only or primary self-report measure of anxiety in National Institute of Mental Health–funded studies of ADHD (Multimodal Study of ADHD) and of selective serotonin reuptake inhibitors (SSRIs; Research Units for Pediatric Psychopharmocology) for children with anxiety (March & Albano, 1998).

The SCARED (Birmaher et al., 1997, 1999) is a self-report measure based on the criteria for anxiety disorders found in the *DSM–IV*. The SCARED is designed to identify symptoms of anxiety in children who also present with many other psychiatric symptoms, such as depression and attention problems (Greenhill, Pine, March, Birmaher, & Riddle, 1998). The most recent version of the scale (Birmaher et al., 1999) demonstrates adequate psychometric properties, including divergent validity. Birmaher et al. report that the SCARED has been effective for differentiating children with anxiety from children without anxiety and from children with depression and disruptive behavior disorders. The scale has also been useful for discriminating between the different anxiety disorders, such as generalized anxiety disorder, social anxiety, and panic disorder. A brief, five-item version of the scale has also shown sound preliminary psychometric properties and may prove to be an effective screening tool for clinicians in the future. The full version of the SCARED has also been effective in monitoring treatment effects for a cognitive–behavioral intervention for children with multiple anxiety disorders, including generalized anxiety disorder, separation anxiety disorder, social phobia, and specific phobias (Muris, Merckelbach, Gadet, Moulaert, & Tierney, 1999).

Adult Reports of Child's Anxiety

Another important source of information about a child's problems with anxiety is the parent and teacher reports of the symptoms and behaviors they see in their natural settings. As mentioned previously, however, it is not uncommon for adults to underrate anxiety symptoms in a child when compared with the child's own ratings. Thus, multiple informants should be used to present an accurate picture of a child's anxiety and level of impairment in the environment. Some of the studies mentioned above have had parents complete the child self-report scale as they see the symptoms presenting in their child. With this method, the SCARED (Birmaher et al., 1999) was found to have moderate correlations with the child's ratings. Parent and child agreement on the MASC (March et al., 1997) was found to be poor to fair. These findings support the idea that children may experience internal anxiety symptoms that are not obvious, and thus not reported, by their caregivers.

Nevertheless, parent and teacher perspectives can add important data to the assessment process for anxiety. Global parent and teacher rating scales with adequate psychometric properties and designed to screen for common emotional and behavioral problems in children often include measures of anxiety. For example, the Child Behavior Checklist (CBCL; Achenbach, 1991) provides broadband discrimination between internalizing and externalizing disorders but does not differentiate between anxiety disorders. The CBCL also has Anxious/Depressed and Withdrawn subscales that may assist in diagnosis or treatment monitoring. The Internalizing and Externalizing factors of the CBCL have frequently been used in the treatment literature as dependent measures (e.g., Barrett, 1998; Kendall, 1994; Silverman, Kurtines, Ginsburg, Weems, Lumpkin, & Carmichael, 1999). The impact of interventions on CBCL subscales such as Anxious/Depressed (e.g., Kendall et al., 1997; Kendall & Southam-Gerow, 1996) and Social Problems (e.g., Kendall, 1994) has also been investigated. The CBCL may be best used as a screening tool for anxiety disorders because of its inability to discriminate between anxiety disorders. Furthermore, there is some evidence that the CBCL is not very valid in discriminating between internalizing disorders such as anxiety and depression (e.g., Jensen, Salzberg, Richters, & Watanabe, 1993).

The Behavior Assessment System for Children (BASC; Reynolds & Kamphaus, 1998) is another psychometrically sound rating scale designed to screen for common mental health problems in children. Similar to the CBCL (Achenbach, 1991), the BASC also offers broadband scores for Internalizing and Externalizing disorders. It provides specific subscale information on Internalizing disorders such as depression, anxiety, somatization, as well as scores on withdrawn behavior, adaptability, and social skills that may provide important information related to anxiety and other disorders. The BASC has four parent forms divided into age groups (toddler, preschool, child, and adolescent) and three teacher forms beginning with preschool age. A child's self-report is also available for children ages 8–18. As mentioned in the previous chapter on disruptive behavior disorders, checklists such as the BASC provide useful information for diagnosis as well as for repeated assessment during and after intervention.

Summary

There are numerous assessment tools available for the clinician to use in evaluating a child for an anxiety disorder. Semistructured interviews such as the ADIS (Silverman & Nelles, 1988) can provide reliable and quantifiable information about symptom history, presentation, and severity. Parent and child versions of these interviews can be useful in evaluating both perspectives on symptomatology and impairment. At times, however, such parent and child interview data may differ, requiring the clinician to obtain more information to assist in reconciling incongruences. Child self-report and adult report rating scales may provide important information to assist in such reconciliation or as part of the recommended comprehensive evaluation. The latest versions of child self-report measures such as the MASC (March et al., 1997) and SCARED (Birmaher et al., 1997, 1999) offer a means of evaluating anxiety symptoms and symptoms of potential comorbid disorders such as depression. Although self-report measures have not had a long history of support as tools for differential diagnosis, more recent studies of these measures are demonstrating adequate discriminant validity (e.g., Birmaher et al., 1999; Weems et al., 1999). Finally, adult reports of the anxiety symptoms they see in the child or student can provide additional information about anxiety symptoms and other possible disorders. These measures, such as the BASC (Reynolds & Kamphaus, 1998), may provide more broadbased evidence of internalizing and externalizing disorders, offering the clinician guidance in areas to explore further during the interview process. Obviously, a single assessment tool does not have the capability for establishing an anxiety disorder diagnosis. The clinician should consider information from various sources, including the child, when evaluating for anxiety and its common comorbid disorders. Finally, once a diagnosis of an anxiety disorder is made, the clinician has many treatment options available, with most being variations of cognitive–behavioral therapy. These interventions are discussed below. Unfortunately, the current state of assessment tools does not directly guide the clinician to the best treatment approach. One exception may be the diagnosis of a specific phobia, which indicates an exposure-based treatment. The treatment of specific phobias is also addressed below.

INTERVENTIONS

Pharmacological Interventions

As with many of the disorders discussed in this book, pharmacological interventions have been investigated as a means of alleviating anxiety symptoms in children. Unfortunately, medical interventions with sufficient documentation of their efficacy and safety are limited for children with anxiety disorders (Kearney & Silverman, 1998; Velosa & Riddle, 2000). The classes of drugs that have been investigated for treating anxiety in children include benzodiazepines, tricyclic antidepressants, SSRIs, and Busipone. None of these medications have definitive evidence of their efficacy or safety for the anxiety disorders discussed in this chapter. Perhaps more important, these medications put children at risk for serious side effects such as dependence and withdrawal for benzodiazepines and rare, but potentially life-threatening, cardiac problems for tricyclic antidepressants (Velosa & Riddle, 2000).

The pharmaceutical studies that have been conducted for children with anxiety are also replete with methodological problems (Kearney & Silverman, 1998). For example, Kearney and Silverman could only identify eight studies published since 1973 that were clearly medication trials with definable outcomes, without the use of other confounding interventions such as psychotherapy. Only three of those eight studies investigated pharmaceutical interventions for the anxiety disorders discussed in this chapter, with the others addressing obsessive–compulsive disorder or panic disorder. Furthermore, most studies of pharmacological interventions with and without psychosocial interventions typically exclude comorbid disorders such as depression that commonly occur with anxiety, significantly limiting the generalizability of any results to many children with anxiety (Kearney & Silverman, 1998).

The practice guidelines offered by the American Academy of Child and Adolescent Psychiatry (1997b) acknowledge the limitations in the state of pharmacological treatment of anxiety for children and suggest that it be used as an adjunctive intervention to nonpharmacological treatments. Similarly, Velosa and Riddle (2000) suggested that medication interventions should also include illness education, support, behavioral components such as relaxation training for the child, and behavior management training for the parents. The practice guidelines also support the continued investigation of medications for anxiety, given their potential for addressing anxiety symptoms in children. They do not suggest which of the drugs mentioned above should be considered "first-line" but do indicate that benzodiazepines such as alprazolom (Xanax) be used only on a short-term basis because of potential for tolerance and dependence. Velosa and Riddle also suggested that benzodiazepines and tricyclic antidepressants only be used after other medications such as SSRIs have not been effective.

The fact that physicians are routinely prescribing medications for anxiety in children, without benefit of empirical studies documenting their efficacy, places an even greater burden on the clinician who is trained in nonpharmacological interventions. A working knowledge of the most commonly prescribed medications, their indications and side effects, as well as their limitations, are valuable aids to the clinician who evaluates and treats children with anxiety disorders. Concern for the health and welfare of a child dictates the use of periodic objective measurement of both the main treatment effects and the side effects of any medication trial. Measures such as the side effects questionnaire developed by Barkley and his colleagues (Barkley et al., 1990) for use with children placed on medication for ADHD need to be developed for use with anxiety and anxiety-related disorders in children. Actual measurement of symptoms before and after starting medication is necessary to document the extent of negative side effects, if any, of medication. Only through such evaluations can the full impact of medications be estimated.

Undoubtedly, studies of pharmaceutical interventions for children with anxiety will continue and may some day demonstrate adequate safety and efficacy. It is our recommendation, however, that at this point in time, nonpharmacological treatments be considered the first-line intervention of choice for the practicing clinician.

Nonpharmacological Interventions

Efficacious, nonmedical interventions are available for treating the anxiety disorders discussed in this chapter. The most well-established treatment reported in the literature for treating anxiety disorders in children has been cognitive–behavioral therapy (CBT). Kendall and his colleagues have been the most productive in developing cognitive–behavioral programs for school-age children with separation anxiety disorder, avoidant disorder (social phobia), and generalized anxiety disorder (Kendall, 1994; Kendall et al., 1997). In addition to CBT programs for children, more recent studies have included parent training as an important part of anxiety interventions. These parental components have addressed the importance of educating parents about how they influence their child's anxiety, as well as how to cope with their own anxiety. A review of CBT and how it applies to anxiety disorders is discussed below. In addition to CBT, there are specific behavioral interventions that are effective in treating specific phobias, and these are also discussed below following a description of CBT for other anxiety disorders.

Cognitive–Behavioral Therapy

To date, CBT has support as a "probably efficacious," nonpharmaceutical intervention for children with the anxiety disorders discussed in this chapter (Ollendick, 2000; Ollendick & King, 1998). Support for other interventions, including play therapy, psychodynamic therapy, and supportive or family therapy as a single intervention, has not been demonstrated (Labellarte et al., 1999). The use of CBT for addressing anxiety in children focuses on how the child learns to be anxious from the models and contingencies in his or her environment, as well as on how the individual child processes and uses that information to form his or her dysfunctional response (Kendall et al., 1997).

As mentioned previously, Kendall and his colleagues have been instrumental in developing effective CBT programs for children with anxiety. Kendall's first reported study of a CBT program, which is described below, investigated the effectiveness of CBT compared with a wait-list control (Kendall, 1994). Participants were diagnosed with overanxious disorder, separation anxiety disorder, and avoidant disorder. A therapist's treatment manual (Kendall, Kane, Howard, & Siqueland, 1990) and a child's treatment workbook (Kendall, 1990) were used for the 16-session intervention. Updated versions of both of these materials are now available (Kendall, 1992, 2000). Kendall (1994) demonstrated that his CBT program was effective in reducing or eliminating the anxiety symptoms of the children in the study. In fact, 64% of the children in the treatment group were "diagnosis-free" at the end of treatment, compared with 5% of the wait-list controls. The treatment gains were maintained at a 1-year follow-up. Further evidence of maintenance of treatment gains at 2 to 5 years postintervention for these children was reported by Kendall and Southam-Gerow (1996). A replication of Kendall's (1994) study demonstrated similar clinically significant results and also explored the effects of comorbid disorders on treatment effectiveness (Kendall et al., 1997). The authors found that the presence of comorbid anxiety or nonanxiety disorders such as depression and ADHD did not influence treatment outcomes. In other words, the CBT program was effective for anxious children with and without comorbid disorders. The investigation of comorbid disorders and their impact on treatment effectiveness is important given the high prevalence of their existence for children diagnosed with anxiety disorders.

Kendall's model for CBT combines the use of educational and exposure strategies to address anxiety in children. A summary of the purpose and sample tasks for the 16 one-hour sessions is provided in Table 2.2. The first 8 sessions introduce concepts to the children for recognizing and managing their anxiety. Children are taught the acronym "FEAR" (Feelings, Expectations, Actions, Reward) to facilitate recall of the steps for coping successfully with anxiety. The second 8 sessions require imaginal and in vivo practice of the skills learned during the first 8 sessions. Throughout the sessions, the clinician develops and refines a hierarchy of anxiety-provoking situations to provide experiences for the child to master. Modeling, role-playing, and reinforcement by the clinician are used throughout the program. The child is also taught a "freeze-frame" technique in Session 3 as a means of communicating to the clinician when he or she is too anxious to continue with the practice. Although parent training is not described as a main component of this CBT program, the parents did meet with the clinician after Session 3 to learn more about the intervention and to have an opportunity to discuss their concerns. Specific ways the parents can be involved, such as helping the child practice relaxation skills, were also reviewed.

Modifications of this program have been investigated as well. For example, the Coping Cat theme was changed to the Coping Koala theme for studies conducted in Australia (e.g., Barrett, 1998; Barrett, Dadds, & Rapee, 1996) and the Netherlands (Muris, Merckelbach, et al., 1999). Barrett also modified the structure to fit the needs of group, individual, and family CBT. Further information on these modified programs is discussed below.

CBT Plus Family Intervention

Because of the potential contribution of parental and family factors, several researchers have added a parent or family training component to

TABLE 2.2
Summary of Kendall's CBT Sessions

	Purpose	Sample Items
Session 1	Build rapport Provide information about treatment Gather information about child's anxieties	Personal facts game Introduction to feelings Learn about homework tasks
Session 2	Review treatment goals Identify different types of feelings; normalize fear/anxiety Begin to construct hierarchy of anxiety-provoking situations	Match faces with feelings Feelings role play Calm, nervous situation cards
Session 3	Distinguish anxiety from other feelings Introduce and identify somatic feelings related to anxiety Introduce "freeze frame" for when child is too anxious to continue with tasks	Questions about anxiety-provoking situations for self and others Modeling and role playing of situations *F* = Feeling Frightened?
Session 4	Review identifying somatic responses to anxiety Introduce tense versus relaxed Introduce relaxation training	Robot vs. rag doll example Discussion of tension and anxiety Progressive muscle relaxation (three muscle groups) through modeling and practice
Session 5	Review relaxation training Introduce thoughts–response connection; self-talk	Role play specific scenarios from child's anxiety hierarchy Cartoons with empty thought bubbles *E* = Expecting bad things to happen?
Session 6	Review anxious self-talk Review relaxation training Introduce active coping strategy—how to change the situation	Make reminder cards of strategies learned so far (recognition, self-talk, attitudes, and actions) Model steps; have child problem solve *A* = Attitudes and actions that will help?
Session 7	Review relaxation training Introduce concept of self-evaluation and reinforcement	Make card for results and rewards Feelings barometer to rate performance List preferred rewards *R* = Results and rewards?

(continued)

TABLE 2.2 *(continued)*

	Purpose	Sample Items
Session 8	Introduce FEAR (Feelings, Expectations, Actions, Reward) acronym Apply skills to low-anxiety situations Practice all skills learned in previous sessions	Have child make own FEAR card Role play and practice various anxiety-provoking situations; imaginal and in vivo
Session 9	Practice FEAR plan with imaginal and in vivo scenarios	Modeling of FEAR to cope with scenario Practice using situation cards of low anxiety arousal created by child
Session 10	Continue practicing skills applied to low level imaginal and in vivo situations	Cartoon strips with empty bubbles Modeling and role play Practice with low-anxiety situation cards
Session 11	Practice skills for imaginal and in vivo scenarios that produce moderate anxiety	Modeling and role play Use imaginal, in office, and first out of office exposure
Session 12	Practice skills for in vivo scenarios that produce moderate anxiety	Role play situation Arrange for child to be transported to anxiety-provoking location Modeling coping skills; practice of skills
Session 13	Practice skills for imaginal scenarios that produce high anxiety	Develop cartoon story of situation and coping strategies Role play situation and coping
Session 14	Practice skills for in vivo scenarios that produce high anxiety	Arrange for high-anxiety situation out of office Practice skills Offer relaxation exercises when needed
Session 15	Continue practicing skills for in vivo scenarios that produce high anxiety	Same as Session 14; develop "commercial" to teach others about anxiety and coping
Session 16	Review and summarize training program Make plans with parents for maintenance and generalization Bring closure to therapeutic relationship	Tape child's commercial Give certificate of achievement Arrange for final session in 1 week

Note. From *Cognitive–Behavioral Therapy for Anxious Children Therapist Manual* (2nd ed.) and *Coping Cat Workbook,* by P. C. Kendall, 1992, Ardmore, PA: Workbook. Copyright 1992 by Workbook. Adapted with permission.

CBT with the hope of enhancing treatment effectiveness. Barrett and her colleagues have added a more structured parent training component to their modified version of Kendall's CBT program for treating children with overanxious disorder, generalized anxiety disorder, and social phobia (Barrett et al., 1996; Dadds, Holland, Barrett, Laurens, & Spence, 1997; Dadds et al., 1999). Barrett et al. compared the effectiveness of an individual CBT program (Coping Koala), CBT followed by a family anxiety management intervention, and a wait-list control condition. The content of the family intervention focused on behavior management strategies such as planned ignoring of anxious behavior, parental awareness of their own emotional responses, and training in problem-solving skills. Both treatment conditions were effective in reducing the anxiety symptoms of the children when compared with wait-list controls. More of the children in the family intervention condition were diagnosis-free at postintervention and at 6- and 12-month follow-up points. The family intervention was also more effective for children ages 7–10. Older children (ages 11–14) did not demonstrate a significant difference in improvements for the CBT or CBT plus family intervention. Overall, the family component enhanced the effectiveness of the CBT based on both child and parent ratings of the child's anxiety symptoms, especially for younger children.

CBT Group Interventions

Perhaps one of the most promising variations of CBT is that of group treatment. A recent study compared the effectiveness of group CBT with a parent training component with a wait-list control condition (Silverman, Kurtines, Ginsburg, Weems, Lumpkin, & Carmichael, 1999). The components of the training were not elaborated on extensively but were described as contingency management and self-control strategies. The intervention lasted 8 to 10 weeks, with 55-minute sessions that allowed for individual instruction for the children and parents, followed by a conjoint activity. Similar to studies of individual CBT, significant improvements were reported in anxiety symptoms for the children who were diagnosed with overanxious disorder, generalized anxiety disorder, and social phobia. Approximately 64% of the children in the treatment group were diagnosis-free at postintervention. Treatment gains were maintained through the 12-month follow-up.

Similar to studies of individual CBT, the specific effects of adding a parent training component to group CBT have also been studied. Barrett (1998) found that group CBT and group CBT plus a family training component were effective in reducing anxiety symptoms in children with overanxious disorder, separation anxiety disorder, and social phobia. The CBT intervention was a modified version of the Kendall program and used the *Group Coping Koala Workbook* (Barrett, 1995a) to address the key components of the program. Those families assigned to the CBT plus family training completed all activities as a family unit with the clinician, and they used the *Group Family Anxiety Management Workbook* (Barrett, 1995b). The intervention took 12 weeks, with weekly 2-hour sessions. Although the children in both treatment groups demonstrated significant improvements over the wait-list controls, the group receiving family intervention showed additional benefits. More of these children showed improvements in externalizing behaviors as well, and more were diagnosis-free at a 1-year follow-up. Similar findings were reported by Mendlowitz et al. (1999), who found that children in a parent and child CBT intervention group had reduced anxiety symptoms and used more active coping strategies than children who only received group CBT without parental involvement.

Preliminary evidence of the effectiveness of group CBT for preventing anxiety disorders has also been reported (Dadds et al., 1997, 1999). Dadds et al. (1997) screened children from eight primary schools for anxiety symptoms using child and teacher reports. Those who were considered at-risk for anxiety disorders were included in the study with parental permission and participation. The authors then implemented a 10-week, school-based CBT intervention based on *The Coping Koala: Prevention Manual* (Barrett, Dadds, & Holland, 1994) that included both child and parent sessions. Results from this study indicated that at 6 months postintervention, the children in the treatment group had lower rates of anxiety than their peers who were simply monitored for anxiety problems. In addition, 54% of the children who were monitored had a diagnosable anxiety disorder at 6 months, compared with only 16% of the children receiving intervention. Data from a 2-year follow-up of these children indicated continuing preventative benefits for the intervention group (Dadds et al., 1999). These studies demonstrate the importance of both monitoring and treating early symptoms of anxiety given the significant number of children that may go on to develop an anxiety disorder. They are also an important first step in attempting to apply an empirically supported intervention to the prevention of anxiety disorders in children. They also attest to the powerful, preventive connection that can exist between clinicians and school district personnel when appropriate funding exists.

Behavioral Interventions for Specific Phobias

The studies discussed above have typically addressed the symptoms of anxiety disorders, such as overanxious disorder, generalized anxiety disorder, and social phobia. Many of the children in these studies who benefited from CBT also had secondary diagnoses of specific phobias (e.g., Barrett et al., 1996; Kendall, 1994; Kendall et al., 1997). CBT has been studied for children with specific phobias as a primary diagnosis and has been supported as "probably efficacious" for this type of anxiety disorder (Ollendick, 2000; Ollendick & King, 1998). Single-subject studies that used combinations of cognitive–behavioral components have also demonstrated success in treating thunderstorm phobia (e.g., Matthey, 1988), fear of injections and medical procedures (e.g., Sanders & Jones, 1990), and fear of the dark (e.g., Heard, Dadds, & Conrad, 1992).

An early study implementing a randomized clinical trial demonstrated the effectiveness of CBT on reducing nighttime fears (Graziano & Mooney, 1980). The children were taught relaxation and verbal coping skills, including statements of bravery, while the parents were asked to reward the children for practice and progress. The authors reported a significant improvement in nighttime fear, sleep onset, and willingness to go to sleep with reduced delay tactics. These gains were maintained at a 2- to 3-year follow-up contact (Graziano & Mooney, 1982). More recently, N. J. King et al. (1998) used a shortened, six-session version of Kendall's (1994) CBT to address school phobia in children ages 5–15. The program also included parent and teacher training in contingency management and strategies for improving school attendance. Children treated with the CBT program had marked improvements in school attendance and scores on self- and parent-reported anxiety measures when compared with children in a wait-list control. In contrast, an investigation of a 12-week CBT program for school phobia found that CBT was not superior to an educational–supportive therapy (Last, Hansen, & Franco, 1998). The educational–supportive therapy consisted of informational presentations and encouragement for the children to talk about their fears. No specific suggestions or recommendations were made by the clinicians. Although the two CBT programs in these studies on school phobia differed in length, parent involvement, and possibly other factors, the study by Last et al. pointed to the need for further research to establish the true efficacy of CBT for simple phobias. In addition, the benefits of simple, supportive therapies should also be explored further.

In addition to studies of the multicomponent CBT, individual behavioral strategies to treat phobias have also been studied. These treatments are often categorized as systematic desensitization, modeling, and operant procedures such as reinforced practice (Ollendick, 2000; Ollendick & King, 1998). A review of treatments of phobia for children by Ollendick and King suggested that systematic desensitization, namely, imaginal and in vivo desensitization, is "probably efficacious," whereas participant modeling and reinforced practice enjoy "well-established" efficacious status. The underlying principle of all of these components is exposure to the feared object in a graduated fashion. All of these components are inherent features of Kendall's (1994) CBT program.

In response to requests in the literature for evaluation of individual intervention components that are part of more comprehensive treatments such as CBT, preliminary research has begun to study the effects of components such as those mentioned above and others on childhood phobias. For example, Silverman, Kurtines, Ginsburg, Weems, Rabian, and Serafini

(1999) compared the effectiveness of reinforced practice (labeled as contingency management) with self-control strategies (identification, self-talk, self-reward) and an educational–supportive condition on children with specific phobias. Silverman et al. reported that all three interventions, which all had treatment manuals to facilitate integrity, were comparable in reducing parent and self-reports of anxiety and fear. Treatment gains for each group were also maintained at a 1-year follow-up. Silverman et al. recognized the possible implications their study may have in our current managed-care environment. Although further research is needed, this study may support a clinician's option to use a simple, "single" treatment depending on his or her client's needs. Furthermore, single treatment may someday also include single-session interventions. Several studies of one-session, therapist-directed exposure have suggested the success of such an approach for adults with simple phobias (e.g., Öst, 1996; Öst, Brandberg, & Alm, 1997; Öst, Hellstroem, & Kaver, 1992). Of course, the fact that such sessions lasted at least 3 hours may present a barrier to third-party reimbursement. Nevertheless, such studies suggest an exciting future direction for the treatment of phobias in children. In fact, current studies are under way using a treatment manual to guide one-session treatments for children with specific phobias (L. Öst & T. Ollendick, personal communication, June 2000). In the event that adequate documentation regarding efficacy of one-session treatments becomes available, it is incumbent on the clinician to seek approval for such services from third-party payers.

Finally, the broad concept of "exposure" as the treatment standard of care has also been compared with other less-established approaches to anxiety disorders. One of these approaches is eye movement desensitization and reprocessing (EMDR). Although most research on EMDR has been used to investigate its effects on symptoms of posttraumatic stress disorder, some interest in its potential for treating other anxiety disorders such as simple phobias is also evident. The conceptualization and treatment protocol for EMDR for simple phobias can be found in Shapiro (1995). In brief, aversive experiences for the child are thought to be reduced by having the child imagine and physically respond to fearful events while engaging in horizontal eye movements. Currently, the two studies for children that compare EMDR with in vivo exposure interventions for children do not support EMDR as an effective intervention (Muris, Merckelbach, Holdrinet, & Sijsenaar, 1998; Muris, Merckelbach, van Haaften, & Mayer, 1997).

Summary

Pharmacological and nonpharmacological interventions have been investigated as strategies for addressing anxiety symptoms in children. The current state of pharmacological treatments does not support their use as a first-line intervention strategy, especially for the disorders discussed in this chapter. The AACAP (1997b) recommended the use of medications as an adjunctive intervention to nonmedical treatments, such as behavioral therapy. Evidence supports the designation of CBT as an empirically supported intervention for anxiety disorders in children. Kendall has contributed significantly with his manualized CBT program for children with separation anxiety disorder, generalized anxiety disorder, and social phobia (e.g., Kendall, 1994; Kendall et al., 1997). His program for individual treatment has been modified for the group setting and to include parent training in contingency management. The clinician may be wise to include the parents as part of a CBT program because environmental factors such as parental response to the child's anxiety behaviors can maintain their expression. Group CBT may be feasible for clinicians in school-based clinics or for those who have their practices set up to address specific diagnoses in a clinic format (e.g., anxiety clinics).

CBT and its individual components, particularly exposure, have also been used to manage specific phobias in children. For example, recent studies have found short (six-session) CBT programs with parent and teacher involvement to be effective in reducing school phobia (N.J. King et al., 1998). Research on one-session treatments with adults has been promising, and similar studies are under way for children with anxiety. The effectiveness of individual behavioral components such as contingency management has also been investigated, with mixed results. Although single behavioral interventions are typically more effective than wait-list control conditions, they have not always been found to be more effective than educational–supportive therapy (e.g., Last et al., 1998). The clinician is advised to judge the severity of the school or other phobia before choosing an approach. A child with mild school phobia may decrease symptomatology with simple support and required attendance (exposure) at school, whereas a child with severe elevator phobia may require each of the systematic steps offered in a more extensive CBT program. This review of interventions offers the clinician options with regard to length, format, and intensity of CBT to address the unique needs of their patients.

CONCLUSION

Many children progress through childhood with fears and worries about developmentally appropriate issues, such as going to school for the first time or academic performance. For the vast majority of the children, these naturally occurring fears may make a child nervous, but they do not impair the child's functioning. However, a significant number of children do suffer from fears and worries that have a negative impact on their daily functioning, resulting in the need for clinical intervention. Because anxiety disorders are often comorbid with other anxiety disorders, as well as with numerous other psychiatric problems such as depression, a comprehensive assessment is essential for an accurate diagnosis. In addition to a detailed interview of caregivers and the child, using either structured or unstructured formats, information should be obtained from rating scales completed by caregivers and the child. Child self-report information may be especially important for diagnosing and treating anxiety disorders given the internal nature of many of the symptoms. Improved methods for the differential diagnosis of anxiety disorders should greatly facilitate the identification and treatment of anxiety as well. Certainly a thorough assessment should include inquiry about possible medical conditions or medication reactions that may mimic anxiety symptoms. The purpose of a comprehensive assessment is to obtain an accurate diagnosis that can guide treatment strategies. The current state of assessment and intervention research does not necessarily dictate which specific treatment is appropriate for each specific diagnosis. Future research on assessment must focus on which treatments are the most effective for which presenting problems. Good specificity in terms of diagnosis, in the absence of similar specificity in terms of intervention strategy, leaves far too much to the discretion of the clinician. Although clinicians need a certain degree of latitude in their approach to childhood anxiety disorders, it would be far better for both clinician and patient if this latitude were in the area of how the intervention strategies are implemented and not on which intervention strategy is implemented.

Despite this shortcoming in the anxiety literature, effective interventions do exist for treating anxiety disorders. Certainly, as more and more outcome studies become available on the pharmacological component of treating anxiety disorders in children, the use of medication in the comprehensive management of anxiety will become a more viable option. The effective treatment of anxiety disorders in children has generally relied on nonpharmacological interventions, such as cognitive and behavioral strategies offered individually or as a comprehensive intervention package such as the one described in this chapter by Kendall (1994). CBTs have had demonstrated effectiveness with various numbers of sessions, in individual and group formats, and with the inclusion of parent training. Preliminary studies show that adding a parent-training component that focuses on contingency management and education may enhance the effects of CBT for individual and group formats. Further exploration of the effects of the parents' own level of anxiety on the intervention is needed, however. For example, Cobham, Dadds, and Spence (1998) found that parents with a high level of anxiety presented a risk factor for child-focused CBT treatment failure. Practical and important suggestions for effectively engaging parents in CBT for their children with anxiety disorders are provided by Siqueland and Diamond (1998).

In the future, the treatment of anxiety disorders in children may focus on even more refined strategies, as some studies suggest that single components of CBT may be effective in reducing anxiety symptoms in children. Group formats, one-session treatments, and prevention efforts may also change the face of anxiety interventions for children in this century. Such strategies may be viewed as proactive efforts to respond to the changing demands of health care, as well as to provide the most efficacious treatment to the children we serve.

3

DIAGNOSIS AND MANAGEMENT OF HABIT DISORDERS

Habit disorders consist of frequent, repetitive behaviors that cannot be explained by physiological causes and appear to serve no identifiable physiological function. These disorders include tics and nervous habits. Tics are recurrent, stereotypic motor movements or vocalizations and may be transient or chronic. Tourette's syndrome is a more complex disorder involving multiple motor tics and one or more vocal tics. In Tourette's syndrome, the tics increase and decrease in frequency and change in typology. For example, eye blinking may increase, then decrease in frequency, then disappear altogether, followed by the emergence of mouth grimacing. During the same time period, one or more vocal tics, such as throat clearing, sniffing, or growling, must also be present, but not necessarily at the exact same time. The diagnostic criteria for tic disorders and Tourette's syndrome as described by the *Diagnostic and Statistical Manual of Mental Disorders* (4th ed., *DSM–IV*; American Psychiatric Association, 1994) are found in Exhibit 3.1. These criteria emphasize the marked distress tics must cause the person. Thus, a motor tic such as occasional eye twitch would most likely be considered within the normal range of behavior.

Exhibit 3.2 lists the *DSM–IV* criteria for stereotypic movement disorders, also known as *habit disorders*, and for trichotillomania (hair pulling). *Stereotypic movement disorders* include common habits such as nail biting,

79

307.22 Chronic Motor or Vocal Tic Disorder	**307.21 Transient Tic Disorder**
A. Single or multiple motor or vocal tics (i.e., sudden, rapid, recurrent, non-rhythmic, stereotyped motor movements or vocalizations), but not both, have been present at some time during the illness.	A. Single or multiple motor and/or vocal tics (i.e., sudden, rapid, recurrent, nonrhythmic, stereotyped motor movements or vocalizations).
B. The tics occur many times a day, nearly every day or intermittently throughout a period of more than 1 year, and during this period there was never a tic-free period of more than 3 consecutive months.	B. The tics occur many times a day, nearly every day for at least 4 weeks, but for no longer than 12 consecutive months.
C. The disturbance causes marked distress or significant impairment in social, occupational, or other important areas of functioning.	C. The disturbance causes marked distress or significant impairment in social, occupational, or other important areas of functioning.
D. The onset is before age 18 years.	D. The onset is before age 18 years.
E. The disturbance is not due to the direct physiological effects of a substance (e.g., stimulants) or a general medical condition (e.g., Huntington's disease or postviral encephalitis).	E. The disturbance is not due to the direct physiological effects of a substance (e.g., stimulants) or a general medical condition (e.g., Huntington's disease or postviral encephalitis).
F. Criteria have never been met for Tourette's Disorder.	F. Criteria have never been met for Tourette's Disorder or Chronic Motor or Vocal Tic Disorder.

307.23 Tourette's Disorder

A. Both multiple motor and one or more vocal tics have been present at some time during the illness, although not necessarily concurrently.

B. The tics occur many times a day (usually in bouts), nearly every day or intermittently throughout a period of more than 1 year, and during this period there was never a tic-free period of more than 3 consecutive months.

C. The disturbance causes marked distress or significant impairment in social, occupational, or other important areas of functioning.

D. The onset is before age 18 years.

E. The disturbance is not due to the direct physiological effects of a substance (e.g., stimulants) or a general medical condition (e.g., Huntington's disease or postviral encephalitis).

Note. Information from *Diagnostic and Statistical Manual of Mental Disorders* (4th ed.), by the American Psychiatric Association, Washington, DC: Author. Copyright 1994 by the American Psychiatric Association. Reprinted with permission.

nail picking, body rocking, and mouthing of objects. To meet the diagnostic criteria for stereotypic movement disorder, the habit must be severe enough to interfere with normal activities or to cause bodily injury. For example, many children bite their fingernails, but most not to the point that they routinely bleed. Similarly, a person's trichotillomania must be severe enough to cause significant distress or impairment. Although the *DSM–IV* includes trichotillomania under impulse control disorders, some authors include trichotillomania with obsessive–compulsive disorder (March & Mulle, 1996), and others have chosen to include it under discussions about habit disorders (D. P. Kohen, 1996). There are no empirical criteria for how these disorders are grouped. Thus, trichotillomania has been included in this chapter because of its similarity to stereotypic movement disorders, both in terms of the presenting symptoms and the treatment procedures that have been effective in managing this disorder in children and adolescents.

EXHIBIT 3.2
DSM–IV Diagnostic Criteria for Stereotypic Movement Disorders
and Trichotillomania

307.3 Stereotypic Movement Disorder	312.39 Trichotillomania
A. Repetitive, seemingly driven, and nonfunctional motor behavior (e.g., hand shaking or waving, body rocking, head banging, mouthing of objects, self-biting, picking at skin or bodily orifices, hitting own body).	A. Recurrent pulling out of one's hair, resulting in noticeable hair loss.
B. The behavior markedly interferes with normal activities or results in self-inflicted bodily injury that requires medical treatment (or would result in an injury if preventive measures were not used).	B. An increasing sense of tension immediately before pulling out the hair or when attempting to resist the behavior.
C. If Mental Retardation is present, the stereotypic or self-injurious behavior is of sufficient severity to become a focus of treatment.	C. Pleasure, gratification, or relief when pulling out the hair.
D. The behavior is not better accounted for by a compulsion (as in Obsessive–Compulsive Disorder), a tic (as in Tic Disorder), a stereotypy that is part of a Pervasive Developmental Disorder, or hair pulling (as in Trichotillomania).	D. The disturbance is not better accounted for by another mental disorder and is not due to a general medical condition (e.g., a dermatological condition).
E. The behavior is not due to the direct physiological effects of a substance or a general medical condition.	E. The disturbance causes clinically significant distress or impairment in social, occupational, or other important areas of functioning.
F. The behavior persists for 4 weeks or longer.	

Note. Information from *Diagnostic and Statistical Manual of Mental Disorders* (4th ed.), by the American Psychiatric Association, 1994, Washington, DC: Author. Copyright 1994 by the American Psychiatric Association. Reprinted with permission.

A summary of diagnostic criteria for the disorders discussed above is found in Table 3.1. This presentation may assist the clinician with differential diagnoses and provides one comprehensive form to use during a diagnostic interview. The criteria included in the *DSM–IV* distinguish habit disorders from organically caused movement disorders, such as the involuntary muscle jerks characteristic of diseases (e.g., Huntington's chorea) or resulting from medications (such as stimulants). In addition, muscular atrophy is not present in habit disorders and nervous tics are not painful, as is sometimes present in such disorders as facial hemispasm (Sindou, Fischer, Derraz, Keravel, & Palfi, 1996). Many children with habit disorders come directly to the attention of the clinician without having seen a physician first. The judgment must then be made whether to refer the family to their primary care physician to rule out possible neurological problems. Nevertheless, a thorough history should always be obtained, and if in doubt, further medical evaluation by a pediatric neurologist should be considered before management as a habit disorder. The interested reader is referred to A. K. Shapiro and Shapiro (1989) for a detailed discussion of the neurological signs, together with the history and clinical course, other neurological abnormalities, and laboratory results used to differentiate tics from other neurological disorders.

PREVALENCE

The prevalence of all nervous tics, which Azrin and Nunn (1977) defined as "a compulsive and persistent muscle movement which is not organic in origin" (p. 17), is estimated at about 1% of the general population. Azrin and Nunn estimated that 40 million people bite their fingernails and more than 8 million people are hair pullers. Although the exact incidence is not known, Erenberg (1999) stated that 24% of children experience tics, but most are of a minor degree and do not lead to a clinical diagnosis. It is only when tics cause marked distress or significant impairment in social, occupational, or other important areas of functioning that they merit a clinical diagnosis. And although most cases of thumb sucking seen in young children do not merit evaluation and treatment, parents usually do seek professional help when their child has a habit that attracts attention in the classroom or at home.

CAUSES AND CORRELATES

The most organized and comprehensive research in the area of habit disorders has been published by Azrin and his colleagues (e.g., Azrin & Nunn, 1977; Azrin, Nunn, & Frantz-Renshaw, 1982; Azrin & Peterson,

TABLE 3.1
Differential Diagnosis of Tic Disorders

Transient Tic Disorder 307.21	Chronic Motor or Vocal Tic Disorder 307.22	Tourette's Disorder 307.23
❑ Single or multiple tic	❑ Single or multiple tic	❑ Both motor and vocal
❑ Many times per day per	❑ Many times per day 4 weeks	❑ Many times per day per year
❑ Not longer than 1 year	❑ Longer than 1 year	❑ Never tic-free 3 months
❑ Causes marked distress	❑ Causes marked distress	❑ Causes marked distress
❑ Onset before age of 18	❑ Onset before age of 18	❑ Onset before age of 18
❑ Not physiological	❑ Not physiological	❑ Not physiological
_____ of 6 (6 = Dx)	_____ of 6 (6 = Dx)	_____ of 6 (6 = Dx)

Stereotypic Movement Disorder 307.3	Trichotillomania 312.39
❑ Repetitive, motor behavior	❑ Recurrent hair pulling
❑ Interferes with normal acts	❑ Tension before pulling
❑ Sufficient severity	❑ Pleasure when pulling
❑ Not OCD, tic, PDD, trichotillomania	❑ Not due to another disorder
❑ Not physiological, or "a general medical condition"	❑ Clinically significant distress
❑ Persists for 4 weeks or more	
_____ of 6 (6 = Dx)	_____ of 5 (5 = Dx)

Note. Information from *Diagnostic and Statistical Manual of Mental Disorders* (4th ed.), by the American Psychiatric Association, 1994, Washington, DC: Author, Copyright by the American Psychiatric Association. Reprinted with permission. Dx = diagnosis; OCD = obsessive–compulsive disorder; PDD = pervasive developmental disorder.

1990). Azrin and Nunn (1973) stated that a nervous habit originally starts as a normal reaction to an extreme event, such as a physical injury or psychological trauma, or it may have started as an infrequent, but normal, behavior that has increased in frequency and has been altered in its form. The behavior becomes classified as a nervous habit when it persists after the original injury or trauma has passed, and when it causes marked distress or significant impairment. In the medical literature, several explanations have been proposed to explain the origin and persistence of stereotypic behavior; none, however, can be supported at the exclusion of the others (Hoder & Cohen, 1992). Therefore, although numerous authors have attributed habit disorders and tics to genetic factors, biochemical factors, or neurological abnormalities, "unfortunately, at present, there is no experimental support for any of the current hypotheses about the etiology of tic and Tourette's disorder disorders" (Hoder & Cohen, 1992, p. 1870).

ASSESSMENT

The initial assessment of a child with a habit disorder or tic should be extensive enough to rule out or identify medical problems (such as a side effect of the use of stimulant medication) and comorbid conditions (such as attention deficit hyperactivity disorder; ADHD) and to determine the extent to which the habit or tic is causing significant distress to the child. At a minimum, this should include an interview with the child, a parent interview, and the completion of standardized rating scales by the parents and teachers that are useful for identifying a variety of presenting concerns. Although none of the rating scales specifically include habit disorders and tics as a subscale, they are useful for identifying behavior problems that could either contribute to the presenting problem or potentially interfere with the management of the problem.

Assessment measures for habit disorders and tics typically have included child or parent reports and direct observation. In research reports, behavioral researchers have frequently used formal observation with an observer either in the natural environment or by watching the behavior on videotape to document the presence, typology, and frequency of habits before, during, and after treatment. These reports are often collaborated by the use of a second observer such as another parent, teacher, or friend (see Azrin & Nunn, 1973). Medical researchers have generally used "severity rating scales" that are designed to be administered during a clinical interview by a trained and experienced clinician. In most clinical practices, clinicians rely on the patient or parent report to assess the efficacy of a clinical intervention.

Behavioral Observations

Some research has involved videotaping patients exhibiting habit disorders and tics. All videotapes are scored by one observer, with at least 20% of the tapes scored, independently, by a second observer. Although the use of daily videotapes of each child is prohibitive in a clinical practice, the participants in Finney, Rapoff, Hall, and Christophersen's (1983) study, for example, were actually brought to the clinic for treatment of their tics. The parents were instructed how to use the video camera to obtain tic rates before, during, and after treatment, including a 1-year follow-up. The videotapes allowed investigators to document the reduction in tic rates for the participants. In our own clinical practices, parents are encouraged to videotape their children's tics before and after treatment. The widespread use of videotaping equipment has made it possible for many parents to do such videotaping.

Tic Severity Rating Scales

Medical researchers have relied on tic severity rating scales as a measure of the frequency of habit disorders and tics. Examples of these scales include the Yale Global Tic Severity Scale (YGTSS; Leckman et al., 1989) and the Yale–Brown Obsessive Compulsive Scale (Y–BOCS; Goodman et al., 1989). Goodman, Rasmussen, Riddle, Price, and Rapoport (1986) reported on a version of the Y–BOCS that was developed for the measurement of children's tics, the Children's Yale–Brown Obsessive Compulsive Scale (CY–BOCS). These rating scales are scored using clinical observations and patient reports. Goodman et al. (1989) made the point that "observer-rated instruments" are necessary because of the poor correlation of patient reports with more objective evaluations. Yet both the YGTSS and the Y–BOCS end up relying in large part on the patient's report because the vast majority of the questions included in these assessment devices, such as "concern with illness or disease," are not observable. Rather, they rely on the patient's or parents' verbal response to the clinician's question.

Walkup, Rosenberg, Brown, and Singer (1992) compared four scales that measure tic severity in Tourette's syndrome, using three independent judges to observe 20 different individuals. They compared the YGTSS (Leckman et al., 1989), the Tourette's Syndrome Severity Scale (A. K. Shapiro, Shapiro, Young, & Feinberg, 1988), the Tourette's Syndrome Clinical Global Impression Scale (Harcherik, Leckman, Detlor, & Cohen, 1984), and the Hopkins Motor and Vocal Tic Scale (Walkup et al., 1992). The instruments were equally effective in determining overall severity and showed good reliability when compared with actual observation of patient's tics by the three judges. Walkup et al. reported that tic symptoms were shown to be independent of symptoms of either ADHD or obsessive–compulsive disorder. Finally, Chappell et al. (1994) published a comparison of videotaped tic counts with the YGTSS and the Clinical Global Impression Scale for Tourette's syndrome and concluded that tic counts were highly reliable for videotapes of at least 5 minutes' duration and correlated significantly with the two rating scales.

When interviewing patients, either in clinical practice or for research studies, clinicians find it impossible to obtain any more than a brief estimate of the frequency of habit disorders, tics, or both. It is equally difficult to determine from an interview the degree to which a habit disorder or tic actually interferes with a patient's day-to-day functioning. Although behavioral researchers have depended on videotapes of patients engaging in the habit or tic, medical researchers have relied on assessment devices such as the YGTSS and Y–BOCS. In the absence of interobserver reliability checks, which are almost always included by behavioral researchers, the tic severity rating scales are sophisticated forms of a patient's report. None of the studies evaluating pharmacological interventions have included social validation components.

INTERVENTION

The interventions available to treat the tic and habit disorders discussed in this chapter are mainly medical or behavioral in nature. The use of pharmacological management has been most extensively researched for Tourette's syndrome. Although relatively little has been written about the medical management of simple habit disorders such as nail biting, Green (1989) recommended that pharmacological treatment is appropriate only in those cases in which habits cause severe physical damage, such as those demonstrated by people with severe retardation. Thus, medication as an intervention in this chapter focuses only on Tourette's syndrome. The behavioral strategies discussed include brief, specific strategies for simple habits such as thumb sucking or nail biting, as well as more comprehensive strategies such as habit reversal and negative practice that can be applied to more complex habits. Other strategies, such as relaxation training, as well as a combination of behavioral strategies, are described as additional effective interventions for tics and habit disorders.

Medical Treatment

As mentioned previously, the use of medical management for habit disorders has been reserved primarily for Tourette's syndrome. Several drugs, including haloperidol, pimozide, and clonidine, have been evaluated for their effectiveness in treating the tics associated with Tourette's syndrome and are reviewed below.

Haloperidol (Haldol)

Haloperidol continues to be the treatment of choice for children with Tourette's syndrome, reportedly relieving symptoms initially in up to 70% (Erenberg, 1999) or 80% (Hoder & Cohen, 1992) of patients. Short-term side effects, such as Parkinsonian symptoms, intellectual blunting, loss of motivation, weight gain, sedation, dysphoria, school phobia, and depression, however, can be more disabling than the tics themselves. Long-term consequences such as tardive dyskinesia also pose serious health threats. Thus, many patients choose to endure the tic symptoms rather than suffer the side effects of haloperidol (Hoder & Cohen, 1992; Silva, Munoz, Daniel, Barickman, & Friedhoff, 1996).

Haloperidol and nicotine. An interesting addition to the literature on the pharmacological management of Tourette's syndrome is the use of nicotine to potentiate the effectiveness of haloperidol. McConville et al. (1991) videotaped 10 patients with Tourette's syndrome before, during, and after they chewed nicotine gum. All of the patients were being treated with haloperidol without adequate control of their Tourette's symptoms, either because of unsatisfactory clinical response or excessive side effects. The results showed a marked potentiation of haloperidol effects by nicotine gum in diminishing tic frequency in Tourette's syndrome. Similarly, Silver, Shytle, Philipp, and Sanberg (1996) examined the use of a transdermal nicotine patch in 16 patients ranging in age from 9 to 15 years. Although there was a broad range of responses on the YGTSS, there was a significant reduction in symptoms. Side effects were reportedly transient.

Haloperidol versus clonidine and pimozide. Peterson, Camprise, and Azrin (1994), in their review of pharmacological treatments for tics, concluded that tics associated with Tourette's syndrome were reduced an average of 50% to 60% with haloperidol, whereas clonidine produced either no effect or only a slight reduction of tics. Sallee, Nesbitt, Jackson, Sine, and Sethuraman (1997) compared haloperidol and pimozide in 22 children with Tourette's syndrome by using a double-blind, placebo-controlled, double crossover study. The primary outcome measure was total score on the Tourette's Disorder Global Scale after 24 weeks of treatment. Pimozide was significantly more effective than the placebo, whereas haloperidol was not. Haloperidol also resulted in a threefold higher frequency of serious side effects and significantly greater extrapyramidal symptoms compared with pimozide. Although the authors concluded that pimozide is superior to haloperidol for controlling the symptoms of Tourette's syndrome in children and adolescents, more research is probably needed before pimozide replaces haloperidol as the drug of choice.

Other Medications

Other medications have also been evaluated for their effects on tics and habit disorders. For example, Bruun and Budman (1996), in a study of 38 patients who failed to respond to conventional treatments (e.g., haloperidol and clonidine), reported that 58% improved when switched to risperidone, as measured by the YGTSS. Eight patients (21%) discontinued the risperidone trial because of "intolerable" side effects. Unfortunately, data were reported for only a 4-week follow-up, limiting information on the long-term usefulness of this medication. A similar study, with similar results, was reported by Lombroso et al. (1995). Although there was an average decrease of 46% on the YGTSS and the CY–BOCS, 100% of the participants had significant weight gains. Data were only reported for a maximum of 4 weeks. Singer et al. (1995) reportedly compared clonidine and desipramine in the management of children with Tourette's syndrome and ADHD. They reported no significant differences in 34 patients, using the Hopkins Motor/Vocal Tic Severity Scale, the Tourette's Syndrome Severity Scale, or the YGTSS. They did note an improvement with desipramine on the hyperactivity subscale of both the parent and teacher form of the Child Behavior Checklist, but not with clonidine. In one of the few well-controlled studies for medical treatment of trichotillomania (with 23 adults), Streichenwein and Thornby (1995) concluded that there were no significant differences between fluoxetine and placebo treatments for trichotillomania. Pollard et al. (1991) reported that 4 patients treated with clomipramine for trichotillomania initially saw a dramatic reduction in symptoms. Three of the 4 patients, however, had relapsed completely at a 3-month follow-up. Iancu, Weizman, Kindler, Sasson, and Zohar (1996) reported similar results with serotonin reuptake inhibitors (clomipramine, fluoxetine, or fluvoxamine) to twelve 14–42-year-old patients with trichotillomania for 6 to 20 weeks. Nine patients relapsed after the initial improvement and 3 patients did not respond at all. Finally, Jaspers (1996) reviewed the literature on pharmacological treatment of trichotillomania, including 3 studies with control groups and 7 without, and concluded that there are no psychopharmacological treatment strategies that can be recommended.

In summary, although some of the newer drugs have produced some encouraging results, the consistent findings of significant side effects limit their widespread use at this time. Thus, although pharmacological interventions have a clear advantage in that they require little, if any, actual "therapy" time, the absence of any data on long-term treatment effects and the presence of adverse side effects limit the usefulness of pharmacology in the treatment of habit disorders and tics. A summary of the results obtained with pharmacological treatments for tic and habit disorders is found in Table 3.2.

TABLE 3.2
Pharmacological Treatments for Habit Disorders and Tics

	Treatments for Habit Disorders and Tics				
Drug	Average Decrease (%)	Maintenance of Tx Effects	Results Replicated?	Negative Side Effects?	Social Validation?
Haloperidol (Haldol)	80%	Yes	Yes	80%	None
Adj. Nicotine Patches	60%	No	Yes	Transient	None
Clonidine	20%	Yes	Yes	20%	None
Flutamide	Sign.	NA	No	Unknown	None
Fluoxetine (Prozac)	None	NA	No	NA	None
Fluoxetine, Clomipramine, Fluvoxamine	None	NA	No	100%	None
Pimozide (Orap)	40%	NA	No	14%	None
Risperidone	41%	11%	Yes	53%	None
	46%	NA	No	100%	None

Note. Adj. = adjunctive; Tx = treatment; NA = not available; Sign. = significant.

Behavioral Treatment

Brief Interventions for Simple Habits

There seems to be general agreement in the literature that simple habits such as thumb sucking and nail biting should not be treated below ages 4 or 5 (see Friman, Barone, & Christophersen, 1986). For children younger than 4, and before any attempts to treat thumb sucking or nail biting, parents should be advised to ignore these habits (Christophersen, 1994). One exception to this suggestion to ignore thumb sucking is for children ages 12–24 months who suck their thumb and pull their hair. The treatment of young children who pull their hair is discussed in the section on *Habit Covariance*. Most informal attempts to stop young children from thumb sucking or nail biting have not been successful and may aggravate the relationship between the parents and the child. Therefore, the parents should not constantly take the child's thumb out of his or her mouth, nag about thumb sucking, punish the child by taking away privileges, or offer rewards that more than likely will not be earned and, thus, become unavailable to the child.

If parents are interested in treating thumb sucking for an older child, some effective and simple interventions are available. For example, Friman et al. (1986) analyzed the effectiveness of a procedure for stopping thumb sucking in children ranging from ages 4 to 12 years. Friman et al. began by briefly instructing the parents to use an increased amount of time-in (Christophersen, 1994) as well as how to paint an aversive-tasting solution on the child's fingers and thumb every time the child moved his or her thumbs or fingers close to his or her mouth. The procedures completely eliminated thumb and finger sucking in all of the children in the study within a matter of weeks. The instructions that were given to parents who participated in the research study are found in Exhibit 3.3.

Friman and Leibowitz (1990) made minor adaptations to these procedures, adding a reward system (a grab bag of tangible reinforcers) to supplement the simple time-in procedures for not thumb sucking. At a 30-month follow-up, none of the 22 children had relapsed to pretreatment levels, and 12 children had completely stopped sucking their thumbs. Friman and Leibowitz also addressed the study's social validity by asking the parents, pediatricians, and pediatric psychologists who participated in the study to rate the acceptability of the procedures. They reported that all of the participants found the procedures "very acceptable."

Habit covariance. A particularly interesting phenomenon in behavioral literature is *covariance*, which refers to behaviors that, although seemingly quite different, will vary together. When something affects one of the behaviors, the other behaviors also change. Friman and Hove (1987) published a report showing that thumb sucking and hair pulling (trichotillomania) can covary. They reported that elimination of hair pulling was obtained

EXHIBIT 3.3
Thumb-Sucking Handout

The use of aversive-tasting substances for the treatment of thumb sucking in young children can be quite successful if the treatment procedures are carefully followed.

1. Approximately 1 week before starting the treatment, begin increasing the number of times that you have brief, nonverbal, physical contact with your child. This may consist of pats on the head, brief back rubs, or roughing up his/her hair. Do not talk during these contacts.

2. Purchase a bottle of StopZit (or a comparable product) at least a couple of days ahead of time, so that you know that it is available when you need it. You should be able to find it in most pharmacies.

3. One or 2 days before you begin the treatment, discuss the situation with your child (taking no more than 2 to 3 minutes), including the fact that he or she is too old to suck his or her thumb, that other kids are beginning to tease him or her, and that both his or her pediatrician and dentist are concerned about the effect that the thumb sucking has on his or her teeth.

4. Begin the procedures on a Friday night. Paint the thumb and/or fingers that he or she sucks immediately prior to bedtime. On Saturday morning, paint the thumb and/or fingers immediately after he or she awakens. Repeat this procedure every time that he sucks his or her thumb and/or fingers, continuing for 1 week after he or she has stopped thumb sucking completely.

5. Never reprimand your child about the thumb sucking. Lectures, explanations, and reasoning are forbidden.

6. If the child refuses to have the "StopZit" applied, place him or her in time-out until he or she agrees to the application. While he or she is in time-out, do not interact with him or her in any way.

7. Keep up the brief, nonverbal, physical contact throughout the treatment procedures and for the next 10 days. Refrain from verbal reprimands.

8. The treatment of a habit, like thumb sucking, requires a diligent effort on the parent's part, primarily because the child is not engaging in the habit on purpose. That means there will be times when he or she is not aware that he or she is sucking his or her thumb and may be upset when you try to apply the StopZit. It's preferable that you go through the treatment procedures only one time, so follow them diligently so you won't have to repeat them.

9. If your child relapses at some future point, institute exactly the same procedures, except for the initial discussion about thumb sucking.

Note. From *Little People: Guidelines for Common Sense Child Rearing* (4th ed., pp. 197–198), by E. R. Christophersen, 1998, Shawnee Mission, KS: Overland Press. Copyright 1987 by Edward R. Christophersen. Reprinted with permission.

concomitantly with successfully treating the thumb sucking of children ages 2–5 who chronically demonstrated both behaviors. Changes in the rates of thumb sucking, which occurred after the parents began using the aversive-taste procedures, were closely followed by similar changes in the rates of hair pulling. Perhaps the most important aspect of the covariance between thumb sucking and hair pulling is evidenced in children who are younger than 12–14 months, who would not normally be considered as candidates for other known hair-pulling treatments. The aversive taste treatment has been successful for reducing both thumb sucking and hair pulling in children who are younger than 1 year. There has been one successful published replication of the strategy of treating thumb sucking as a treatment for trichotillomania (Watson & Allen, 1993). They used response prevention (the application of a "thumb-post" that made thumb sucking virtually impossible) to reduce thumb sucking and reported complete elimination of the thumb sucking and the covarying trichotillomania.

The most important consideration in deciding whether to use treatment of thumb sucking for children who also pull their hair is whether the two behaviors always occur together. Friman and Hove (1987) reported that the children were always sucking their thumbs while pulling their hair, but they did suck their thumbs without pulling their hair. When this is true, treatment of the thumb sucking is certainly a viable treatment option to address both problems. Because thumb sucking almost always occurs more often than hair pulling, it is usually easier to treat. Because the majority of very young children (ages 10 months to 2 years) we see suck their thumbs *and* pull their hair, we have been successful in eliminating both habits by treating the thumb sucking.

Habit reversal. For most habit disorders other than thumb sucking and nail biting, the solutions are not as simple as using an aversive tasting solution. Azrin and Nunn (1973) published research on the use of a comprehensive approach to eliminate a variety of habit disorders, which they called *habit control* or *habit reversal*. Their original habit reversal procedures consisted of 13 components that focused on awareness, motivation, correction, and prevention. These components were introduced in one counseling session that lasted about 2 hours, with some variation in time depending on the type of tic or habit being treated. Second sessions were not provided unless the client experienced difficulties after many days or weeks had lapsed. Azrin and Nunn (1977) reported treating more than 300 patients, with an average habit reduction of 99.5% at the 6-month follow-up.

Since Azrin and Nunn (1977) published their original work on habit reversal, several researchers have demonstrated that not all of the 13 components are necessary for habit reversal procedures to be effective. For example, Finney et al. (1983) provided a systematic replication of Azrin and Nunn's (1973) study while improving on their measurement by conducting the assessment in the patient's home and by assessing social validity. They reported using only 5 of the original 13 components of Azrin and Nunn's (1977) habit reversal procedures—awareness training, situations and habit inconvenience review, relaxation, a competing response, and social support—to treat several different tics and habit disorders, including eye blinking and hair pulling. The procedures were taught to parents, who were instructed to practice them with their children daily. In each case, the child was interviewed first to ascertain the child's level of motivation to use the habit reversal procedures. Then the parent and child were instructed to practice the habit reversal procedures in front of a mirror during the office visit. Their results, which included 12-month follow-up data, used video-taped data to document the efficacy of the use of habit reversal for the treatment of tics and habits. They reported a decrease from 48% of the intervals observed to 4%. The simplified habit reversal procedures have been used successfully with children as young as 5 years. Miltenberger, Fuqua, and McKinley (1985) reported using the same five components used by Finney et al. They reported that 3 out of 4 participants showed substantial decreases in their tics, which were maintained at 7- and 15-week follow-ups. Miltenberger et al.'s study also concluded that effective treatment of tic disorders can be achieved with fewer components of the habit reversal procedures than the 13 components initially used by Azrin and Nunn.

In more recent literature, only 4 of the original 13 components were found to be necessary to obtain significant treatment effects (Azrin & Peterson, 1990; Woods & Miltenberger, 1996; Woods, Miltenberger, & Lumley, 1996). For example, Azrin and Peterson (1990) reported on the effectiveness of habit reversal training on 10 children and adolescents ages 6–16 diagnosed with Tourette's syndrome, 3 of whom were taking the same dose of medication throughout the study. Using awareness training, relaxation training, competing-response training, and social support provided by each child's parents, the researchers showed a reduction from 89% to 100% in motor and vocal tics at home and from 88% to 100% in tics in the clinic. Follow-up data at 8 and 12 months showed a mean percentage reduction for all 10 children of 93% at home and 93.5% in the clinic. These data were impressive—better than the data that have been published using pharmacological management of Tourette's syndrome. Woods et al. (1996) reported similar results in 4 children with motor tics. They reported that simplified habit reversal, similar to the procedures used by Azrin and Peterson, resulted in virtual elimination of the motor tics. The parents of the children who participated in the study rated the treatment as acceptable and reported satisfaction with the results, which supported the social validity of the treatment as well. Finally, Rapp, Miltenberger, Long, Elliott, and Lumley (1998) reported successful use of simplified habit reversal procedures, including awareness training, competing response, and social support, in the treatment of hair pulling. The use of these procedures resulted in an almost immediate reduction to near-zero levels of hair pulling, with one to three booster sessions required to maintain these levels. The results were reportedly maintained from 18 to 27 weeks posttreatment. An example of simplified habit reversal procedures including only awareness training, competing response training, parental support, and relaxation is presented in Exhibit 3.4.

Many studies have shown that habit reversal procedures can be effective with as few as four components. Further simplification of the procedures, however, has not produced consistent results. For example, Silber and Haynes (1992) used self-monitoring and competing response to reduce nail

EXHIBIT 3.4
Habit Reversal Training for Reducing Children's Tics

Habit reversal is a set of treatment procedures that have been used very success-fully with trichotillomania, nail biting, thumb sucking, transient and chronic motor tics, and the tics associated with Tourette's syndrome. After your physician or psy-chologist has demonstrated the procedures in the office, use the following outline for your daily practice sessions at home.

Step 1: Increase Your Child's Awareness of the Habit on a Daily Basis

1. Have your child look in a mirror while performing the habit on purpose. Help your child become aware of how her body moves and what muscles are being used when she performs the habit.

2. Have your child identify each time he or she engages in the habit, by either rais-ing his or her hand when the habit occurs, or by saying, "that was one," when the habit occurs. If you see the habit occur but your child does not appear to be aware that it occurred, use a prearranged gesture or expression to make him or her aware.

3. Self-monitoring: Your child should record each occurrence of the habit on a 3 x 5 card. Keeping track of how often the habit occurs is the only way that you and your child can tell when progress is being made.

Step 2: Competing Response Should be Practiced Daily

1. Have your child practice his or her competing response in the mirror. This helps your child become comfortable with the response and assures him or her that the competing response is not noticeable socially.

2. Encourage your child to use the competing response when he or she feels the urge to engage in the habit.

3. Encourage your child to use the competing response in situations where the child has a history of engaging in the habit.

4. Encourage your child to use the competing response for 1 minute following the occurrence of the habit.

Step 3: Stress/Anxiety Reduction Procedures
(all should be practiced daily)

1. Progressive muscle relaxation training.

2. Visual imagery.

3. Breathing exercises.

Step 4: Parent Involvement

1. Feedback: Work with your child to increase awareness of the habit by helping him or her identify the habit when it occurs.

2. Support and encouragement: Encourage your child to use the competing re-sponse and praise him or her when he or she does so. Praise any noted de-crease in the habits.

3. Remember, although many children and adolescents will notice a decrease in their habit within a couple of days, the greatest change from using these habit-reversal procedures occurs during the second and third month. Don't give up after only a couple of days or weeks.

Note. From *Habit Reversal Training for Reducing Children's Tics,* by S. Swansen and E. R. Christophersen, 1997. Copyright 1997 by Sara Swansen and Edward R. Christophersen. Reprinted with permission.

biting behavior in children and compared the results with those from the use of a mildly aversive solution painted once on the child's fingers. Although both procedures resulted in marked increases in their outcome measure of nail length, the habit reversal procedures resulted in more significant reductions in damage to the skin around the nails. These results were only partially replicated by K. W. Allen (1996), who reported a similar comparison between a bitter substance and the use of a competing response for the management of nail biting. Allen reported a significant improvement in nail length for the group that used the bitter substance compared with the competing response, which failed to show a significant effect.

Finally, two studies investigating the use of relaxation training only with Tourette's syndrome have produced conflicting results. D. P. Kohen and Botts (1987) reported on the use of relaxation-mental imagery (RMI) with 4 children, 2 of whom were already taking haloperidol for frequent tics. Their results showed an almost immediate reduction in the frequency of tics in all 4 children, particularly when they were using their RMI procedures. In a study using only relaxation therapy in 23 patients (mean age = 12 years) with Tourette's syndrome, Bergin, Wranch, Brown, Carson, and Singer (1998) reported little difference between patients trained in relaxation procedures and a control group. These findings suggest that although relaxation procedures may be a component of the habit reversal procedures, they are probably insufficient as the only form of therapy.

Group habit reversal training. There has only been one published report on the effectiveness of conducting habit reversal training in a group format for the treatment of trichotillomania. Mouton and Stanley (1996) reported that all 5 patients (ranging in age from 17 to 44 years) had decreases at treatment termination, with 2 patients maintaining the treatment gains at a 6-month follow-up. It is clear that more research is needed to support this innovative approach to the treatment of habit disorders such as trichotillomania.

Negative Practice

One of the earliest studies on the treatment of nail biting was by M. Smith (1957). Smith reported that 49% of the college students who performed the negative practice procedures either broke their nail-biting habit or showed a marked improvement compared with 3% of the untreated control students. The negative practice procedures involved having the students stand in front of a mirror once an hour and act out the motions of nail biting (without doing any damage) for 30 seconds. They were instructed to maintain the exercises for 4 days after entirely breaking their habit and then to gradually decrease the exercises over a 2-week time period. The therapist emphasized the principles of satiation and heightened awareness.

Azrin, Nunn, and Frantz (1980) published a comparison of habit reversal and negative practice procedures to treat trichotillomania in 34 patients with a mean age of 28 years (range = 13–48 years). All patients in Azrin et al.'s study were asked to monitor and record their daily progress. Their results showed a reduction of 58% in hair pulling for the negative practice group on the first day after training, which was generally maintained during the 3-month follow-up. The habit reversal patients showed a 99% reduction on the first day after training and that same general level of reduction (97–99%) for 4 weeks. At the 22-month follow-up, hair pulling was reduced by 87% for the habit reversal group. For the negative practice group, 3 of the 8 (37%) patients exhibited fewer than two episodes of hair pulling per day at the 22-month follow-up; of these 8 patients, 2 (25%) exhibited no hair pulling.

Azrin et al. (1982) focused on the treatment of 10 patients (including 3 children) with self-destructive oral habits who were randomly assigned to either habit reversal or negative practice. After a single 2-hour session, the habit reversal patients had reduced their oral habits by 97% during the first week of treatment and by 99% at the 22-month follow-up. The negative practice group showed a mean reduction of 66% during the first week after treatment and remained at a 60% reduction over the 4-week follow-up period. In summary, the research to date has demonstrated that habit reversal procedures are more effective than negative practice. In fact, the components of the negative practice procedures are actually included in the habit reversal procedures. Both procedures involve the patient regularly practicing the habit in front of a mirror. Table 3.3 compares the results obtained with the behavioral intervention procedures discussed above.

Other Strategies

Hypnotherapy and cognitive–behavioral therapy are two strategies with promising results for habit disorders, specifically trichotillomania. For example, a combination of self-monitoring, hypnotic techniques, and relaxation/mental imagery for the child and education plus supportive strategies for the parent has reportedly been successful in decreasing trichotillomania in 5 children and adolescents ages 3 years 10 months to 15 years (D. P.

TABLE 3.3
A Comparison of Behavioral Treatments for Habit Disorders and Tics

	Average Decrease (%)	Maintenance of Treatment Effects (%)	Results Replicated?	Negative Side Effects?	Social Validation?
Negative practice	66	60	Yes	None	No
Full habit reversal	99	99	Yes	None	No
Simplified habit reversal	99	95	Yes	None	Yes

Kohen, 1996). Kohen concluded that, in children, trichotillomania may be similar to a habit disorder and as such is relatively benign and analogous to habits such as nail biting and thumb sucking. Kohen's is the first study that reported the successful application of hypnotic techniques for children and adolescents with trichotillomania. H. A. Cohen, Barzilai, and Lahat (1999), in a study of 3 children with trichotillomania, reported complete resolution of their complaints after 7–8 weeks and 1 patient after 16 weeks. There were no recurrences during a mean follow-up period of 16 months.

Lerner, Franklin, Meadows, Hembree, and Foa (1998) reported on the effectiveness of a cognitive–behavioral therapy for trichotillomania. Immediately following treatment, 12 of the 14 patients showed at least a 50% improvement on the Trichotillomania Severity Scale. However, only 4 of the 13 patients were classified as "responders" at follow-up at 3 years 9 months later. Learner et al. concluded that there was a significant risk for relapse and recommended the use of relapse prevention strategies.

Long-Term Follow-Up

Most of the studies that have examined habit reversal and negative practice procedures for the management of habit disorders have reported follow-up data for periods of time ranging from several months up to 1 year. The longest follow-up data in the literature was the 22-month follow-up reported by both Azrin et al. (1982) and Azrin et al. (1980). These 22-month follow-ups on habit reversal and negative practice, using a prospective design, far exceed the length of prospective studies that have examined pharmacological approaches to the management of habit disorders. Clearly, more long-term data are needed to provide further support for the effectiveness of the interventions described above.

CONCLUSION

A variety of medical and behavioral treatments are available for managing tics and habit disorders. Although pharmacological management of simple habit disorders has not received much study, there have been numerous studies reporting the effective medical management of children with Tourette's syndrome. Unfortunately, many of the pharmacological options also have significant side effects. Such side effects certainly reduce the acceptability of these options for the management of Tourette's syndrome in children. The flurry of research studies on the effects of drugs with Tourette's syndrome, however, offers the promise of a breakthrough for effective and less aversive medical management of this disorder in the future.

At this time, however, the use of nonpharmacological interventions, particularly habit reversal procedures, is still the treatment of choice for tics,

Tourette's syndrome, and habit disorders. The treatment of simple habit disorders can be implemented by the clinician with adequate training. The procedures typically take from 1 to 2 hours to introduce to the parents and children, thus increasing their feasibility for use in the office setting as well as acceptability to both professionals and parents. Many of the behavioral researchers who have reported on interventions with habit disorders and tics have objectively measured social validity. The combination of actual videotapes of patient behavior before and after treatment, combined with a social validation component, provides a reasonable estimate of the acceptability and significance of an intervention strategy.

Finally, because there has been no standard treatment modality for more serious habit disorders, a variety of providers have used a wide array of treatment modalities to deal with such habit disorders as hair pulling and muscle tics. The recent extensions of habit reversal procedures to include Tourette's syndrome demonstrates the utility of these intervention procedures. The adaptations of the early work of Azrin and Nunn (1977) are providing feasible and effective treatment protocols to address such disorders. Probably the most pressing need in the treatment of habit disorders and tics is for more well-controlled studies, including data on the maintenance of treatment effects over time. None of the studies on pharmacological treatments and only a small percentage of the behavioral treatments included data on long-term follow-up. Without adequate controls and long-term follow-up, the possibility exists that the patients would have shown an improvement without any treatment. Nevertheless, the clinician can be helpful in managing the often distressing and disruptive symptoms of tic and habit disorders.

4

DIAGNOSIS AND MANAGEMENT
OF SLEEP PROBLEMS

Before we discuss common sleep problems in children, it is important to understand what is considered to be normal sleep behavior. Several studies have been conducted to determine typical sleep patterns in children, including common bedtime hours, onset of sleep, the usual number of hours a child sleeps, and the prevalence of nighttime awakenings. An early study by Anders (1979) used time-lapse videotape recordings to examine the typical bedtimes of children and patterns of sleep onset. His sample consisted of 2- and 6-month-old children from a suburban, middle-class population. Anders found that approximately 60% of the children were put to bed awake, generally between the hours of 7:00 p.m. and 10:00 p.m. Anders also reported that once in bed, 2-month-old children took approximately 28 minutes to fall asleep, whereas 9-month-olds' average time decreased to 16 minutes. Anders found that for older children, approximately 70% fell asleep in less than 1 hour, and 80% can be expected to sleep through the night.

Typical sleep requirements have been offered by Ferber (1985), based on his clinical experience and a review of the sleep literature. From his review, he reported that newborns typically need the greatest amount of sleep, approximately 16 hours 30 minutes, with a decline in the need for sleep through adolescence. Such guidelines can assist parents and health care providers in having appropriate expectations for the amount of sleep a child needs and help them identify sleep problems.

99

In addition to establishing the typical amount of sleep children need, researchers have made efforts to understand how often children, especially infants, awake during the night. Moore and Ucko (1957) conducted a longitudinal study of the night-awakening habits of more than 100 infants ranging in age from 1 to 12 months. They defined regular sleep as sleeping from midnight to 5:00 a.m. By age 3 months, 71% of the children had established a regular sleep pattern; by age 6 months, 83% of the children were sleeping regularly. Moore and Ucko also reported that 10% of the children never established a regular sleep pattern.

Finally, A. W. Wolf and Lozoff (1989) found that most young children need something to assist them with sleep onset. They surveyed the bedtime practices of the parents of more than 100 healthy children younger than age 4 who had visited their pediatrician. On the basis of a structured parent interview, Wolf and Lozoff reported that 60% of the children used thumb sucking or a transitional object such as a blanket, toy, or both to help them fall asleep. The majority of children who did not use such a transitional object required adult company for sleep onset. The research suggested that children who readily soothe themselves with thumb sucking or transitional objects have an easier time of falling asleep when left alone than children who do not use such methods.

SLEEP PROBLEMS

Most of the research that has been published on common childhood sleep problems has been on either sleep onset, including sleep resistance, or night awakenings (Mindell, 1993). In fact, sleep research involving toddlers represents merely 3% of all the published research on sleep. Several common sleep problems in children have been reported by Blader, Koplewicz, Abikoff, and Foley (1997). In their study of more than 900 children ranging in age from 5 to 12 years, Blader et al. found that bedtime resistance (at least 3 nights per week) was the most prevalent sleep problem. Morning wake-up problems, fatigue complaints, sleep-onset delays of up to 1 hour or more, and night awakening were also common. Among children with sleep-onset problems, 80% also displayed bedtime resistance. Sleep problems also tend to persist, especially from infancy to later childhood. Kataria, Swanson, and Trevathan (1987) reported that 84% of their sample of children had persistence of sleep disturbances after 3 years. Similarly, Pollock (1992, 1994) reported in a longitudinal study that sleep problems were more likely at ages 5 and 10 in those children who had sleep problems before age 6 months. Thus, sleep problems are quite common for the typical child and may persist over time.

When should parents be concerned about their child's sleep behavior? Some general guidelines include excessive delay of sleep onset, numerous night awakenings, or if most nights present a constant struggle for parents who are trying to get their child to bed. Richman (1981) described sleep problems for 12-month-olds more specifically as either frequent sleep-onset periods associated with fussing of 30 minutes or longer or night-waking episodes that occur at least 4 nights a week and require parental intervention. It is also important to remember that during the toddler period, sleep disturbance rates may increase with the common onset of fears, such as fear of parental separation or fear of the dark.

The *Diagnostic and Statistical Manual of Mental Disorders* (4th ed., *DSM–IV*; American Psychiatric Association, 1994) provides criteria for various sleep disorders. Each of the major diagnostic categories for sleep problems includes the criteria that the disorder not be due to any other mental health disorder, that it not be due to any known substance, and that it causes clinically significant distress. Most of the research on children's sleep problems appearing in either psychology or pediatric literature deals with the initiation of sleep, maintenance of sleep, or both, and falls under the general category of primary insomnia (see Exhibit 4.1). Primary hypersomnia is also described in Exhibit 4.1 and refers to excessive sleepiness. The vast majority of cases of excessive sleepiness in young children during the day are secondary to poor or inadequate sleep schedules or poor sleep habits at night.

The areas of nightmare disorder, sleep terror disorder, and sleepwalking disorder have received far less attention in the published literature. See Exhibit 4.2 for a description of the *DSM–IV* criteria for these disorders. Nightmares occur in about 10–50% of all children between the ages 3 and 6 years (Mindell, 1993). After a gradual onset, nightmares typically decrease in frequency over time. A small percentage of children continue having nightmares throughout adolescence and even possibly into adulthood (Mindell, 1993).

Night terrors are characterized by recurrent episodes of abrupt awakening from sleep, typically including intense fear and signs of autonomic arousal, during which the child is relatively unresponsive to efforts of others to comfort him or her. The parents are aroused from sleep by the child's piercing screams or cries. They usually occur within 2 hours of sleep onset and are characterized by agitation after awakening. The child is often unresponsive to attempts at soothing and may be confused and disoriented if awakened. Sleep terrors are most common in children who range in age from 4 to 12 years and tend to resolve by adolescence (Mindell, 1993). Sleep terrors (or night terrors) are reported to have a genetic component (Kales, Soldatos, & Caldwell, 1980) and are considered a disorder of impaired arousal (Broughton, 1968, as cited in Mindell, 1993).

Finally, approximately 1–6% of children experience chronic sleepwalking, with as many as 15% of all children having experienced at least one such episode (Anders, 1982). The behavior may range from simply

EXHIBIT 4.1
DSM–IV Criteria for Primary Insomnia and Primary Hypersomnia

Primary Insomnia 307.42

A. The predominant complaint is difficulty initiating or maintaining sleep, or non-restorative sleep, for at least 1 month.

B. The sleep disturbance (or associated daytime fatigue) causes clinically significant distress or impairment in social, occupational, or other important areas of functioning.

C. The sleep disturbance does not occur exclusively during the course of Narcolepsy, Breathing-Related Sleep Disorder, Circadian Rhythm Sleep Disorder, or a Parasomnia.

D. The disturbance does not occur exclusively during the course of another mental disorder (e.g., Major Depressive Disorder, Generalized Anxiety Disorder, a delirium).

E. The disturbance is not due to the direct physiological effects of a substance (e.g., a drug of abuse, a medication) or a general medical condition.

Primary Hypersomnia 307.44

A. The predominant complaint is excessive sleepiness for at least 1 month (or less if recurrent) as evidenced by either prolonged sleep episodes or daytime sleep episodes that occur almost daily.

B. The excessive sleepiness causes clinically significant distress or impairment in social, occupational, or other important areas of functioning.

C. The excessive sleepiness is not better accounted for by insomnia and does not occur exclusively during the course of another Sleep Disorder (e.g., Narcolepsy, Breathing-Related Sleep Disorder, Circadian Rhythm Sleep Disorder, or a Parasomnia) and cannot be accounted for by an inadequate amount of sleep.

D. The disturbance does not occur exclusively during the course of another mental disorder.

E. The disturbance is not due to the direct physiological effects of a substance (e.g., a drug of abuse, a medication) or a general medical condition.

Note. Information from *Diagnostic and Statistical Manual of Mental Disorders* (4th ed.), by American Psychiatric Association, 1994, Washington, DC: Author. Copyright 1994 by the American Psychiatric Association. Reprinted with permission.

sitting up in bed to actual sleepwalking. The child is often difficult to awaken and, upon awakening, appears confused (Mindell, 1993). Sleepwalking is most prevalent in children between ages 4 and 8 years and usually resolves by adolescence. The frequency can vary from infrequently to several times a week.

Table 4.1 summarizes the diagnostic criteria of the *DSM–IV* for the various sleep problems discussed above. This checklist format can assist the clinician in making a differential diagnosis by providing a list of symptoms to question the parents about during the initial interview.

EXHIBIT 4.2

Nightmare Disorder 307.47

A. Repeated awakenings from the major sleep period or naps with detailed recall of extended and extremely frightening dreams, usually involving threats to survival, security, or self-esteem. The awakenings generally occur during the second half of the period.

B. On awakening from the frightening dreams, the person rapidly becomes oriented and alert (in contrast to the confusion and disorientation seen in Sleep Terror Disorder and some forms of epilepsy).

C. The dream experience, or the sleep disturbance resulting from the awakening, causes clinically significant distress or impairment in social, occupational, or other important areas of functioning.

D. The nightmares do not occur exclusively during the course of another mental disorder (e.g., a delirium, Posttraumatic Stress Disorder) and are not due to the direct physiological effects of a substance (e.g., a drug of abuse, a medication) or a general medical condition.

Sleep Terror Disorder 307.46

A. Recurrent episodes of abrupt awakening from sleep, usually occurring during the first third of the major sleep episode and beginning with a panicky scream.

B. Intense fear and signs of autonomic arousal, such as tachycardia, rapid breathing, and sweating, during each episode.

C. Relative unresponsiveness to efforts of others to comfort the person during the episode.

D. No detailed dream is recalled and there is amnesia for the episode.

E. The episodes cause clinically significant distress or impairment in social, occupational, or other important area of functioning.

F. The disturbance is not due to the direct physiological effects of a substance (e.g., a drug of abuse, a medication) or a general medical condition.

Sleepwalking Disorder 307.46

A. Repeated episodes of rising from bed during sleep and walking about, usually occurring during the first third of the major sleep episode.

B. While sleepwalking, the person has a blank, staring face, is relatively unresponsive to the efforts of others to communicate with him or her, and can be awakened only with great difficulty.

C. On awakening (either from the sleepwalking episode or the next morning), the person has amnesia for the episode.

D. Within several minutes after awakening from the sleepwalking episode, there is no impairment or mental activity or behavior (although there may initially be a short period of confusion or disorientation).

E. The sleepwalking causes clinically significant distress or impairment in social, occupational, or other important areas of functioning.

F. The disturbance is not due to the direct physiological effects of a substance (e.g., a drug of abuse, a medication) or a general medical condition.

TABLE 4.1
The *DSM–IV* Differential Criteria for Primary Insomnia, Primary Hypersomnia, Nightmare Disorder, Sleep Terror Disorder, and Sleepwalking

Primary Insomnia 307.42	Primary Hypersomnia 307.44	Nightmare Disorder 307.47
❏ Difficulty initiating/ maintaining sleep for 1 month	❏ Excessive sleepiness for at least 1 month	❏ Repeated awakening
❏ Causes clinically significant distress	❏ Causes clinically significant distress	❏ Rapidly oriented
❏ Not during other sleep disorder	❏ Not accounted for by insomnia	❏ Causes clinically significant distress
❏ Not due to other mental disorder	❏ Not due to other mental disorder	❏ Not due to other mental disorder
❏ Not due to a known substance	❏ Not due to a known substance	
_____ of 5 (5 = Dx)	_____ of 5 (5 = Dx)	_____ of 4 (4 = Dx)

Sleep Terror Disorder 307.46	Sleepwalking Disorder 307.46
❏ Abrupt awakening beginning with a panicky scream	❏ Repeated episodes of rising from sleep and walking about
❏ Intense fear and signs of autonomic arousal	❏ Has a blank, staring face, is relatively unresponsive to communication or awakening
❏ Unresponsiveness to attempts to comfort	❏ On awakening, amnesia for the episode
❏ No detailed dream is recalled	❏ No impairment of mental activity or behavior
❏ Causes clinically significant distress	❏ Causes clinically significant distress
❏ Not due to a known substance	❏ Not due to a known substance
_____ of 6 (6 = Dx)	_____ of 6 (6 = Dx)

Note. Information from *Diagnostic and Statistical Manual of Mental Disorders* (4th ed.), by the American Psychiatric Association, 1994, Washington, DC: Author. Copyright 1994 by the American Psychiatric Association. Reprinted with permission. Dx = diagnosis.

PREVALENCE

Clinical sleep problems in the absence of pathological central nervous system (CNS) functioning or maturational lags in CNS development are common in the first years of life (Anders, 1982). For example, parents report in many surveys that from 10% to 40% of infants experience difficulties in "settling to bed" or in "night waking" (e.g., Anders, 1982; Ferber, 1985). Similarly, Lozoff, Wolf, and Davis (1985) surveyed parents of children ranging in age from 6 months to 4 years; approximately 30% of the parents surveyed reported bedtime struggles with their children three or more nights a week. Blader et al.'s (1997) study of school-age children suggests that older children also demonstrate a variety of sleep problems. The most prevalent reported sleep problem in the study was bedtime resistance (27%), followed by sleep-onset delays (11%). Bedtime resistance was associated with an inconsistent bedtime and the child falling asleep away from his or her bed. Finally, there is also evidence that adolescents suffer from sleep problems. In a study of 484 male and 459 female adolescents from the general population, Morrison, McGee, and Stanton (1999) reported that 25% needed a lot more sleep than they were getting, with 10% complaining of difficulty falling asleep. They also reported that adolescents who reported having sleep problems showed more signs of anxiety, depression, inattentiveness, and conduct disorder than those who had no or only occasional sleep problems. Neurological conditions such as narcolepsy, which affects only from 0.03% to 0.16% of children, are rarely diagnosed in preadolescent children (Kotagal, Hartse, & Walsh, 1990) and are not discussed in this chapter.

In general, bedtime problems appear to be very common and disruptive to parents. In fact, during the first 2 years of an infant's life, the most frequent complaint of parents during pediatric health supervision visits is sleep problems (Ferber, 1986). Furthermore, sleep and bedtime problems are the second most frequently encountered behavior problem in primary care (42% occurrence rate), exceeded only by oppositional behavior (60% occurrence rate; Arndorfer, Allen, & Aljazireh, 1999). The high incidence rate of sleep problems suggests the need for effective, and preferably simple, intervention strategies that improve children's sleep behavior. Such interventions do exist and are reviewed in the "Intervention" section of this chapter.

CAUSES AND CORRELATES

One factor associated with sleep problems in children has been the extent of parental presence and involvement in the sleep process. Infants whose parents are present when they fall asleep typically wake up more often during the night than infants who are put to bed awake and then left alone. For example, Adair, Bauchner, Philipp, Levenson, and Zuckerman (1991) examined whether parents who reported being present when their infant fell asleep at bedtime were more likely to report increased frequency of night awakening by the infant. More of the infants whose parents were present at sleep onset experienced frequent night awakenings than infants whose parents were not present. Similarly, Rapoff, Christophersen, and Rapoff (1982) reported on 4 children who had no problems with sleep onset—all 4 children were placed in the cribs awake by their parents. After 1 to 4 minutes of talking, babbling, cooing, or fussing, they each fell asleep on their own. Finally, Anders, Halpern, and Hua (1992) reported that by the age of 3 months, infants who were put to bed awake and allowed to fall asleep on their own were also more successful at returning to sleep when they awoke during the night. Conversely, infants who were put to bed already asleep were significantly more likely to be identified by their mothers as problem sleepers requiring parental intervention, such as picking them up from their cribs when they woke up during the night. Anders et al. concluded that infants' pattern of initial sleep onset is related to their ability to fall back to sleep following an awakening in the middle of the night.

There may also be a correlation between sleep problems at night and behavior problems during the day. For example, in a study of 510 children (ages 2–5 years), children who received less night sleep and less sleep in a 24-hour period had more behavior problems and more externalizing problems on the Child Behavior Checklist (CBCL; Achenbach & Edelbrock, 1988) than children who received more sleep (Lavigne et al., 1999). Furthermore, when Minde, Faucon, and Falkner (1994) treated 28 children ages 12 to 36 months for severe sleep disturbances, there was a correlated improvement in the children's daytime behavior, sleep patterns, and interactions with their mothers during feeding. Thus, given the possible association between sleep problems and daytime behavior disorders, thorough assessment of both of these problems should be obtained by the clinician.

ASSESSMENT

Medical Assessment

Common sleep problems, such as recurrent night waking and sleep refusal, are rarely, if ever, caused by an underlying medical problem. For instance, an acute medical problem that either interferes with sleep onset or contributes to night awakening, such as an ear infection, is often easily discernible by parents and the physician (Blum & Carey, 1996). Despite the very low likelihood that a sleep disturbance is caused by a medical problem, parents may want to discuss their concerns with their physician to receive reassurance or assistance with intervention strategies. Furthermore, during an assessment for sleep problems by the clinician, disorders such as diabetes should be considered if, for example, frequent night awakenings are accompanied by frequent urination.

Behavioral Assessment

Numerous procedures are available to interview parents about their child's sleep behaviors. In our opinion, questions about sleep onset and night awakening should be included in all initial interviews with parents, regardless of the presenting problem. Screening questions should also be asked by the child's primary-care physician during regularly scheduled child health supervision visits. Parents should also be questioned about the amount of assistance they give the child at bedtime. Zuckerman (1995) recommended asking key clinical questions, including the following:

- During infancy:
  a. How do you know when your child is awake?
  b. How do you put your child to sleep?
  c. Do you feed your infant when he or she awakens? How much?
  d. Have you been away from your baby? Have you and your spouse gone out by yourselves? When you are away, do you think and worry about your baby all of the time?

- Toddlers:
  a. Do you have other problems with your child?
  b. Are you frustrated about not being in control? Do you believe your child is in charge? Do you get into power struggles with your child?
  c. Are you afraid that your child's sleep problem is part of a larger, more significant problem?
  d. How much of a problem is this for you?

An alternative to including such questions in the interview is to request that the parent or parents complete a Sleep Intake Form, either in the office waiting room or in the exam room while waiting for the primary-care provider. A Sleep Intake Form is shown in Exhibit 4.3.

In addition to parents' completing an interview with the clinician, information from a standardized behavior rating scale may also provide useful information in the assessment of a child's sleep problems and related difficulties. Of the most widely used parent rating scales, only the CBCL (Achenbach & Edelbrock, 1988) includes questions about and norms on toddlers' sleep problems. Neither the Conners Parent Rating Scale (Goyette et al., 1978) nor the Behavior Assessment System for Children (Reynolds & Kamphaus, 1998) includes questions about sleep or norms on toddlers' sleep problems. The printout from the computerized scoring program for the CBCL for the 2- to 3-year-old child has a Sleep Problems scale that includes "not wanting to sleep alone," "trouble sleeping," "nightmares," "resists bed," "sleeps little," "talks, cries in sleep," and "wakes often." Thus, of the parent rating scales, only the CBCL can be used to routinely aid in the assessment of children's sleep problems.

Finally, when the parents express significant concerns about their child's sleep or night waking, Zuckerman (1995) suggested asking the parents to complete a sleep diary similar to the one found in Exhibit 4.4 for a

EXHIBIT 4.3
Intake Form for Children With Sleep Problems

Child's Name: _____ Date of Birth: _____

Mother's Name: _____ Age: _____

Father's Name: _____ Age: _____

What is the present problem? _____

Breast-Fed? _____ Bottle-Fed? _____ Solids? _____

Where did your child sleep as a newborn? _____

Where does he/she sleep now? _____

Number of night feedings as a newborn? _____

Age when slept through the night the first time? _____

Length and time of morning nap? _____

Length and time of afternoon nap? _____

Time put down for the night? _____

Where put down for the night? _____

Number of night awakenings? _____

How/where does your child fall asleep for naps? _____

How/where does your child fall asleep for the night? _____

Is sleep any different for sitters/relatives? _____

What have you tried before? _____

    Breast-feeding _____   Rocking _____

    Crying to sleep _____   Lying down with child _____

    Alone with bottle _____   On sofa/parents' bed _____

    Medication _____   Other devices _____

From whom have you sought help before? _____

When did the present problem start? _____

What do you think is going on? _____

Other children and their ages _____

1-week period before any discussion of the child's sleep problem. The parents should be asked to complete such a diary in the time period between when they schedule their appointment and the actual date of their appointment. The completion of a sleep diary and standardized rating scales will provide the clinician with a comprehensive history before discussion of the child's sleep disturbance.

In summary, given the prevalence of sleep problems and the comorbidity between sleep problems and externalizing problems, parents should routinely be asked several questions about their child's sleep routines. Par-

EXHIBIT 4.4
Sleep Diary

	Mon.	Tues.	Weds.	Thurs.	Fri.	Sat.	Sun.
Time awoke in morning							
Times and lengths of naps during day							
Time went to bed in the evening							
Time settled in bed in evening							
Issues in settling in bed and what you did							
Where child fell asleep and with whom?							
Times and lengths of waking at night and what you did (What was successful and what was not?)							

Note. From "Sleep Problems," by B. Zuckerman. In S. Parker and B. Zuckerman (Eds.), *Behavioral and Developmental* Pediatrics, p. 292, 1995, Boston: Little, Brown. Copyright 1995 by Little, Brown. Adapted with permission.

ents should be questioned specifically about the amount of assistance they give their child at bedtime. As Ferber (1987) elucidated, although parents may not report problems at bedtime, they may be intimately involved in the process of sleep initiation (through rocking, nursing, lying down with the child, or replacing the pacifier), suggesting the development of less-than-optimal sleep habits for the child. Of the available parent rating scales, only the CBCL can be routinely used to assess children's sleep problems.

INTERVENTION

Preventing Sleep Problems

Some studies have found that prevention of sleep problems in children may be facilitated by simply providing parents with written instructions about sleep. For example, Adair, Zuckerman, Bauchner, Philipp, and Levenson (1992) evaluated a brief intervention to treat infant nighttime awakenings, which involved providing mothers with a written instruction sheet for dealing with infant sleep. The instructions advised the mother to establish a bedtime routine that included putting her infant into the crib partially awake so the child could learn to go to sleep without an adult being present. Infants in the intervention group were reported to experience 36% fewer nighttime awakenings than those in an untreated control group. Parental presence at bedtime was significantly less common in the intervention group compared with the control group. Kerr, Jowett, and Smith (1996) conducted a similar experimental study on preventing sleep problems. The intervention group received a booklet that addressed two major areas: settling methods and the importance of routine. Kerr et al. reported significant differences between the intervention and control groups 6 months later in the following areas: settling difficulties, night awakening, nights per week of awakenings, and times of awakenings per night. Unfortunately, although they reported using a "health education booklet" as a part of their intervention, no reference is made to the specific contents of the booklet in their publication.

Pinilla and Birch (1993) examined the efficacy of a prevention approach focused on the timing of breast feedings to reduce night awakenings in breast-fed infants. Twenty-six first-time parents and their newborns were randomly assigned to either a treatment group or a control group. The parents in the treatment group were instructed to offer a "focal feed" to their infants every night between 10:00 p.m. and 12:00 a.m., gradually lengthen the interval between middle-of-the-night feedings, and maximize environmental differences between daytime and nighttime feedings. At each night awakening, mothers were instructed to go to their baby immediately but to try soothing the baby by rocking or cuddling prior to breast feeding. Over time they were instructed to wait longer before breast feeding. They referred to this as "stretching" the time. The control group received the same amount of time with their providers but were not given any information about regulating their breast feeding. By age 8 weeks, 100% of the intervention infants were sleeping through the night (defined as being from midnight to 5:00 a.m.) versus 23% of the control infants. Breast milk intake per 24-hour period did not differ between the two groups. Additionally, the intervention infants were rated as having a more predictable temperament. The authors concluded that parents can have a profound influence on the development of their infants' sleep patterns. Exhibit 4.5 is a summary of the procedures used by Pinilla and Birch (1993).

Medical Treatment for Sleep Problems

Several authors have reported using sleep-inducing medications to help children with their sleep problems. For example, Russo, Gururaj, and Allen (1976) examined the effects of Benadryl Elixir (diphenhydramine hydrochloride) as a bedtime sedative for 41 children (from ages 2 to 12 years) with such problems as not falling asleep or waking up in the night. Russo et

Teaching Your Baby to Sleep Through the Night

Getting on the Right Track

When you come home from the hospital with your baby:

1. Try not to hold, rock, or nurse your baby to sleep.
2. Concentrate your baby's waking times in the daytime hours. Do not entertain your baby at night. When you go into your baby's room, do not turn on the light (a hall light or night light should work fine).
3. Start a *focal feeding time* around Day 3 of your baby's life. You should wake your baby for this feeding between 10:00 p.m. and midnight.
4. At night, be sure to wait to pick up your baby until he or she is really complaining (not merely a nondistressful whimper).

When Your Baby Is 3 Weeks Old, Steadily Gaining Weight, and Has No Major Health Problems

If baby wakes up in the middle of the night (between midnight and 5:00 a.m.):

1. Wait a few minutes until he or she is *really complaining.*
2. Check to see if he or she is physically okay. Change your baby, wrap baby up, and try to settle baby back to sleep. Do not pick baby up at this time. Go back to bed.
   a. If your baby goes back to sleep—so do you!
   b. If your baby does not go back to sleep or wakes up again:
      – It's *stretching* time
      – Change baby, if necessary, wrap your baby
      – Take a walk with your baby, or sit in a chair
      – Hold your baby, but *not in a feeding position.*
   c. At this point, you have stretched your baby from 10 to 45 minutes. Congratulate yourself for successful stretching. You are beginning to extinguish the stimulus–response pattern: wake-up and expect to eat. When your baby complains (after 45 minutes), it's time to feed him or her.
3. If you are lucky to have your baby waking only once between midnight and 5:00 a.m. before he or she is 4 weeks old, give yourself a present (e.g., a night out for you and your spouse alone).

Note. From "Help Me Make It Through the Night: Behavioral Entrainment of Breast-Fed Infants' Sleep Patterns," by T. Pinilla and L. L. Birch, 1993, *Pediatrics,* 91, pp. 436–444. Copyright 1993 by American Academy of Pediatrics. Adapted with permission.

al. used a double-blind, placebo-controlled design with random assignment to treatment groups. The results indicated that Benadryl Elixir was statistically better than the placebo in reducing the time to fall asleep and for reducing the number of awakenings per night. These improvements seemed to be small, however, and the actual weekly means were not reported. Improvement in the amount of sleep was only marginally significant. One side effect noted from a parent's report was minimal drowsiness of 1 child during the day. Unfortunately, Russo et al. did not report any reliability measures on the parents' completion of the nightly sleep diary.

Another drug that has been studied is trimeprazine tartrate. Richman (1985) investigated the effects of trimeprazine tartrate in reducing sleep problems in a random sample of 22 children ranging in age from 1 to 2 years. On the basis of parental diaries, Richman's double-blind drug trial compared the effects of the drug (1 mg/kg) with those of a placebo. A composite score of sleep problems revealed that the drug produced no permanent effects on sleep, and a follow-up of 14 children 6 months later showed that the sleep problems persisted. On the basis of these findings, Richman concluded that strong sedatives are of extremely limited use for most children with sleep-onset problems. In a similar follow-up study, however, Simonoff and Stores (1987) reached a different conclusion on the basis of the effects of using a higher dose of trimeprazine tartrate (6 mg/kg) for night awakening in children. Their double-blind crossover design randomly assigned 18 children with sleep problems to either a drug or placebo group. The children, who ranged in age from 1 to 3 years, had been referred from general practitioners. The researchers found that children taking the drug had statistically fewer awakenings, less time awake at night, and more nighttime sleeping compared with those on the placebo. They did note the limitation that children continued to have some night awakenings on these higher doses, suggesting this treatment may be viewed as a temporary aid in reducing nighttime wakefulness rather than a cure. They reportedly observed no adverse effects at this dose, and the often-cited side effects of daytime sleepiness and irritability almost always ceased after several days of treatment with this drug.

Medical Treatment for Sleep Terrors

Glick, Schulman, and Turecki (1971) treated 3 children, ages 8–11, with diazepam (Valium). In all three cases, a reduction in sleep terrors was evident. However, in two of the cases, relapse occurred when the drug was stopped, and recovery occurred again when the medication was resumed. A second study (Fisher, Kahn, Edwards, & Davis, 1973) also found diazepam to be effective in the treatment of night terrors (as long as the child was taking the medication). Weissbluth (1984) cautioned that night terrors are a benign disorder of arousal that is not associated with psychopathologic symptoms in prepubertal children, and that there are no data that drugs are indicated for the night terrors commonly encountered in pediatric practice.

Because medication can help initiate and maintain sleep in adults, intuitively it seems medication administered to help children sleep should be more effective than indicated by these studies. Thus, questions clearly remain concerning the effectiveness of medication in treating sleep difficulties among young children. One possible explanation for the findings reported in these studies lies in their methodologies. Although the double-blind crossover is a good design to help alleviate any bias the parents may have about a child being on medication, questions still remain about the accuracy of parental reports concerning their child's nighttime behaviors. Reliability checks are therefore needed to reveal the clear effects of medications (cf. Christophersen, 1983; Edwards & Christophersen, 1993). An additional issue related to all medication for children is the potential for side effects.

Finally, one of the most recent "advances" in the management of sleep problems involves the use of melatonin, an over-the-counter product. Masters (1996) reported, in an uncontrolled study, that all 20 children using melatonin for a range of 7 to 90 days were successful in correcting their sleep disorders. If replicated in a well-controlled study, without any negative side effects, melatonin could become an important "drug" available to the clinician. In the absence of further study, however, melatonin should not be recommended.

Dietary Treatments

Dietary treatments have also been investigated as solutions to sleep problems in children. Macknin, Medendorp, and Maier (1989) investigated the old folklore notion that feeding infants solids before bedtime increased the length of uninterrupted sleep. They randomly assigned 106 infants seen at a well-child-care center before the age of 1 month to begin a diet that included feeding the infant rice cereal at either age 1 month or 4 months. The main measure was a comparison of parental reports of sleeping between the two groups at ages 4, 8, 12, 16, and 20 weeks. Although they found children to sleep more as they got older, there were no significant differences between the groups in the number of hours or duration of sleep based on the addition of rice cereal. Thus, the notion that feeding solids before bedtime will improve sleep was not supported by the results of their study.

Milk allergies have also been considered as a contributor to sleep problems. For example, Kahn et al. (1987) drew the conclusion that infants with clinically evident milk allergy may suffer from sleeplessness and that when no evident cause for chronic insomnia can be found, the possibility of milk allergy should be given serious consideration. Similarly, Kahn, Mozin, Rebuffat, Sottiaux, and Muller (1989) found that 12% of the young children with sleep problems in their study had normalized sleep patterns when cow's milk was eliminated from their diets. The majority of the children, however, had sleep problems as a result of poor sleep habits.

Behavioral Interventions

Behavioral interventions have been offered as effective solutions for the sleep problems discussed in this chapter. In a review of the literature on 41 studies of empirically supported treatments for bedtime refusal and night wakings in young children, Mindell (1999) concluded that evidence exists indicating that extinction (ignoring) and parent education on the prevention of sleep problems can be considered well-established treatments, and graduated extinction and scheduled awakenings are probably efficacious treatments, with positive routines being a promising intervention.

Primary Insomnia

As mentioned earlier, the vast majority of research on children's sleep problems has addressed either the initiation (sleep onset) or maintenance of sleep. A number of different behavioral interventions are reported in the literature. Each of the procedures identified below, which have been used to deal with sleep-onset problems, is addressed in turn:

- ignoring
- graduated extinction
- scheduled awakenings
- establishment of bedtime routines
- treatment of sleep disorder and daytime behavior
- relaxation
- treatment with white noise

Ignoring. Some researchers have suspected that children's sleep problems are related to parental reactions; specifically, they assume that parents' attention to their child's night fussing makes it occur more often. Consequently, researchers have emphasized ignoring procedures in the treatment of sleep problems. Most ignoring procedures involve some variation of trying to teach parents to refrain from all forms of attention to their children after bedtime and if they awaken during the night. For example, Rapoff et al. (1982) empirically evaluated ignoring procedures with 6 children with a mean age of 36 months. The components of their treatment program included the following routine to prepare the child for bed:

1. Turn off the light.
2. Ignore the child's crying or requests.
3. If the child leaves the bed, return him or her to bed.

Their results were inconclusive. Inappropriate vocalizations decreased and remained near zero for 3 children but not for the other 3. The parents of the 3 children who showed substantial improvements followed the treatment recommendations. The parents of the 3 children who did not improve did not follow the treatment recommendations; instead, they intermittently responded to their children. It has been noted that some parents find it difficult to ignore their children's crying and requests at night. Drabman and Jarvie (1977) cautioned that ignoring often results in a temporary increase in the behavior being ignored. The study by Rapoff et al. (1982) provides evidence of how parents may not adhere to a plan to ignore their child's crying and also indicates the need for measuring treatment integrity as well as treatment outcome.

France and Hudson (1990) found that ignoring worked with the 7 children (ages 8–20 months) in their study. The components of their treatment program included telling parents to follow their usual bedtime routine, and, after they said "good night," parents were not to return to the room. The results of this study indicated that the frequency of night awakenings decreased from a mean of 3.31 to near zero for each child and maintained at 3-month and 24-month posttreatment checks. These data would be more convincing if reliable measurements had been used to verify the parents' reports.

Given the knowledge that ignoring usually results in at least a temporary increase in children's fussing at bedtime, France, Blampied, and Wilkinson (1991) examined the use of sedative medication (trimeprazine tartrate) combined with ignoring, to determine whether the medication might blunt the initial increase in fussing at bedtime usually associated with ignoring. The medication was phased out during a 10-day period. In this study, 35 children, ranging in age from 7 to 27 months, were assigned to one of three groups (ignoring alone, ignoring plus medication, or ignoring plus placebo). Although night awakenings were reduced in all three groups, sleep problems in the ignoring plus medication group were reduced more quickly than in the other groups. France et al. (1991) reported several of the parents' negative comments about the medication, such as their children seemed "doped-up" (p. 313) during the day. In addition, when the medication was stopped, there was a temporary increase in nighttime awakenings. Thus, the medication did not eliminate the child's fussing at bedtime; it more accurately postponed it until the medication was stopped.

Graduated extinction. Rolider and Van Houten (1984) investigated a variation of ignoring procedures by teaching parents to ignore bedtime crying for as long as they felt comfortable, in a procedure called *graduated extinction*. Over several nights, the time of ignoring was increased before checking on the child. During treatment, the parents were instructed to put their child to bed and leave the room. Parents were instructed not to go to the child immediately; instead, they were to wait a specified period of time (e.g., 5 minutes) before going to their child. Every 2 days, the length of the ignoring period was increased by 5 minutes. Results indicated that over a period from 4 to 9 nights, crying was reduced to near zero for each child. Follow-up data indicated the bedtime crying did not return.

Although the data are persuasive, intuitively it seems this approach could teach a child to cry for longer periods of time to bring back the parent. The parents were instructed to make minimal contact when checking on their children, however. Thus, it appears that the minimal contact was not what the children wanted, therefore, crying did not produce a reward for them. These procedures are very similar to those Ferber (1985) recommended in his popular book, *Solve Your Child's Sleep Problems*.

Recently, Reid, Walter, and O'Leary (1999) compared graduated ignoring with standard ignoring in 49 young children with bedtime refusal and nighttime awakenings. They reported that both treatments were superior to a wait-list control group. There was actually no difference between the two treatments in the resolution of children's bedtime refusal, but the mothers in the standard ignoring group reported less stress in parenting.

Scheduled awakenings. Rickert and Johnson (1988) compared scheduled awakenings and ignoring for reducing the occurrence of night awakenings and crying episodes in 33 young children (ages 6–54 months) whose parents were recruited by newspaper advertisements. These children were randomly assigned to one of three groups: scheduled awakenings, ignoring, or control. The control group was told to handle the problem in their usual way and that a treatment would be provided later. Parents in the scheduled awakening group were instructed to awaken their child at scheduled times during the evening and to do things like soothe the child or change a diaper. Parents in the systematic ignoring group were instructed to check on their child after a night awakening; ensure that there were no physical reasons for the child's crying; and respond to the crying in a stereotypic, mechanical fashion and to not provide any soothing while the child was crying. Then they were to leave the child. Statistically and clinically, children in the scheduled awakenings group and the systematic ignoring group awoke and cried less frequently than children in the control group during the 8 weeks of treatment and at 3- and 6-week follow-up checks after treatment.

Ignoring reduced the problem more rapidly, taking approximately 3 weeks. Rickert and Johnson (1988) suggested that although scheduled awakenings may not be as rapid as ignoring, it is a viable alternative. They made a clear point, however, that many parents do not find ignoring an acceptable procedure: Five parents refused to implement the ignoring, and many others declined to participate in the study because they might have been assigned to this condition.

Bedtime routines. Other interventions have emphasized the actual bedtime routines and schedules followed by parents. For example, Adams and Rickert (1989) compared routines and graduated extinction for reducing bedtime tantrums in 36 children ranging in age from 18 to 48 months. They were randomly assigned to one of three groups: positive routines (consisting of four to seven quiet activities lasting no longer than a total of 20 minutes), graduated extinction, or control. The control group was told that treatment would be provided if there was no improvement. Graduated extinction involved the parent putting the child to bed and ignoring tantrums for increasingly longer spans of time throughout the treatment. From parental reports, children in both treatment groups had tantrums less often and for shorter periods of time than the control children, but routines produced the fastest improvements, taking 4 weeks. The accuracy of data was verified by comparing mothers' report with fathers' report once for each condition. In a comparison of schedule awakenings and systematic ignoring, Rickert and Johnson (1988) found essentially similar outcomes. The parents who participated in the study, however, reportedly did not want to "ignore" their child's crying, usually because they had tried it before and found ignoring unpleasant.

Treatment of sleep problems and daytime behavior. Minde et al. (1994) investigated the effects of a treatment program for severely sleep-disturbed children on their daytime interaction with their mothers. They concluded that helping families to manage children with sleep disturbances can generalize to daytime mother–infant interactions. Their results, based on interventions with 28 children with serious sleep problems and 30 matched control children ages 12–36 months, showed improvements in their general behavior, in their sleep patterns, and during feeding interactions with their mothers.

Edwards and Christophersen (1994) described preliminary data, using time-lapse videotape recordings, to suggest that parents can be instructed to encourage the development of sleep-onset skills by setting occasions for their child to learn "self-quieting skills" during the day; they refer to this procedure as "Day Correction of Bedtime Problems" (see Exhibit 4.6). They reported that the majority of the toddlers, after the day component was completed, would settle themselves, at bedtime or upon night awakening, within 3 nights. Although intriguing, these results need to be replicated.

Relaxation. One alternative to ignoring a child's crying is the use of relaxation techniques. The rationale cited in the relaxation studies was that children were learning strategies they could use to reduce "fears" that were presumably interfering with their sleep. Giebehain and O'Dell (1984) evaluated the effectiveness of a treatment package that included teaching 6 children how to relax and say such positive statements as, "I am brave and I can take care of myself when I'm alone or when I'm in the dark." The researchers also had the children practice setting the light level lower with a rheostat control in their own bedroom; the goal was to set the light level lower each night and have the child remain in the room for 5 minutes. Additionally, the children were rewarded each morning for staying the whole night in a room darker than the night before. Reinforcement was phased out over time. The main measure in this multiple-baseline design was the setting of the light control. Results showed that all of the children were sleeping at a low light level after 2 weeks. This improvement was maintained at 3-, 6-, and 12-month follow-up checks.

McMenamy and Katz (1989) taught 5 young children relaxation skills that involved taking deep breaths while in a comfortable position, imagining a pleasant image, and saying such brave statements as, "I can take care of myself in bed at night." Additionally, parents read a story to their child about two children overcoming their fear of the dark. At home, the children

EXHIBIT 4.6
Day Correction of Bedtime Problems

There are three important components to getting a child to go to sleep at night. The child must be 1. tired 2. quiet 3. relaxed.

When these three components are in place, children who have adequate "self-quieting skills" will be able to go to sleep rather easily.

1. **Tired.** The easiest way to make sure that your child will be tired when he or she goes to bed is by getting him or her up at the same time every day and by getting him or her an adequate amount of exercise during the day—vigorous exercise that requires a good deal of energy. For an infant, this might include several long periods of time when he or she is on the floor and can see what you are doing, but the infant must hold his or her head up in order to really see much. For almost any child, 20 minutes of good exercise each day, after a nap, is usually adequate.

2. **Quiet.** You can elect to either quiet down the entire house or quiet down your child's room. Quieting down your child's room by closing the door and keeping it closed is probably the easiest (and the one that is recommended by the vast majority of professional firefighters). You might need to turn on the furnace or air conditioning fan as a masking noise for the first few nights.

3. **Relaxed.** Children can relax only if they have learned self-quieting skills. Self-quieting skills refer to a child's ability to calm himself or herself, with no help from an adult, when the child is unhappy, angry or frustrated. Whereas older children (at least age 6 years) can be taught relaxation procedures, infants and toddlers need to practice self-quieting skills in order to know what works for them. Perhaps the easiest way to teach self-quieting, during the day, is by allowing your child to self-quiet during naturally occurring times of frustration.

Self-quieting behaviors. The baby who goes to sleep with help from one of his or her parents by nursing, rocking, or holding learns only adult transition skills and needs an adult present in order to fall asleep. The baby or toddler who goes to sleep alone cuddling a stuffed animal, holding his or her favorite blanket, or sucking his or her thumb learns valuable self-quieting skills that can be used for many years to come.

How they feel. Children who go to bed easily and sleep through the night uninterrupted get a good night's sleep. They will feel better during the day, just as the adults in their household will feel better during the day. It may take from several nights to 1 week to teach a child the skills he or she needs for going to sleep alone, but this is one behavior that the child will be able to use for the rest of his or her life.

These three components described here have the added advantage that they can be taught during the day, which removes many of the fears parents have about handling behavior problems at bedtime. Even parents who choose co-sleeping can allow their infant or toddler the opportunity to fall asleep on their own, with the parent joining the child at the parents' regular time for retiring. In this way, the infant or toddler gets the perceived advantages of co-sleeping and the known advantages of learning self-quieting skills.

Note. From *Beyond Discipline: Parenting That Lasts a Lifetime* (2nd ed., pp. 127–128), by E. R. Christophersen, 1998, Shawnee Mission, KS: Overland Press. Copyright 1998 by Edward R. Christophersen. Reprinted with permission.

earned stickers for practicing their relaxation skills; the stickers were exchanged weekly for such items as toys or ice cream. At the end of the study, all of the children were given a special T-shirt as a reward. McMenamy and Katz reported an overall reduction of 40% in fearful behaviors for all the children but noted that children throughout the study had "'good' nights and 'bad' nights" (p. 147). There were no reported steps taken to determine if the parents were accurately recording, nor were any measures reported to determine whether the child followed the procedures as described.

Friedman and Ollendick (1989) examined a relaxation treatment package to reduce severe nighttime fears in 6 children ranging in age from 7 to 10 years. The package included the following instructions to practice relaxing muscles:

1. Have the child imagine pleasant scenes while relaxing.
2. Have the child use "brave words."
3. Give the child up to four tokens each night for appropriate bedtime behaviors.

Tokens were earned when the children went to bed without complaining, slept in their own room, went to bed within 15 minutes of being told to go to bed, and did not call out to their parents once during the entire night. In general, the results indicated that for 5 of the 6 children, the problem behaviors were reduced, although 1 child continued to be fearful. Additionally, on some of the measures, several of the children improved during the extended baseline before the treatment began. Improvements before treatment, however, cast doubts on whether the study procedures were solely responsible for the changes reported.

The effectiveness of relaxation therapy leaves unanswered questions because the studies did not include objective measures of the child's behavior before or after treatment. In the absence of such data, it is difficult to truly evaluate the efficacy of relaxation procedures in the treatment of children's fears associated either with sleep onset or night awakenings. It is clear, however, that relaxation procedures have been demonstrably effective with many other types of childhood fears.

White noise as a treatment. Several researchers have investigated electronic equipment as a means of helping infants sleep. Spencer, Moran, Lee, and Talbert (1990) used a commercially available white-noise generator to produce sound intensities from 67 to 72.5 decibels with 2- to 7-day-old infants. The noise level corresponded to a vacuum cleaner or a small car traveling at 50 kilometers per hour. One group of 20 neonates received the noise, whereas 20 other infants served as a control group. Data were collected by an observer who watched the babies for 5 minutes and judged whether or not they were asleep. The researchers found that 80% of the infants fell asleep within 5 minutes with the noise, whereas only 25% of the infants in the control group fell asleep in that amount of time. They also found that heart rates decreased from a range of 120–180 beats per minute before the noise to 100–110 beats after the noise. Furthermore, when the white noise was turned on for the babies still awake in the control group, 73% consequently fell asleep.

Finally, Mailman-Sosland and Christophersen (1991) evaluated the efficacy of a commercially available device ("SleepTight") that gently vibrated an infant's crib and produced white noise. The use of SleepTight was associated with a decrease in crying in 4 of 6 infants with colic. The outcome data notwithstanding, the combination of parents not recording severe crying episodes and mixed reports from parents about their satisfaction with SleepTight suggested that SleepTight may not be a viable means of managing infant crying. It is clear that more studies are needed to evaluate the effectiveness of white noise in the treatment of children's sleep problems.

Nightmare Disorder

Treatment strategies for nightmares have focused on anxiety reduction, often combined with other behavioral strategies, such as systematic desensitization (Cavior & Deutsch, 1975) or response prevention (Roberts & Gordon, 1979). Krakow et al. (1993) reported significantly fewer nightmares in a group of children who were trained to use imagery rehearsal, compared with the control group who were instructed to record nightmares only. At a 3-month and 30-month follow-up, both groups had significantly fewer nightmares, but only the rehearsal group had less total distress. One 13-year-old girl was successfully treated for nightmares with reinforcement and anxiety management techniques (Kellerman, 1980). For most families, reassurance that nightmares are part of normal child development is beneficial and all that is necessary, especially to decrease the likelihood that the child may be considered psychologically disturbed.

Sleep Terror Disorder

Unfortunately, little controlled outcome research has been published on sleep terrors. Scheduled awakenings and a combination of reinforcement, desensitization, and reduction of attention are the only effective procedures that have been reported in the literature.

Scheduled awakenings. C. M. Johnson, Bradley-Johnson, and Stack (1981) reported that two out of three families that used scheduled awakenings with the children (the third family chose to withdraw from the study rather than use the treatment procedures) gradually reduced and eventually eliminated their child's nighttime crying episodes.

Reinforcement, desensitization, and reduction of attention. Kellerman (1979) demonstrated a significant reduction in the night terrors of a 3-year-old girl with acute lymphocytic leukemia, using a combination of positive reinforcement, systematic desensitization, and reduction of parental attention. Using similar techniques, Kellerman (1980) also successfully treated a 5-year-old boy with a 7-month history of sleep terrors.

Sleepwalking Disorder

Typically, parents can also be reassured that sleepwalking is usually a benign, self-limited occurrence that most children outgrow (Mindell, 1993). For more reassurance, parents are told to safety proof the house by making sure all doors leading to the outside of the house are locked. The only outcome study that we were able to locate that shows promise for sleepwalking is that of scheduled awakenings.

Frank, Spirito, Stark, and Owens-Stively (1997) evaluated the use of scheduled awakenings in 3 children (ages 6, 7, and 12 years) with persistent sleepwalking. The treatment procedure involved instructing the parents to awaken the child several hours after the child went to sleep and just before the time a sleepwalking episode typically occurs. The treatment was immediately successful in eliminating sleepwalking in all 3 children. Treatment effects were maintained at a 3- and 6-month follow-up.

CONCLUSION

With between 20% and 25% of children between ages 1 and 5 years experiencing sleep problems, they are one of the most common complaints that parents have about their children. Sleep problems, with the possible exception of sleepwalking, also tend to persist from infancy to adolescence and adulthood.

Although medication has been shown to help adults fall sleep quickly, there are few empirical studies demonstrating its effectiveness with children. In most cases, the possible side effects of medications that help children fall asleep outweigh the usefulness of the drugs. Additionally, the early years probably lay the foundation for a person learning how to fall sleep; dependency on medications to sleep could result in delays in learning this important skill, or conceivably in a dependency on drugs for sleep onset.

There are many strategies available to assist parents with the common problem of sleep disturbances in their children. Behavioral procedures, relaxation procedures, changes in routines, medication, changes in diet, and the use of electronic equipment are all possible choices in treating children's sleep problems. On the basis of the many successful reports with reliable measures, behavioral procedures have shown that children's sleep difficulties are often related to how their parents interact with them at bedtime.

Ignoring children after they are put to bed usually works relatively quickly but can be distressing to the parents. Other behavioral treatments that emphasize positive routines and schedules have been effective but do not show improvements as quickly as does ignoring.

So, what can be done to help most infants and children learn to fall asleep? The most practical recommendation is for parents to follow a bedtime routine. Before or while the bedtime routine is being established, the parents can work on opportunities during the day to encourage the child to develop self-quieting skills (Christophersen, 1998a). Although many parents find it difficult to ignore their child who is fussing at bedtime, it may be much more realistic to instruct parents to refrain from trying to ignore their child at bedtime until after the child has consistently exhibited good self-quieting skills during the day. The difference between parents who have successfully allowed their children to "cry themselves to sleep" and those parents who have been unsuccessful may be the presence or absence of self-quieting skills. That is, children who lacked self-quieting skills fuss so much that their parents are unable to cope. Thus, the strategy of teaching self-quieting skills during the day may offer promise for parents of children who lack sleep onset skills. White-noise generators may be of use to parents in helping their children establish good sleeping habits, particularly in those cases in which the child has a difficult time with sleep onset.

Getting children to bed and asleep remains a widespread problem for parents and an important area for researchers. There are numerous studies supporting the idea that parents can actually prevent sleep problems by refraining from practices that result in poor sleep habits. The absence of evidence to support the use of medication as a viable alternative should lead future researchers and clinicians to further explore parenting strategies that facilitate the development of better sleep habits.

5

DIAGNOSIS AND MANAGEMENT OF ENCOPRESIS

Encopresis is the involuntary loss of formed, semiformed, or liquid stool in inappropriate places, such as underwear, in children older than age 4 (Loening-Baucke, 1996). Primary or continuous encopresis applies to children who have been incontinent their entire lives. Secondary or discontinuous encopresis applies to children who, at some point, were fully bowel trained (Levine, 1975). The diagnostic criteria for encopresis as indicated in the *Diagnostic and Statistical Manual of Mental Disorders* (4th ed., DSM–IV; American Psychiatric Association, 1994) are found in Exhibit 5.1.

Other definitions that are important to the understanding of encopresis are Hirschsprung disease, constipation, and toileting refusal. *Hirschsprung disease* (congenital megacolon) is a congenital anomaly wherein the furthest part of the child's large intestine lacks appropriate innervation. Forty percent of children with Hirschsprung disease are diagnosed in the first 3 months, 61% by 12 months, and 82% by age 4 years (Loening-Baucke, 1994). Hirschsprung disease in older children causes chronic constipation and abdominal distention. The stools, when passed, may consist of small pellets, be ribbonlike, or have a fluid consistency; the large stools and fecal soiling of patients with functional constipation are absent. In the vast majority of cases, the primary care physician has already ruled out Hirshsprung disease prior to a child being seen by a mental health professional. Nevertheless,

EXHIBIT 5.1
DSM–IV Criteria for Encopresis

Encopresis

A. Repeated passage of feces into inappropriate places (e.g., clothing or floor) whether involuntary or intentional.

B. At least one such event a month for at least 3 months.

C. Chronological age is at least 4 years (or equivalent developmental level).

D. The behavior is not due exclusively to the direct physiological effects of a substance (e.g., laxatives) or a general medical condition except through a mechanism involving constipation.

Code as follows:

797.6 With Constipation and Overflow Incontinence: there is evidence of constipation on physical exam or by history

307.7 Without Constipation and Overflow Incontinence: there is no evidence of constipation on physical exam or by history

Note. Information from *Diagnostic and Statistical Manual of Mental Disorders* (4th ed.), by the American Psychiatric Association, 1994, Washington, DC: Author. Copyright 1994 by the American Psychiatric Association. Reprinted with permission.

further information about how to distinguish Hirschsprung disease from encopresis is found in the "Assessment" section of this chapter.

Constipation has been defined as the passage of large or hard stools at a frequency of less than three times per week (Sutphen, Borowitz, Hutchison, & Cox, 1995). Luxem and Christophersen (1999, p. 199) defined constipation as "hard stools that are difficult to pass" rather than referring to the frequency of stooling. They also reported that constipation in children may be accompanied by complaints of abdominal discomfort; infrequent bowel movements (e.g., fewer than three bowel movements a week); a palpable abdominal mass; emotional upset, including crying and screaming before, during, and after defecation; vigorous attempts at bowel movement withholding; nausea and vomiting; poor appetite; weight loss; sadness; and irritability. Occasionally, children with encopresis (secondary to constipation) pass amounts of feces so large that they can plug up toilets. A history of constipation in one or both parents may also predispose the child to constipation by means of an abnormally long colonic transit time, overly efficient intestinal absorption of water, or both.

The term *toileting refusal* is used to refer to children who refuse to have a bowel movement in the toilet but who will willingly have a bowel movement in a diaper or a pull-up (Luxem, Christophersen, Purvis, & Baer, 1997). Children with encopresis may come to the attention of the clinician through a referral from the child's pediatrician or physician for assistance with bowel retraining or during the history obtained from a diagnostic interview for a different referring problem. The differential diagnosis of these toileting disorders is discussed in the "Assessment" section of this chapter.

PREVALENCE

The prevalence of encopresis in the child population has been estimated to range from 1% to 2%, affecting boys three to six times more often than girls (Bellman, 1966). Levine (1975) reported a slightly higher prevalence rate of clinic-referred cases at 3%. Levine also reported that the mean age of onset for secondary encopresis is 7 years 4 months. Despite the prevalence of encopresis, it has been called the "hidden disease" in at least one published report (Brody, 1992). Parents of children with encopresis often think that they are the only family that has a child with encopresis. In addition, the fact that encopresis is rarely mentioned in the popular press may contribute to this misconception.

It is important to report the prevalence of constipation, given its direct relationship to encopresis. In fact, as many as 95% of children referred for the treatment of encopresis present with functional constipation (Loening-Baucke, 1996). Sonnenberg and Koch (1989) reported that between 1958 and 1986 there was a twofold increase in physician visits for constipation in children ranging in age from birth to 9 years. The prevalence of constipation, and thus possibly encopresis, appears to be increasing, although no apparent explanation has been reported in the literature for this increase.

CAUSES AND CORRELATIONS

Over the years, both biological and psychiatric factors have been explored as causes of encopresis in children. Historically, encopresis was deemed a psychiatric disorder (Richmond, Eddy, & Garrard, 1954). Davidson (1958) was one of the first authors to challenge the long-standing notion that the cause was psychogenic. Davidson's work was also instrumental in recognizing the important role that constipation plays in the etiology of encopresis. Essentially, the focus of the treatment program was on managing the child's constipation first and toilet training second. His program has been labeled the *pediatric approach* and is described further in the "Intervention" section of this chapter.

Since Davidson's (1958) seminal work, others have also found that constipation plays a major role in encopresis as well as in other toileting problems, such as withholding, that can create and exacerbate stooling difficulties. For example, one study of over 200 children who presented at a gastroenterology clinic found that 85% of children over 3 years old had encopresis, the majority of which also suffered from stool withholding, fecal impaction, and pain on defecation (Partin, Hamill, Fischel, & Partin, 1992). They reported that over 70% of the children younger than age 3 also withheld stools and had fecal impaction and painful defecation, all suggestive of constipation. The majority of these children (71%) also suffered from fecal impaction, a condition in which the colon is so full of stool that peristalsis is inhibited. Of the children older than age 3, 96% exhibited stool withholding, 57% with pain on defecation, 73% with fecal impaction, and 85% presented with encopresis. Constipation plays a major role in encopresis and in other toileting problems, such as withholding, that can create and exacerbate stooling difficulties.

Constipation-related stooling abnormalities, such as frequent small or pebbly stools, infrequent large stools, or both, are not always distressing to the child. Therefore, the significance of such episodes may be overlooked or underestimated by parents. Constipation may also be misinterpreted by parents and consequently treated improperly. For example, Christophersen (1991) wrote that a constipation cycle may be confusing for parents because of the child's "paradoxical diarrhea," which refers to the seepage of feces around hard stool in the colon rectum that the child has been unable to pass. Although the child is actually constipated or impacted, symptomatically, it appears to the parents as though the child has diarrhea, producing numerous watery, foul-smelling stools. Some parents attempt to treat this type of diarrhea with over-the-counter antidiarrheal agents, an approach that potentially exacerbates the condition.

In addition to suffering from constipation, children with encopresis may also have a rectum that is less sensitive to the "call to stool" than is needed for appropriate elimination. For example, anal manometry·has been used to determine the rectum sensitivity of children with and without normal bowel histories (Meunier, Mollard, & Marechal, 1976). Anal manometry is a laboratory procedure in which a small tube is inserted into the patient's rectum. One or more portions of the tube can be inflated until the patient subjectively reports that he or she feels as though he or she is about to have a bowel movement. The amount of pressure necessary to create that feeling is noted. This procedure allows the researcher to simulate the increased pressure in the rectum that normally signals an individual of the need to have a bowel movement. In Meunier et al.'s study, most of the children with normal bowel histories required a small amount of pressure in the rectum. In contrast, most of the children with encopresis required two to four times as much pressure before they felt the call to stool. The data presented here support the comment often heard from children with encopresis that they "couldn't feel the bowel movement coming."

Further support for the role of biological factors in encopresis is provided by Ingebo and Heyman (1988), who conducted a study to determine if children with encopresis retained more stool in their rectum than children without encopresis. They conducted a clinical trial using an oral solution, GoLytely (polyethylene-glycol-electrolyte), with 24 children ages 9 months to 17 years with severe constipation. Approximately 50% of the children were being treated for encopresis, whereas the other half were being prepared for colonoscopy. The children with encopresis required almost three times as much medication, administered over three times as long a period of time, to clean out the colon. These results lend support to the notion that children with encopresis are retaining more stool, as they required more medication over a longer period of time than children who did not present with encopresis. Ingebo and Heyman reported no clinically important changes in the laboratory values measured before and after the intestinal clean out in either group of children, suggesting that the use of enemas to "clean out" the colon is not detrimental to children.

As mentioned previously, encopresis has been viewed as a psychiatric disorder or a symptom of emotional disturbance. Consequently, a number of studies have specifically examined the notion that children with encopresis have emotional or behavioral problems. The use of child-behavior rating scales, such as the Achenbach (1991) Child Behavior Checklist (CBCL), has revealed no systematic differences between children with encopresis and normal children of the same age and gender. Rating scales also show that children with encopresis tend to be better adjusted than same-age, same-sex samples of "behavior problem" children (Gabel, Hegedus, Wald, Chandra, & Chiponis, 1986; Loening-Baucke, Cruikshank, & Savage, 1987).

For example, Friman, Mathews, Finney, Christophersen, and Leibowitz (1988) demonstrated that children referred for management of encopresis did not differ significantly from the standardization sample for the Eyberg Child Behavior Inventory (E. A. Robinson, Eyberg, & Ross, 1980). Furthermore, both the children with encopresis and the standardization sample differed significantly from children who were referred for diagnosis and management of behavior problems. Similarly, Ling, Cox, Sutphen, and Borowitz (1996), in comparing children with encopresis with their nonsymptomatic siblings, found the two groups were essentially identical in terms of their self-perceived psychological functioning, behavioral problems, and parent–child relations.

Loening-Baucke et al. (1987) examined the social competence and behavioral profiles of 38 children with encopresis, with specific interest in children who were resistant to treatment. They concluded that the persistence of encopresis at 6-month and 12-month follow-ups after the initiation of treatment was not related to social competence or behavior scores. Given the research that clearly demonstrates the presence of significant physical findings and the absence of research demonstrating consistent behavior problems in the vast majority of children diagnosed and treated for encopresis, the conclusion seems warranted that encopresis can and should be treated primarily as a dysfunction of the bowel.

ASSESSMENT

Medical Assessment

To effectively treat encopresis, one should obtain a thorough history of the child's stooling habits since infancy, with special attention paid to any evidence of prior or current constipation. Such history information should include stooling frequency, stool size, stool consistency, any prior problems such as bleeding, and any prior interventions attempted by professionals or by parents using home remedies. Many parents fail to recognize constipation in their child, apparently assuming that as long as a child has a bowel movement on most days, he or she "couldn't have constipation." In actuality, children can have daily bowel movements and still be constipated. The child who is having daily bowel movements but is not actually expelling all of the waste matter from the rectum can gradually accumulate larger and larger amounts of fecal matter (Christophersen, 1994). Also, although some children only defecate every 3 to 5 days, their parents might assume that the child is not constipated because they are having bowel accidents, probably assuming that on the days without any bowel accidents their child used the toilet appropriately. Soiling accidents tend to occur at home, typically after school, between 3:00 p.m. and 7:00 p.m. (Levine, 1976), although children with histories of chronic and frequent soiling may have accidents outside the home and at various times throughout the day. Only rarely do children soil during their sleep. Parents report that the child is often observed to be standing upright, walking, or engaged in vigorous play when soiling occurs (Luxem & Christophersen, 1999).

A number of medications, such as pain medications and some anticonvulsants, relax the intestine and may produce or aggravate constipation as a side effect. For this reason, asking parents to complete and bring a detailed history form with them to the first office visit helps identify any medication-related constipation problems. The history form can include questions about the family medical history, the child's stooling habits, the child's diet history, and information about any previous attempts to deal with the encopresis, including rewards or punishment (Christophersen, 1994). Health care providers may find that mailing out a detailed history form before the child's first appointment will increase the efficiency of the initial intake interview. Exhibit 5.2 contains a bowel problem intake form that can be used to facilitate the parent interview regarding encopresis (Christophersen, 1994).

Although many pediatric textbooks recommend a digital rectal examination by a physician to assess for constipation and impaction (see Davidson, Kugler, & Bauer, 1963; Levine, 1982), the procedure is not performed in the majority of children evaluated for chronic constipation. For example, in a study of 128 children with chronic constipation, Gold, Levine, Weinstein, Kessler, and Pettei (1999) reported that only about 23% of the children were given a rectal examination. Negative findings of constipation at the time of physical examination do not, however, necessarily rule out constipation because evidence of constipation may be intermittent. In cases in which the history is consistent with constipation, but constipation cannot be confirmed by the physical examination, a plain X-ray of the abdomen

EXHIBIT 5.2
Bowel Problem Intake Form

What word does your child use for a bowel movement? _____

Has your child ever been "potty trained"?   Yes _____   No _____

If yes, bladder trained: Age started _____   Age accomplished _____

If yes, bowel trained: Age started _____   Age accomplished _____

Does your child wet the bed at night?   Yes _____   No _____   If yes, how long has bedwetting occurred? _____   Has he ever been dry for 3 months? _____

If your child was potty trained, what methods were employed to train the child? ___

_____

If your child was potty trained, when did soiling first occur after training? Age _____

Number of daily soilings _____   Does this occur at the same time each day? _____
　　If yes, note the time(s) _____

Note the amount (circle 1):   Very small   Small   Moderate   Large   Very Large

Note the consistency (circle 1):   Hard/Pebbles   Soft   Runny

Does your child have a history of constipation?   Yes _____   No _____
　　If yes, for how long? _____ Previous treatment for constipation? _____
　　What treatments for constipation? _____

Does your child wipe clean after a bowel movement? Yes _____   No _____.

How is the soiling discovered? Describe: _____

_____

What action is taken with your child after soiling has been discovered? _____

_____

What is verbally said to the child? Supply the quotes used.

Father _____

Mother _____

Have you been able to correlate any traumatic experience happening in your child's life with the onset of soiling?   Yes _____   No _____

If yes, please describe _____

Food List: Does your child like and eat the following foods? (Circle all foods eaten regularly)

Lettuce	Broccoli	Oranges	Pop Tarts®
Spinach	Cauliflower	Grapes	Candy
Cabbage	Green Beans	Raisins	Ice Cream
Peas	Green Peppers	Dried Figs	Cheese
Asparagus	Fresh Plums	Prunes	Milk
Tomatoes	Fresh Peaches	Honey	Cottage Cheese
Onions	Fresh Apples	Bran	Yogurt
Celery	Pears	Bran Products	Custard
Carrots	Grapefruit	Whole Wheat Bread	
Corn	Pineapple	White Bread	

(continued)

EXHIBIT 5.2 *(continued)*

Questions asked of the child during the clinic visit:

Can you always feel it when you are about to have a bowel movement? _____

How do you feel when you soil your pants? _____

Why? Describe in the child's words _____

What do you do when you soil your pants? Describe in the child's words _____

_____

What do your mom and dad do when they find out you've soiled your pants? _____

_____

Do you want to stop soiling your pants?   Yes _____   No _____

What have you tried to help you to stop soiling your pants? _____

Note. From *Pediatric Compliance: A Guide for the Primary Care Physician* (pp. 223–224), by E. R. Christophersen, 1994, New York: Plenum. Copyright 1994 by Plenum. Reprinted with permission.

may be necessary (Levine, 1982). Barr, Levine, Wilkinson, and Mulvihill (1979) reported on the use of X-rays to assess the degree of retention. They reported significant differences between pre- and posttherapy X-rays of treatment successes and no differences between pre- and posttherapy X-rays of treatment failures. These findings lend further support to the fact that the vast majority of children with encopresis have physical findings related to their colon that should be reviewed by the child's physician.

Another purpose of obtaining a thorough history is to rule out the possibility of Hirschsprung disease (Levine, 1982). Children with encopresis usually appear well-nourished and healthy during the school years. In contrast, a child with Hirschsprung disease is likely to look wasted and chronically ill and to have had intermittent obstructive symptoms. Although children with encopresis often have a history of passing very large stools (sometimes large enough to plug up the plumbing), children with Hirshsprung disease are more apt to have thin, ribbonlike stools. Furthermore, incontinence is the most prominent symptom of encopresis, whereas heavy soiling is uncommon in Hirschsprung disease. Table 5.1 lists the symptoms of encopresis and Hirschsprung disease, two conditions that produce very different, almost mutually exclusive symptoms, in a format that is readily incorporated into the clinical interview for a child who presents with encopresis.

In the vast majority of cases, the primary-care physician has already ruled out Hirshsprung disease prior to a child being seen by a mental health practitioner. If a child has not been seen by a primary care physician, such a referral is probably indicated.

To facilitate a differential diagnosis of encopresis, Table 5.2 provides a list of the symptoms of toileting refusal, encopresis, and Hirshsprung's dis-

TABLE 5.1
Symptoms of Encopresis and Hirschsprung Disease

Characteristic	Encopresis	Hirschsprung Disease
Stool incontinence	Always	Rare
Constipation	Common, may be intermittent	Always present
Symptoms as newborn	Rare	Almost always
Infant constipation	Sometimes	Common
Late onset (after age 3)	Common	Rare
Problem toilet training	Common	Rare
Avoidance of toilet	Common	Rare
Failure to thrive	Rare	Common
Anemia	None	Common
Obstructive symptoms	Rare	Common
Stool in ampulla	Common	Rare
Loose or tight sphincter tone	Rare	Common
Large-caliber stools	Common	Never
Preponderance of males	86%	90%
Incidence	1.5% at age 7	1:25,000 births
Anal manometry	Sometimes abnormal	Always abnormal

Note. From "Encopresis," by M. D. Levine. In M. D. Levine, W. B. Carey, & A. C. Crocker (Eds.), *Developmental–Behavioral Pediatrics* (2nd ed., p. 393), 1983, Philadelphia: Saunders. Copyright 1983 by Saunders. Reprinted with permission.

ease. Although toileting refusal and Hirshsprung disease are not included in *DSM–IV*, these conditions must be ruled out as part of the diagnosis of encopresis. The symptoms listed for Hirschsprung's disease are rarely, if ever, seen in children with either encopresis or toileting refusal.

Behavioral Assessment

Assessment of the child's toilet-training history should include a review of the onset and duration of the child's bowel and bladder training; methods used; and the behavioral responses of the child, the parents, and others involved in the training process (Luxem & Christophersen, 1999). Evaluation of previous treatments for the child's constipation and soiling, including behavioral and psychological interventions, can reveal telling evidence of the parents' and child's ability and willingness to adhere to treatment recommendations. For example, it is common for parents to report their child "hides soiled underwear," which is suggestive of a prior history of punishment for soiling. When there is such a history, it is imperative that

TABLE 5.2
DSM–IV Diagnostic Criteria for Toileting Problems in Children

Toileting Refusal	Encopresis 307.7	Classic Symptoms
		R/O behavior problems
❏ Regular stools	❏ Repeated soilings	Large-caliber stools
❏ Never in toilet	❏ At least one per month	Paradoxical diarrhea
❏ In diaper or pull-ups	❏ Not physiological	Hide soiled clothing
❏ Age 3 or over	❏ Age 4 or over	Foul-smelling stools
❏ Hx of constipation	❏ Hx of constipation	Days without stools
_____ of 5 (4+ = Dx)	_____ of 5 (4+ = Dx)	
		Hirschprung's
		Anemia as an infant
		Easy to toilet train
		Failure to thrive
		Family history of colon Dx

Note. Information from *Diagnostic and Statistical Manual of Mental Disorders* (4th ed.), by the American Psychiatric Association, 1994, Washington, DC: Author. Copyright 1994 by the American Psychiatric Association. Reprinted with permission. R/O = rule out; Dx = diagnosis; Hx = history.

the parents be thoroughly educated about the most common causes of encopresis, so they understand the child is not soiling intentionally and that punishment for soiling is rarely effective.

Although studies have documented the absence of significant behavior problems in children with encopresis, it is prudent to have both parents and teachers complete a standardized rating scale, such as the CBCL (Achenbach, 1991) or the Behavior Assessment System for Children (Reynolds & Kamphaus, 1998), to document that the child does not present with significant behavior problems. If the history and the rating scales are significant for behavior problems, the treatment of the encopresis may be more complicated. The clinician must then decide whether to first treat the encopresis or the problems with behavior management. Christophersen (1994) suggested that this determination can be made on the basis of whether the history and rating scales document significant problems with behaviors such as defiance and difficulty following instructions. Such behavior problems may interfere with the parent or the child's ability to adhere to the treatment recommendations. If adherence has been or is expected to be a problem, Christophersen usually recommends introducing small changes, such as slight modification of the diet (described later in this chapter), then concentrates on dealing with the adherence issues using the procedures discussed in chapter 1 on disruptive behaviors.

INTERVENTION

The pediatric and child psychology literature reveal two main approaches to the treatment of encopresis: medical management and medical–behavioral (Luxem & Christophersen, 1999).

Medical Treatment

The pediatric approach to the treatment of encopresis, originally described by Davidson (1958) and Davidson et al. (1963), includes a three-phase treatment protocol. The first phase involves cleaning out the child's colon with enemas and giving the child large doses of mineral oil to help the child continue passing stools. The second phase involves decreasing the child's dietary intake of milk and dairy products to the equivalent of 1 pint of whole milk daily. (Davidson made the observation that milk, because of its low residue and high calcium content, may cause or aggravate constipation.) The objective of this phase is to eliminate enemas and encourage regular bowel habits. The third phase involves continuation of the stool habit while gradually fading out the use of mineral oil. In 12 weeks of clinical trials with 119 severely constipated children, Davidson et al. (1963) found that parents reported a 90% success rate when using this regimen.

Similar procedures have been used in a number of other studies in the pediatric literature. Levine (1976) presented outcome data on 127 children with primary encopresis, with an average age of 8 years 2 months. The children, mainly boys, were treated with a program that included counseling and education; initial bowel catharsis; and a supportive maintenance program to potentiate optimum evacuation, retraining, and careful monitoring and follow-up. Of those children for whom 1-year outcome data were available, 51% were in remission, 27% showed marked improvement, 14% showed some improvement, and 8% were unchanged. Levine reported that 11 difficult cases were referred for psychiatric help at the end of the treatment year. After 1 year of psychotherapy, 10 of these patients remained in treatment. Levine's experience as well as ours indicates that although psychotherapy may be effective for psychological problems other than the encopresis, no controlled studies have documented the effectiveness of psychotherapy as the primary intervention for encopresis.

Rockney, McQuade, Days, Linn, and Alario (1996) reported long-term outcome data on 45 children treated for encopresis using a treatment regimen essentially the same as Levine's (1976). At a mean of 53 months after treatment, 58% of the children were in remission and 29% had improved. Only 13% showed no improvement. The major risk factors for treatment resistance were previous treatment for encopresis and nonretentive encopresis (i.e., no history of constipation). The longest reported follow-up data on the medical management of childhood constipation is for 6.8 years (Sutphen et al., 1995). In their study, Sutphen et al. reported follow-up data on 43 children treated with an initial clean-out to remove impactions, prompted toilet sits, and laxatives, including enemas prescribed anytime a child went 24 hours without a bowel movement. The majority (70%) of the children were entirely asymptomatic at follow-up, and the remaining 30% of the children experienced mild intermittent constipation. It appears, both from the treatment literature and our own clinical experience, that continued reliance on a medical treatment program, in the absence of clear and contributing psychopathology, is the treatment of choice. Although psychotherapy may be effective for psychological problems other than the encopresis, no controlled studies have documented the effectiveness of psychotherapy as the primary intervention for encopresis.

In contrast, in a study of children resistant to treatment, Landman, Levine, and Rappaport (1983) reported that continued management with a pediatric approach resulted in 57% of the children no longer soiling at the 1- to 2-year follow-ups. Thus, it appears, both from the treatment literature and our own clinical experience, that continued reliance on a medical treatment program, in the absence of clear and contributing psychopathology, is the treatment of choice.

Levine (1982) advocated a "demystification" process in which the child and his or her family learn that encopresis is a common ailment in children. See Levine's (1982) study for details of his medical treatment of encopresis. He reported that parents often benefited from viewing a simple drawing or diagram to explain how abnormal bowel functioning can lead to encopresis. It was also important that both the parent and the child be told that the child was not to blame for his or her abnormal bowel functioning and that effective treatment methods were available. Figure 5.1 is a diagram that has been used by Levine (1982) to help parents understand that their child's bowel "problem" is not intentional soiling. The clinician can use this diagram to explain to the child and the parents the factors that are present in encopresis, including the "muscles that are thin, weak and stretched" (p. 326), which refers to the fact that the majority of children with encopresis have a larger diameter rectum than children without encopresis, as well as the "warning nerves that don't work"(p. 395), which refers to the fact that children with encopresis often report, correctly, that they cannot feel the "call to stool."

Because the pediatric approach to the treatment of encopresis typically involves the use of a lubricant such as mineral oil as well as increased dietary fiber, several studies have examined the safety of such treatment components. J. H. Clark, Russell, Fitzgerald, and Nagamori (1987) monitored 25 children for 3 months of therapy using mineral oil. They concluded that treatment that included mineral oil therapy had no adverse effect on the children in the study. Clark et al. stated that the concern for possible deleterious effects of mineral oil therapy could be traced to a study from the

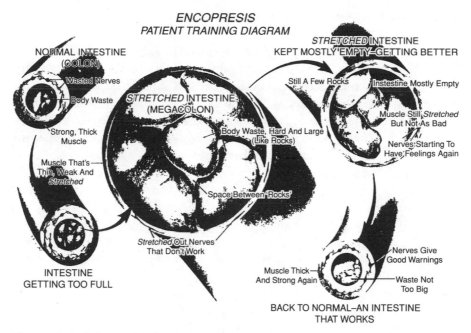

ENCOPRESIS
PATIENT TRAINING DIAGRAM

STRETCHED INTESTINE
KEPT MOSTLY EMPTY—GETTING BETTER

NORMAL INTESTINE
(COLON)

Wasted Nerves

Body Waste

STRETCHED INTESTINE
(MEGACOLON)

Still A Few Rocks

Instestine Mostly Empty

Strong, Thick
Muscle

Body Waste, Hard And Large
(Like Rocks)

Muscle Still Stretched
But Not As Bad

Muscle That's
Thin, Weak And
Stretched

Nerves Starting To
Have Feelings Again

Space Between 'Rocks'

Stretched Out Nerves
That Don't Work

Nerves Give
Good Warnings

INTESTINE
GETTING TOO FULL

Muscle Thick
And Strong Again

Waste Not
Too Big

BACK TO NORMAL—AN INTESTINE
THAT WORKS

Figure 5.1. Schematic representation of a normal colon and a megacolon.

From "Encopresis: Its Potentiation, Evaluation, and Alleviation," by M. D. Levine, 1982, *Pediatric Clinics of North America, 29*(2), p. 326. Copyright 1982 by Pediatric Clinics of North America. Reprinted with permission.

1930s (Curtis & Ballmer, 1939). The recent research has not supported the earlier concerns for deleterious effects from using mineral oil.

McClung et al. (1993) evaluated the safety of combined high-fiber, laxative, and lubricant therapy on bowel movement frequency, fecal soiling, and nutritional status over a 6-month period. Biochemical and anthropometric measures indicated that nutritional status was not adversely affected by therapy. The therapy was also effective in eliminating soiling for 75% of the children. The remaining children demonstrated reduced soiling episodes to a frequency of less than once a week. Thus, although historically there has been some concern in the literature for the safety of using mineral oil, increased dietary fiber, and a laxative regimen for ameliorating problems with constipation, recent research has not detected any negative effects.

As further testament to the medical approach to the management of encopresis, the North America Society for Pediatric Gastroenterology and Nutrition recently published its Medical Position Statement on constipation in infants and children (Baker et al., 1999). Included in the statement is a summary of recommendations for the history, initial "clean out," and dosages for a variety of pharmacological agents that have been empirically supported for use in children with encopresis.

Medical–Behavioral Treatment

One of the earliest behavioral treatment programs for encopresis was offered by Wright (1975). His treatment program consisted of an initial enema, daily glycerin rectal suppositories if the child did not have a bowel movement that day, and behavioral procedures designed to enhance treatment adherence, such as daily symptom and regimen recording. Variations of this medical and behavioral treatment program have also been successful. For example, O'Brien, Ross, and Christophersen (1986) evaluated a treatment program that was based on Wright's (1975) program, using a multiple baseline design across 4 children who were ages 4 to 5. For 2 of the children, treatment with cathartics and special time with their parents, as a reinforcer for appropriate toileting, remedied their soiling accidents and increased their independent toileting in 8–11 weeks. The other 2 children achieved independent toileting after 32 and 39 weeks of treatment, which included positive practice, time-out, and hourly toilet sits added to the treatment regimen.

The importance of parent education about encopresis, along with medical and behavioral management, has been demonstrated as having a positive effect on improving encopresis in children. Information about encopresis has been presented in a parent group format, with some evidence of success for resolving encopresis (e.g., Stark et al., 1997). Stark et al. reported on the outcome of a parent group intervention for 59 children who had previously been treated unsuccessfully for encopresis. They met with the parent group on a weekly basis to discuss standard medical management strategies such as enema clean outs, increased dietary fiber, and daily toilet-sitting, as well as child behavior management strategies of differential attention, contingency management, and behavioral contracting. Stark et al. reported a significant improvement in the encopresis symptoms in 85% of the children.

Stark, Owens-Stively, Spirito, Lewis, and Guevremont (1990) treated 18 children (ranging in age from 4 to 11 years), using parent education about encopresis and integrating behavioral parenting procedures with medical management. Their results showed that the children who had increased their intake of dietary fiber by 40% increased appropriate toileting by 116% and decreased their soiling accidents by 83%. Furthermore, the treatment gains were maintained or improved at the 6-month follow-up.

Stark et al. (1990) discussed the benefits of such group interventions. First, numerous parents can be given essentially the same information at the same time, so a group setting provides cost-effective treatment. Second, the parents who had participated in the study reported feeling a great deal of relief and support in meeting other families who had children with encopresis. In addition, the children reportedly enjoyed the group and had feelings of relief on meeting other children with the same problem.

Stark et al.'s (1990) study furthers the research of Houts, Mellon, and Whelan (1988), who, among others, recognized the importance of the role of dietary fiber in the treatment of encopresis. Williams, Bollella, and Wynder (1995) provided a convenient summary of the recommendations of the American Academy of Pediatrics for intake of dietary fiber. They recommend a daily intake of dietary fiber equivalent to the child's age plus five; for example, a 5-year-old child should be eating 10 grams of dietary fiber (5 + 5) per day. Owens-Stively (1995) also published an excellent educational guide for parents to help them in selecting foods that are high in fiber for their children. To assist in that process, Table 5.3 summarizes the fiber content of many common household foods.

Finally, Cox, Sutphen, Borowitz, Kovatchev, and Ling (1998) published a comparison of three treatment procedures:

1. intensive medical care (IMC), in which children received enemas for disimpaction and laxatives to promote frequent bowel movements
2. enhanced toilet training (ETT), in which children received the IMC, instruction, and modeling to promote appropriate muscle straining and relaxation, as well as reinforcement and scheduling to promote response-to-defecation urges
3. biofeedback (BF), in which children received enemas and laxatives, in addition to biofeedback training that taught them how to tense and relax the muscles used to defecate.

Cox et al. reported that 3 months following treatment, the ETT and BF procedures resulted in similar reductions in soiling that were superior to just the IMC. The ETT training benefited significantly more children, while using fewer laxatives and fewer treatment sessions at a lower cost. Exhibit 5.3 is a summary of their recommendations for ETT.

Choosing Between Treatment Options

There are no published outcome studies that have compared the use of individual versus group treatment or the implementation of a simple medical–behavioral treatment with more extensive behavior treatment, such as the procedures reported by O'Brien et al. (1986). The strategy followed by O'Brien et al., however, is a reasonable one. They began with a standard medical–behavior treatment with all of the children in the study. Within about 2 months, 2 of the children's encopresis had improved substantially, whereas 2 had not. The "child time" and mild "punishment" procedures were added after 2 months, when the children had not shown a significant improvement. Finally, the few studies that have specifically addressed the issue of treatment resistance have documented the efficacy of

TABLE 5.3
Dietary Fiber Content of Selected Foods

The following table may help you obtain the recommended amount of dietary fiber in your child's diet. Many new high-fiber foods are coming on the market each week. Watch for them! Check food labels for actual grams of dietary fiber per serving.

	Serving Size	Dietary Fiber (Grams)
Breads and crackers		
Fiberich bread™	1 slice	3.2
Seven grain bread	1 slice	3.0
High bran "health bread"	1 slice	3.0
Cornbread	1 square (2 1/2")	3.0
100% whole wheat bread	1 slice	2.4
Cracked wheat bread	1 slice	2.1
Whole wheat crackers	6	2.0
Rye crackers	3	2.0
Whole wheat croutons	1/4 cup	1.5
Rye bread	1 slice	1.2
White bread	1 slice	0.8
Cereals		
Fiber One™	1 cup	24.0
100% bran cereal	1 cup	20.0
Corn Bran™	1 cup	8.0
Cracklin' Oat Bran™	1 cup	8.0
Fruit n' Fiber™	1 cup	8.0
Granola	1 cup	7.0
Shredded Wheat and Bran™	1 cup	6.0
Raisin Squares™	1 cup	6.0
Bran Muffin Crisp™	1 cup	6.0
Raisin Nut Bran™	1 cup	6.0
Grape Nuts™	1 cup	5.3
40% Bran Flakes™	1 cup	5.0
Most™	1 cup	5.0
Raisin Bran™	1 cup	4.0
Oatmeal, cooked	3/4 cup	3.0
Shredded Wheat™	1 biscuit	3.0
Wheat Chex™	1 cup	3.0
Ralston™, cooked	3/4 cup	2.7
Wheaties™	1 cup	2.0
Cheerios™	1 cup	1.8
Flours		
Bran (millers)	1 cup	48.0
Cornmeal, stoneground	1 cup	16.5
100% whole wheat	1 cup	14.4
100% rye	1 cup	14.4
Rolled oats	1 cup	12.0
All purpose white flour	1 cup	1.6
Fruits (fresh, unless otherwise indicated)		
Figs, dried	2	8.0
Apricots, dried	8	7.8

(continued)

TABLE 5.3 *(continued)*

	Serving Size	Dietary Fiber (Grams)
Dates, dried	10	7.0
Raisins	1/2 cup	5.4
Prunes, dried	4	5.2
Orange	1 medium	4.5
Banana	1 medium	4.0
Apple, with peel	1 medium	3.3
Strawberries	1 cup	3.3
Pear	1 medium	3.1
Cantaloupe	1/4 medium	2.5
Plums	2	2.5
Apricots	3	2.4
Nuts and seeds		
Brazil nuts	10	5.5
Peanuts	1/2 cup	5.5
Almonds	10	3.6
Soy nuts	2 tbsp.	3.0
Sunflower seeds	2 tbsp.	3.0
Corn nuts	2 tbsp.	3.0
Walnuts	1/2 cup	3.0
Peanut butter	2 tbsp.	2.3
Poppy seeds	2 tbsp.	2.0
Sesame seeds	2 tbsp.	2.0
Vegetables (fresh, raw, unless otherwise indicated)		
Baked beans	1 cup	18.6
Peas	1 cup	11.3
Corn	1 cup	9.3
Broccoli	2 spears	7.0
Yams, baked with skin	1 medium	6.8
Brussels sprouts	1 cup	6.5
Green beans	1 cup	3.5
Spinach	1 cup	3.5
Carrots	1 cup	3.2
Potatoes, baked with skin	1 medium	3.0
Tomato	1 medium	3.0
Cauliflower	1 cup	2.5
Cabbage, shredded	1 cup	1.9
Lettuce	1 cup	0.8
Celery	1 stalk	0.7
Miscellaneous		
Kidney beans	1 cup	20.0
Chili	1 cup	17.0
Macaroni and pasta (whole wheat, cooked)	1 cup	5.7
Brown rice	1 cup	4.0
Coconut, shredded	2 tbsp.	3.0
Popcorn, popped	1 cup	1.0

Note. From *Childhood Constipation and Soiling: A Practical Guide for Parents and Children* (pp. 23–24), by J. Owens-Stively, 1995, Minneapolis, MN: Children's Health Care. Copyright 1995 by Children's Health Care. Reprinted with permission.

Many children who have difficulty with soiling (encopresis), when they are trying to have a bowel movement, tighten up both their abdominal muscles (which is appropriate and necessary to push a bowel movement out) and the muscles in their bottom. It may be necessary for them to practice before they can relax the muscles in their bottom at the exact same time that they tighten the muscles in their abdomen.

Wearing a reasonably tight-fitting shirt or blouse, sit on a small chair with your feet parallel and flat on the floor. Demonstrate to the child how to relax and tense your legs and feet, how to take a deep breath and hold it while sitting up straight, and how to push down with the held breath and pull in from the lower abdomen in order to propel a stool out. Place your hand on your abdomen so that you can demonstrate which muscles you are tensing and relaxing. Place the child's hand over your hand to demonstrate how to do the muscle exercised properly.

The child should replicate this while sitting on the same chair. The child should receive "hand feedback" by placing one hand on the abdomen just below the navel to feel it move out when the breath was pushed down and placing the second hand just below the first hand to feel it go in with the contraction of the abdominal muscle.

Caregivers should practice these "muscle exercises" at least once each day. Spend several minutes with the child tightening up and relaxing the muscles in the leg and feet separately from the muscles in the abdomen. Additionally, 8 to 12 minutes of toilet time should be scheduled daily, beginning 15 to 30 minutes after the same two meals. During these times, children should be instructed to practice tensing and relaxing their bottom for the first 4 minutes with the objective of being able to localize control of and fatigue of the muscles in their bottom, as well as to mechanically stimulate the rectum. In order to desensitize the child to toilet sitting, the second 4 minutes should be spent having fun while being read to or playing games. During the final 4 minutes, the child should be encouraged to strain and attempt to have a bowel movement while relaxing the legs and feet. This routine toilet sitting should be discontinued after the child no longer experiences regular episodes of incontinence.

Note. From "Contribution of Behavior Therapy and Biofeedback to Laxative Therapy in the Treatment of Pediatric Encopresis," by D. J. Cox, J. Sutphen, S. Borowitz, B. Kovatchev, and W. Ling, 1998, *Annals of Behavioral Medicine, 20*(2), pp. 70–75. Copyright 1998 by the Society of Behavioral Medicine. Adapted with permission.

continuing with the treatment procedures (Landman et al., 1983), adding more treatment components (O'Brien et al., 1986) and adding more of an educational component (Stark et al., 1990). There are no studies to support the use of one of these interventions over the other.

Enhancing Treatment Adherence

Patients and families need to know that encopresis treatment is a long-term treatment. In general, 4 to 6 weeks of consistent treatment may be required before a substantial improvement in encopretic symptoms is observed. Furthermore, long-term maintenance is needed to prevent recurring constipation and impaction. For these reasons, provisions need to be made for follow-up care that includes, at least during the first month of treatment, daily record keeping of treatments and treatment effects.

A parent-report Symptom Rating Sheet (e.g., Christophersen, 1994) can facilitate record keeping and, when used reliably and mailed to the treatment provider's office on a weekly basis, is helpful for assessing patient progress, making treatment plan modifications, and encouraging treatment adherence. The Symptom Rating Sheet, if completed each day by the child's caregiver and brought to each follow-up appointment, provides the health care provider with a great deal of information about the child's symptoms without taking up unnecessary clinic time. The completed sheet can be photocopied, with the original returned to the caregiver and the copy archived in the child's medical record (see Exhibit 5.4).

EXHIBIT 5.4
Bowel Symptom Rating Sheet

Date												Comments
1												
2												
3												
4												
5												
6												
7												
8												
9												
10												
11												
12												
13												
14												
15												
16												
17												
18												
19												
20												
21												

(continued)

EXHIBIT 5.4 *(continued)*

Date												Comments
22												
23												
24												
25												
26												
27												
28												
29												
30												
31												

KEY:

Mineral Oil	No. of tablespoons
Size/Consistency	Approx. no. of cups; H = hard, S = soft formed, D = diarrhea
Amt. of liquids	No. of glasses of water or juices per day
Activity	3 = very active, 2 = moderately active, 1 = little activity
Time	Indicates how parent spent reward time with child

Note. From *Pediatrics Compliance: A Guide for the Primary Care Physician* (pp. 229–230), by E. R. Christophersen, 1994, New York: Plenum. Copyright 1994 by Plenum. Reprinted with permission.

CONCLUSION

Clinicians who provide medical or psychological services to children are almost certain to encounter patients who have a history of encopresis. As Brody (1992) pointed out, encopresis has come to be known as the "hidden disease." An extensive search of the popular literature, including parenting magazines and newspapers, revealed very few articles that address the topic of encopresis. Given the number of children who suffer from encopresis, it is interesting that popular literature, which is often a source of child health information for parents, contains almost no discussion of it.

The diagnosis and treatment of encopresis is a relatively straightforward procedure. The history and initial presentation are typically quite similar across cases. After ruling out behavior and emotional problems that may have contributed to the toileting problem, either the primary care physician or the clinician treating the child must arrive at a clinical judgment regarding whether the child is constipated. If the child is constipated, procedures must be used to relieve the constipation, which can take anywhere from 1 day to 2 weeks. These procedures are well detailed in the Medical Position

Statement of the North American Society for Pediatric Gastroenterology and Nutrition (Baker et al., 1999).

In addition to relieving the child's constipation, the clinician or primary care physician must institute procedures to reduce the probability that the child will become constipated again by making dietary modification recommendations and through the use of stool softeners. Procedures to increase the parents' adherence with treatment procedures, such as written treatment summaries and symptom recording sheets, are often helpful. Adequate education for the parents and the child is a valuable aid in the treatment of encopresis. In the vast majority of cases, the encopresis does resolve within a predictable time frame. Treatment-resistant cases have been adequately investigated by several researchers. Typically, the management of such cases involves further efforts and education and further persistence in the implementation of the treatment regimen.

6

DIAGNOSIS AND MANAGEMENT OF NOCTURNAL ENURESIS

Enuresis is the repeated voiding of urine into the bed or clothes, whether involuntary or intentional, according to the *Diagnostic and Statistical Manual of Mental Disorders* (4th ed., *DSM–IV*; American Psychiatric Association, 1994). The behavior is clinically significant when manifested either by a frequency of twice a week for at least 3 consecutive months or by the presence of clinically significant distress or impairment in social, academic, or other important areas of functioning. The child must be at least 5 years old or at an equivalent developmental level, and the enuretic behavior must not be due exclusively to the direct physiological effect of a substance such as a diuretic or general medical disorder (e.g., diabetes, spina bifida, or a seizure disorder). The *DSM–IV* diagnostic criteria are listed in Exhibit 6.1.

PREVALENCE

Approximately 40% of children wet the bed at age 3. The prevalence declines slowly thereafter, with 22% wetting the bed at age 5, 10% at age 10, and 3% at age 15 (Binderglas, 1975). Despite the prevalence of enuresis in young children, it is a primary concern for parents (Richman, Stevenson, & Graham, 1982a), who may not have realistic expectations. For example,

Shelov et al. (1981) found that parents thought children should be dry at night by age 2.75 years, compared with their pediatricians' estimate of 5.13 years.

In addition to nocturnal enuresis, day wetting is also a problem for many children. In a survey of more than 3,000 students who were 7, Hjalmas (1992) reported that day wetting of any kind occurred in 6% of students. Day wetting at least once a week was found in 3.1% of girls and 2.1% of boys. Over 70% of the children who wet during the day also had increased urgency. Combined daytime and nighttime incontinence was reported by 17% of the children, whereas 22% wet only during the day and 61% wet only at night. None of the students had a previously indicated organic cause for their incontinence. Hjalmas did report a strong correlation between bacterium and day wetting in girls, but not in boys. Such research shows that both day and night wetting can be a common occurrence in young children.

CAUSES AND CORRELATES

A number of etiologic factors have been proposed for enuresis, including food allergies, deep sleep, small bladder capacity, developmental delays, and faulty training habits (M. W. Cohen, 1975; McKendry & Stewart, 1974; Simonds, 1977). No definitive cause of enuresis has been identified, however. There is general agreement that enuresis is not primarily a psychopathological disorder (Olness, 1975; Perlmutter, 1976; Werry & Cohrssen, 1965). Secondary emotional and behavioral problems may develop, however, as a result of trying to cope with enuresis. Enuresis is generally a self-limiting condition with a spontaneous cure rate of 12–15% per year (Binderglas, 1975).

A positive family history of clinical enuresis has been frequently noted. For example, when both parents had a history of enuresis, M. W. Cohen (1975) found that 77% of children had enuresis; when one parent did, 42% of children did; and when neither parent did, only 15% of children did.

ASSESSMENT

Medical Assessment

The assessment of enuresis typically involves ruling out significant pathology, both medical and behavioral. In the vast majority of referrals, the primary care physician has already ruled out most of the more common organicities. For example, a urinary tract infection, which produces such physical symptoms as burning during urination, a discharge from the urinary meatus, and perhaps a low-grade fever, can also cause enuresis. Only urinalysis and a urine culture, however, however, can accurately identify a urinary tract infection, because children can have a urinary tract infection with no symptoms. In many areas of the United States, psychologists can order both a urinalysis and urine culture either on their own or through the child or adolescent's primary care physician. A request can be made for the written lab reports to be sent to both the primary care physician and the psychologist. Despite the occasional medical problem, however, Hurley (1990) and others have taken the position that day wetting is mainly a behavioral problem, whereas night wetting is mainly a developmental problem that will resolve in most children without intervention.

Behavioral Assessment

Most patients can be adequately screened for behavioral and emotional problems through the use of a thorough interview and common rating scales such as the Achenbach Child Behavior Checklist (Achenbach, 1994) or the Behavioral Assessment System for Children (Reynolds & Kemphaus, 1998) without any initial need for an extensive psychological evaluation (Friman, Handwerk, Swearer, McGinnis, & Warzak, 1998). To obtain a comprehensive history, the clinicians at Children's Mercy Hospital in Kansas City, Missouri, rely on both general and specific intake forms. Exhibit 6.2 shows an Enuresis Intake Form completed by parents who scheduled an appointment to have their child evaluated and treated for enuresis.

EXHIBIT 6.2
Enuresis Intake Form

PARENTS

1. What word does your child use for urinating? _____

2. Has your child ever been potty trained? _____ .

	Age Started	Age Accomplished
Bladder trained?	_____	_____
Bowel trained?	_____	_____

3. What potty-training method did you use? _____

4. Was there ever a time when your child did not wet the bed? Yes ____ No ____

5. If so, when did bed-wetting begin? _____

6. When did you decide that it was a problem? _____

7. Your spouse? _____ Your child? _____

8. What about bed-wetting makes it a problem for you? _____
   For your spouse? _____ For your child? _____

9. Does your child wet the bed every night? _____ If not, how often? _____

10. Has your child ever gone for 2 months without wetting the bed? _____ How long? _____ How often? _____

11. What methods have you used in the past to stop the bed-wetting? _____
    _____

12. Are you still using any of these methods? _____

13. What is your child's responsibility when he or she wets the bed? _____

14. Does your child ever wet his or her pants during the day? _____

15. How much ? Small _____ Medium _____ Large _____

16. Does your child ever dribble in his or her pants during the day? _____

17. Does your child ever complain of burning when he or she urinates? _____

18. Does your child have to go more frequently than you think is normal? _____

19. Does your child complain that it doesn't feel like he or she has completely emptied his or her bladder when finished? _____

20. When your child has to urinate, can he or she wait a while or does he or she have to go right then or have an accident? _____

21. Have you ever noticed any irritation around the end of his penis or her meatus? _____

22. Has your child ever had a work-up for a urinary tract infection or any other urinary problem? _____

23. When ? _____

24. By whom? _____ Where ? _____ Results? _____

25. Is your child a sound sleeper? _____

26. When your child stays overnight with relatives or a friend, does he or she wet the bed? _____

27. What do you believe causes bed-wetting ? _____

28. Has your child ever had problems with constipation ? Yes _____ No ? _____

(continued)

EXHIBIT 6.2 *(continued)*

29. Has your child ever had a problem with soiling?
30. To your knowledge, did anyone in either the biological mother's or father's family wet the bed? If so, who ? _____

CHILD
1. Tell me why you're here. _____
2. Do you want to stop wetting the bed? _____
3. Does wetting the bed cause you any problems? _____
4. What do Mom and Dad say or do when you wet the bed ? _____
5. Have you ever gone without wetting the bed? _____
6. When you wet the bed, what do you do about it ? _____

Note. From *Pediatric Compliance: A Guide for the Primary Care Physician* (pp. 235–237), by E. R. Christophersen, 1994, New York: Plenum. Copyright 1994 by Plenum. Reprinted with permission.

Daytime wetting, which involves essentially the same medical and psychological evaluation, has received much less attention in medical and psychological literature than night wetting, perhaps because day wetting may be considered incomplete toilet training rather than a separate clinical entity. The diagnostic criteria in the *DSM–IV* do not differentiate between day wetting and night wetting, although the treatment of these two types of enuresis is usually quite different. Hudziak et al. (1993) demonstrated that the actual use of *DSM–IV* diagnostic criteria was beneficial for training medical students in a primary care clinic to make a diagnosis.

INTERVENTION

Numerous treatments for enuresis have been suggested, including diet restrictions, psychotherapy, retention-control training, drugs, and behavioral methods. For example, assuming that enuretic children have a smaller bladder capacity than nonenuretic children, it has been suggested that small bladder capacity may be due to spasms of the smooth muscle in the bladder wall. This spasm may have an allergic basis, and therefore removal of substances that irritate the bladder wall may arrest enuresis (Christophersen & Purvis, 2001). Recent promotion of the drug desmopressin (DDAVP) has included the speculation that enuresis is the result of a hormone deficiency. The use of this drug as a treatment option for enuresis is discussed below.

Although both psychological and pharmacological interventions have reported outcomes superior to those reported in control groups, children receiving psychological treatments were more likely to have ceased enuresis at posttreatment and follow-up than children given pharmacological treatments (Houts, Berman, & Abramson, 1994). Short-term psychotherapy has been recommended by some clinicians for treatment of enuresis (Sperling, 1965). The few comparative studies that have been done, however, have shown that short-term psychotherapy is no more effective than no treatment and that more direct methods such as use of a urine alarm are more effective. Psychotherapy may be desirable, however, in those few cases in which significant psychopathology is suspected in addition to the fact that the child has enuresis (M. W. Cohen, 1975; Lovibond, 1964).

Medical Treatment

The most common drug used to treat enuresis is imipramine (Tofranil), a tricyclic antidepressant. Imipramine resolved the symptoms in 43% of the patients, whereas other tricyclics had a success rate of 33%, but the relapse rate was high and the final outcome was no better than a placebo or baseline treatment (Moffatt, 1997). The Food and Drug Administration recommends that imipramine be used only as contemporary adjunctive therapy for children with enuresis who are ages 6 or older (*Physician's Desk Reference*, 1995). Like any other powerful pharmacological agent, imipramine has potentially serious side effects and should be reserved for cases in which more conventional therapies are not practical or effective.

The efficacy and safety of the use of DDAVP, a hormonal nasal spray used to treat diabetes insipidus, has been examined as a cure for nocturnal enuresis. Moffatt (1997) reported that, for studies that had not preselected for DDAVP response, the best estimate for dryness was approximately 25%. The relapse rate, when reported, also was high. Only 5.7% of the test participants remained dry after withdrawal of the drug. Moffatt, Harlos, Kirshen, and Burd (1993) reported on a total of 689 participants from 18 studies of DDAVP; an average of only 24% of the participants achieved short-term dryness. In three studies reporting on long-term dryness, only 5.7% maintained dryness after stopping DDAVP. Moffatt et al. concluded that on the basis of current knowledge, DDAVP is inferior to conditioning alarms as a primary therapy. An article in a Danish journal (Ankjaer & Sejr, 1994) reported a cost-effectiveness analysis of the use of DDAVP for enuresis. The authors estimated that the use of urine-alarm training would save the socialized medical care system DKK19.2 million annually (US $3.3 million), whereas the use of DDAVP would cost the system DKK44.8 million (US $7.8 million). This is the first article to actually address the cost–benefit considerations of widespread DDAVP use.

As Moffatt (1997) concluded, DDAVP and antidepressants are a second line of management when the alarm has failed or is impractical. For children who are known responders to medication, it can be used for special occasions, such as sleepovers and camps, or on a longer term basis.

S. Thompson and Rey (1995) arrived at essentially the same conclusions about desmopressin from their review of 61 published articles, which indicated an average of only 25% of patients becoming dry with the use of desmopressin.

Behavioral Treatment

Bell-and-Pad or Urine-Alarm Training

For six decades, the standard behavioral treatment for enuresis has been the bell-and-pad or urine-alarm procedure originally reported by Mowrer and Mowrer (1938). In general, studies have shown that the urine-alarm treatment initially eliminates enuresis in approximately 75% of children with the problem, with treatment duration ranging from a mean of 5 to 12 weeks (Doleys, Ciminero, Tollison, Williams, & Wells, 1977). Relapse rates are generally high and occur in 46% of cases, although reinstatement of the procedures usually results in a complete cure (Taylor & Turner, 1975). The urine-alarm treatment has also been shown to be superior to no treatment, short-term psychotherapy, and imipramine (McKendry, Stewart, Khanna, & Netley, 1975; Werry & Cohrssen, 1965). For the interested reader, Forsythe and Butler (1989) published an interesting summary of 50 years of research on enuresis alarms, including a discussion of some rather bizarre (by today's standards) procedures.

Overlearning

The term *overlearning* refers to the process of training children to a higher criterion than is normally thought to be necessary, with the hope of reducing the relapse rate. For example, Houts, Liebert, and Padawer (1983) reported on 60 primary children with enuresis (ages 4–12 years) who were treated using a package including a bell and pad, cleanliness training, retention control, and overlearning. Overlearning refers to a procedure in which a child, after he or she is dry at night from using a bed-wetting alarm, is encouraged to drink extra liquids before retiring for the night until the child attains 14 additional consecutive dry nights (Houts, 1996). Drinking such extra fluids should make it more difficult for the child to avoid bedwetting, thereby training them to a higher criterion. Forty-eight children achieved initial arrest of enuresis, and only 11 had relapsed at 1-year follow-up. These results, using 1-hour group training sessions, supported the efficacy of the overlearning and retention-control training procedures, in addition to using the bell and pad. Overlearning usually results in a relapse of wetting, but in the majority of cases, that only lasts a week or so (Moffatt, 1997).

Moffatt (1997) provided some "Practical Tips," listed in Exhibit 6.3, for implementation of bed-wetting alarm treatment; although not empirically

EXHIBIT 6.3
Practical Tips for Successful Use of an Enuresis Alarm

- Contract with the parent and child for a 3-month trial.
- Have the child keep a diary, starting at least 2 weeks before the first visit, that includes the number of wet nights, the number of episodes per night, and the size of the wet spot.
- The parent must be part of the alarm system (many children will not arouse on their own to the alarm initially but after a few weeks of parental help will begin to respond on their own).
- Emphasize and reward arousal.
- See the child at least every 3 weeks initially.
- Use a decreased frequency of wet nights, a decreased number of episodes per night, and a decreased size of wet spot as signs of improvement.
- Continue until the child achieves 14 consecutive dry nights (no alarm sound for even a spot of urine).
- After initial goal is achieved, use overlearning, that is, either 16 oz of fluid before bed or gradual 2-oz increments, increasing as each step is mastered, until 16 oz is reached.
- Continue overlearning until the child achieves 14 consecutive dry nights.
- When overlearning is completed, stop the alarm and extra drinking.
- Relapses can be retreated successfully in the same manner, in many cases.

Note. From "Nocturnal Enuresis: A Review of the Efficacy of Treatments and Practical Advice for Clinicians," by M. E. Moffatt, 1997, *Journal of Developmental and Behavioral Pediatrics, 18,* p. 52. Copyright 1997 by Lippincott Williams & Wilkins. Reprinted with permission.

evaluated, these tips do not contradict published research on the use of bed-wetting alarms.

Dry-Bed Training

The most promising adaptation of the urine-alarm treatment is dry-bed training (Azrin, Sneed, & Foxx, 1974). Dry-bed training combines a number of behavioral procedures, including cleanliness training, positive practice, nighttime awakening, retention-control training, and positive reinforcement. Success with dry-bed training approaches 85%, with relapse rates reported between 7% and 29% (Azrin et al., 1974). As with urine-alarm treatment, relapsed children were cured when the training procedures were reinstated, although Azrin et al. did not provide data on the length of reinstatement time required.

A study conducted by Duke University Medical Center ("Determining Reasonable Expectations," 1990) reported that only 5% of physicians were trained in the use of urine-alarm or dry-bed training, as opposed to almost 100% of physicians who were trained in the pharmacological management of enuresis. Perhaps physicians do not recommend urine-alarm or dry-bed training because they are not acquainted with it during their residency training. In a more recent study, however, Vogel, Young, and Primack (1996) reported a much higher percentage of physicians (80%) recommending the use of nonpharmacological treatments for enuresis than had been reported in previous studies. Interestingly, dry-bed training has also been shown to be effective with adults, with higher cure rates and lower relapse rates than

EXHIBIT 6.4
Dry-Bed Training Procedures

I. Recording: Use calendar progress chart to record dry or wet for each night
   A. Parent praises child if dry
   B. Parent encourages child to keep working if wet

II. At bedtime
   A. Child feels sheets and comments on their dryness
   B. Child describes what he or she will do if he or she has the urge to urinate
   C. Child describes current need to urinate and does so
   D. Parent expresses confidence in child and reviews progress
   E. Alarm is placed on bed or on child
   F. Alarm is connected and turned on
   G. Child goes to sleep

III. Nightly awakening
   A. Awaken child once during the night
      1. Use minimal prompt in awakening, but be sure the child is awake
      2. Child feels sheets and comments on dryness
      3. Parent praises child for dry sheets
      4. Child goes to bathroom, urinates as much as possible, returns to bed
      5. Child feels sheets again
      6. Child states what he or she will do if he or she feels urge to urinate
      7. Parent expresses confidence to child
      8. Keep alarm on bed if it has not sounded before awakening
      9. If alarm has sounded more than 30 minutes before scheduled awakening, awaken at schedule time
      10. If alarm has sounded less than 30 minutes before scheduled awakening, awaken at the scheduled time
   B. Adjust time of nightly awakening
      1. On first night, awaken child 5 hours before his or her usual time of awakening
      2. After child has 6 consecutive dry nights, awaken him or her 1 hour earlier the next night. Continue to move the awakening time 1 hour earlier after each 6 dry nights until the awakening time is 8 hours before the usual time of awakening
      3. When dry for 14 nights at 8-hour awakening, discontinue awakening and discontinue alarm

(continued)

EXHIBIT 6.4 *(continued)*

IV. When alarm sounds

    A. Awaken child and give mild reprimand for wetting
    B. Child feels sheets and comments on wetness
    C. Child walks to bathroom and finishes wetting
    D. Child takes quick bath
    E. Child changes into dry clothes
    F. Child removes wet sheets and places them in laundry
    G. Child remakes bed with dry sheets
    H. Child feels bed sheets and comments on dryness
    I. Do not reconnect alarm
    J. Child returns to sleep

V. During day

    A. Child and parents describe progress to relevant friends or family members
    B. Parents repeatedly express confidence in child and praise him or her
    C. Parent calls therapist at set times to report progress

Note. From "Dry-Bed Training: Rapid Elimination of Childhood Enuresis," by N. H. Azrin, T. J., Sneed, and R. M. Foxx, 1974, *Behaviour Research and Therapy, 12,* p. 150. Copyright 1974 by Elsevier Science. Adapted with permission.

have been reported with children (van Son, Mulder, & van Londen, 1990). Exhibit 6.4 is a summary of the dry-bed training procedures.

Cendron (1999) provided a convenient listing of some of the bed-wetting alarms, their manufacturer and contact information, and approximate cost. This information is reproduced in Table 6.1. Cendron also included a review of the prescription medications that are recommended for enuresis and their approximate monthly cost.

Arousal Training

Arousal training, a combination of a urine-alarm and rewarding the child for awakening, has recently been credited with a success rate of 98%, with no dropouts from treatment (van Londen, van Londen-Barentsen, van Son, & Mulder, 1993). Data reported 2.5 years after the arousal training intervention indicated that the arousal training group was still dry 92% of the mornings, compared with 77% for the urine-alarm with specific instructions and 72% with the urine-alarm only (van Londen et al., 1993).

Hypnosis

Through the years, various authors have reported on the use of hypnosis as a treatment for enuresis. The first such report by Olness (1975) showed almost an 80% cure rate with hypnosis. D. P. Kohen, Olness, Colwell, and Heimel (1984) reported on the use of self-hypnosis with 505 pa-

TABLE 6.1
Some Alarm Devices for the Treatment of Primary Enuresis

Device	Manufacturer	Cost (Approximate)
Wet-Stop	Palco Labs Santa Cruz, CA 800-346-4488	$65.00
Nytone Enuretic Alarm	Nytone Medical Products Salt Lake City, UT 801-973-4090	$53.50
Potty Pager	Ideas for Living Boulder, CO 800-497-6573	$49.95
Nite Train'r	Koregon Enterprises Beaverton, OR 800-544-4240	$69.00
Sleep Dry	Star Child Labs Aptos, CA 800-346-7283	$45.00

Note. From "Primary Nocturnal Enuresis: Current Concepts," by M. Cendron, 1999, *American Family Physician, 59,* pp. 1205–1218. Copyright 1999 by American Academy of Family Physicians. Reprinted with permission.

tients ranging in age from 3 to 20 years. They reported that approximately 50% were completely dry and another 32% showed a significant improvement at least 4 months later. Banerjee, Srivastav, and Palan (1993) compared hypnosis with imipramine drug treatment in people with enuresis ranging in age from 5 to 16 years. After treatment and at the 9-month follow-up, the hypnosis group reported vastly superior results: 68% of the hypnosis group were still dry, whereas only 24% of the imipramine group were still dry. Although implementation of hypnosis procedures for the treatment of conditions such as enuresis requires substantial advanced training, it is an option available to the interested practitioner. Referral to a properly trained hypnotist may be another alternative.

Positive Practice

The toilet-training procedures described in Azrin and Foxx's (1974) book, *Toilet Training in Less Than a Day,* were based on research they published that described almost 100% cure rates. In their book, Azrin and Foxx described a procedure for day wetting that they called *positive practice,* which involves having the toddler practice going to the bathroom, on the potty, 10 times after each accident. Clinicians at Children's Mercy Hospital have

EXHIBIT 6.5
Positive Practice for Toileting Accidents

After they have been toilet trained, some children occasionally have periods of frequent wetting or soiling. The children should first be examined by a physician to rule out physical conditions, such as urinary tract infections, that may be causing the accidents.

When you find your child with wet or soiled pants, use the following guidelines:

1. Show verbal disapproval for the wetting or soiling.
   a. Tell your child why you are displeased, saying something like, "You wet your pants."
   b. Express your disapproval of the accident by saying something like, "You shouldn't wet your pants. You should use the toilet."

2. Have your child do positive practice of self-toileting.
   a. Tell your child what you are doing and why by saying something like, "Bobby wet his pants. Bobby has to practice going to the bathroom."
   b. Guide your child quickly to the toilet or potty chair.
   c. Guide your child to quickly lower his or her pants and sit on the toilet or potty.
   d. After sitting 1 or 2 seconds (do not allow urination), guide your child to quickly raise his or her pants.
   e. Guide your child back to the area where you discovered the accident for a total of five positive practices from where your child had the accident. Then, guide your child to practice from five other parts of the house (e.g., from the front door, from the back door, from the kitchen) to the bathroom or potty chair.
   f. If your child refuses to do the positive practice trials, or if he or she has a temper tantrum, direct him or her to time-out. After he or she completes the time-out, begin the positive practice from where you left off.

3. Make your child responsible for cleaning up.
   a. If there is urine on the floor, guide your child to get a cloth and wipe up the spot.
   b. With a minimum of guidance, require your child to remove his or her soiled pants.
   c. Guide your child to put his or her soiled clothing in an appropriate place.
   d. If your child has had a bowel movement, guide him or her to clean himself or herself up or to take a quick partial bath.
   e. Guide your child to put on clean clothes.

4. After the accident has been corrected, do not continue to talk about it. Your child should start with a clean slate.

5. Remember to praise and hug your child when he or she eliminates in the toilet or potty chair.

Note. Information from *Toilet Training in Less Than a Day,* by N. H. Azrin and R. M. Foxx, 1974, New York: Pocket Books. Copyright 1974 by Pocket Books. Adapted with permission.

recommended positive practice procedures for toileting accidents, during toilet training with children up to 5 years of age, as the treatment of choice, based on the positive results reported by parents in Azrin and Foxx's book (Christophersen, 1994). Exhibit 6.5 is the written treatment protocol for positive practice with toileting accidents that was adapted by Christophersen (1994) from Azrin and Foxx's work.

Social and Interpersonal Treatments

Negative psychosocial consequences of enuresis are common (Warzak, 1993), secondary to the impact of enuresis on family members and others. The child with enuresis may be at increased risk for emotional or even physical abuse from family members and may experience stress related to fear of detection by peers. These factors may contribute to the loss of self-esteem that the child often experiences (Warzak, 1993). Thus, children with enuresis should be evaluated for common emotional responses, such as embarrassment, fear, and concern about being punished.

Comments About Treatment Options

The prevalence of nocturnal enuresis, combined with the availability of several treatment modalities (drugs, urine alarm, dry-bed training, and hypnosis), has produced a rather large body of literature on the topic. Parents and clinicians must choose between the ease and expense of medications that are marginally effective versus the difficulty of urine-alarm procedures that are far more effective but require significantly more effort on the part of the caregiver. The vast majority of caregivers can implement both drugs and urine-alarm procedures. The use of hypnotherapy, however, requires rather extensive training, results in fewer patients stopping their bed-wetting, and is moderately expensive. Clearly, the clinician who is aware of the many treatment modalities available can better inform the client and family of the options, including the degree of difficulty, the cost, and the expected level of effectiveness. The family members can then choose for themselves which treatment is most suitable for their lifestyle and needs. There are varying recommendations regarding the age at which nocturnal enuresis becomes a clinical problem requiring treatment. Although Azrin et al. (1974) suggested that children older than age 4 are ready for treatment, Christophersen (1994) recommended waiting until the child is older than age 7 and is concerned about his or her wetting. Mellon and McGrath (2000) recommended the combination of urine-alarm training and the use of DDAVP to push the already high success rates of alarm approaches closer to 100%.

CONCLUSION

When a family presents with a child who has nocturnal enuresis, both the child and parents should be given information about enuresis, including its prevalence, in an effort to alleviate some of their concerns. The choices for treatment and the respective outcomes can be described, and the family can chose to try a treatment or wait for the child to outgrow the enuresis. Regardless of the choice made by the family, there may need to be a reassessment mechanism, or waiting period, to see if the child or parent has become discouraged or is interested in exploring other available options.

Great strides have been made over the past 20 years in the treatment of enuresis. Clinicians now have the information to make informed decisions regarding the diagnosis and treatment of enuresis. Although at one time these problems were not well understood and treatment was only marginally successful, we now have the technology to intervene effectively with the vast majority of patients with enuresis. Although current pharmacological agents for enuresis can produce undesirable side effects, future agents may not have that disadvantage and may become as effective as behavioral treatments. At this time, however, nonpharmacological behavioral procedures are available that are easy to implement and are extremely effective in addressing enuresis in children.

7

ASSESSMENT AND MANAGEMENT OF PAIN

Many children will experience pain in their childhood as a result of medical procedures, recurrent medical conditions, or chronic disease. Pain has been defined as a complex construct comprised of a sensory and response component (P. A. McGrath, 1990). According to McGrath, the sensory component, called *nociception*, is the direct response of the neural pathway to actual tissue damage. The response component to the nociception involves physiological and emotional experiences, as well as the cognitive interpretation and behavioral manifestations of the person in pain. Responses to pain can also be influenced by individual characteristics of the child and by external sources such as parental reactions. These sources and their contribution to a child's pain experience are described more thoroughly later in this chapter.

Pain has also been defined with respect to its duration and etiology. Acute pain, such as that experienced during medical procedures, often has an adaptive component as a warning signal for recent tissue damage. Recurrent and chronic pain may be associated with physical injury, illness, disease, or an unidentifiable medical cause and may be present even after the original cause of the pain has been identified and alleviated. Children who experience such pain often also suffer from sleep problems and emotional problems such as depression or anxiety, may demonstrate developmentally inappropriate behaviors, and may restrict common activities such as attending school or playing with friends (P. A. McGrath, 1990; Varni & Walco, 1988). Pain management strategies, as well as assistance in addressing pain-related problems such as those mentioned above, may be requested of clinicians by the child's primary care doctor or medical specialist. Many major medical centers also have clinicians who address pain issues for specific groups of children, such as those with cancer. The management of pain related to medical procedures, recurrent medical conditions, and chronic disease are also discussed in this chapter.

DSM–IV AND PAIN DISORDER

Psychological factors play an important role in one's experience of pain. Consequently, the American Psychiatric Association, with some fairly significant revisions over the years (S. A. King, 1995), has included diagnostic criteria for pain disorders in the current version of the *Diagnostic and Statistical Manual of Mental Disorders* (4th ed., *DSM–IV*; American Psychiatric Association, 1994). This category has become separate from somatoform disorders, which are beyond the scope of this chapter. The pain disorders category was developed to avoid the pejorative adjectives often associated with "somatoform" disorder and to avoid the inference that pain associated with psychological factors is less "real" than pain from a known physiological source (S. A. King, 1995). The diagnostic criteria for pain disorders are found in Exhibit 7.1. The diagnostic criteria for somatization disorder are also included in Exhibit 7.1 to assist with differential diagnosis.

PREVALENCE OF PAIN EXPERIENCES IN CHILDREN

The prevalence of pain experiences in children has been reported in many different ways. First, epidemiological studies have been conducted to help determine how prevalent significant pain is for children who have experienced medical procedures or who have chronic medical conditions. The results from these studies suggest that approximately 40% or more of children hospitalized for medical procedures or chronic illness experience significant pain (Cummings, Reid, Finley, McGrath, & Ritchie, 1996; Finley, McGrath, Forward, McNeill, & Fitzgerald, 1996; Johnston, Abbott, Gray-Donald, & Jeans, 1992). More specifically, a comparison of pain for various medical procedures was conducted by Finley et al. (1996), who found that pediatric tonsillectomies, circumcisions, and dental extractions produced the most significant pain for 1 to 3 days postsurgery, compared with pain after procedures such as the insertion of myringotomy tubes.

Prevalence rates for medical conditions that have a high incidence of recurrent or chronic pain are also available. For example, the prevalence of

EXHIBIT 7.1

Pain Disorder	Somatization Disorder

Pain Disorder

A. Pain in one or more anatomical sites is the predominant focus of the clinical presentation and is of sufficient severity to warrant clinical attention.

B. The pain causes clinically significant distress or impairment in social, occupational, or other important areas of functioning.

C. Psychological factors are judged to have an important role in the onset, severity, exacerbation, or maintenance of the pain.

D. The symptom or deficit is not intentionally produced or feigned (as in Factitious Disorder or Malingering).

E. The pain is not better accounted for by a Mood, Anxiety, or Psychotic Disorder and does not meet criteria for Dyspareunia.

Code as follows:

307.80 Pain Disorder Associated With Psychological Factors: Psychological factors are judged to have the major role in the onset, severity, exacerbation, or maintenance of the pain. (If a general medical condition is present, it does not have a major role in the onset, severity, exacerbation, or maintenance of the pain.)

This type of Pain Disorder is not diagnosed if criteria are also met for Somatization Disorder. Specify if acute (duration of <6 months) or chronic (duration of ≥6 months).

307.89 Pain Disorder Associated With Both Psychological Factors and a General Medical Condition: Both psychological factors and a general medical condition are judged to have important roles in the onset, severity, exacerbation, or maintenance of the pain. The associated general medical condition or anatomical site of the pain is coded on Axis III. Specify if acute (duration of <6 months) or chronic (duration of ≥6 months).

Somatization Disorder

A. A history of many physical complaints beginning before age 30 years that occur over a period of several years and result in treatment being sought or significant impairment in social, occupational, or other important areas of functioning.

B. Each of the following criteria must have been met, with individual symptoms occurring at any time during the course of disturbance:

(1) Four pain symptoms: a history of pain related to at least four different sites or functions (e.g., head, abdomen, back, joints, extremities, chest, rectum, during menstruation, during sexual intercourse, or during urination).

(2) Two gastrointestinal symptoms: a history of at least two gastrointestinal symptoms other that pain (e.g., nausea, bloating, vomiting other than during pregnancy, diarrhea, or intolerance of several different foods).

(3) One sexual symptom: a history of at least one sexual or reproductive symptom other than pain (e.g., sexual indifference, erectile or ejaculatory dysfunction, irregular menses, excessive menstrual bleeding, vomiting throughout pregnancy).

(4) One pseudoneurological symptom: a history of at least one symptom or deficit suggesting a neurological condition not limited to pain (conversion symptoms such as impaired coordination or balance, paralysis or localized weakness, difficulty swallowing or lump in throat, aphonia, urinary retention, hallucinations, loss of touch or pain sensation, double vision, blindness, deafness, seizures; dissociative symptoms such as amnesia; or loss of consciousness other than fainting).

(continued)

EXHIBIT 7.1 *(continued)*

Pain Disorder	Somatization Disorder

	C. Either (1) or (2):
	  (1) after appropriate investigation, each of the symptoms in Criterion B cannot be fully explained by known general medical condition or the direct effects of a substance (e.g., a drug of abuse, a medication).
	  (2) when there is a related general medical condition, the physical complaints or resulting social or occupational impairment are in excess of what would be expected from the history, physical examination, or laboratory findings.
	D. The symptoms are not intentionally produced or feigned (as in Factitious Disorder or Malingering).

Note. Information from *Diagnostic and Statistical Manual of Mental Disorders* (4th ed.), by the American Psychiatric Association, 1994, American Psychiatric Association. Copyright 1994 by the American Psychiatric Association. Reprinted with permission.

pediatric headaches was estimated at 2.5% of the child population, from a nationally representative sample of children younger than age 18 (Newacheck & Taylor, 1992). Estimates of recurrent abdominal pain in school-age or younger children range from 9% to 17% (Rappaport & Leichtner, 1993; Zuckerman, Stevenson, & Bailey, 1987). Abdominal pain and headaches are the two most frequently researched recurrent pain disorders in pediatric pain literature, possibly because of their frequent occurrence during childhood. Pain is also frequently a characteristic of disease states such as AIDS, cancer, cystic fibrosis, sickle cell disease, juvenile rheumatoid arthritis (JRA), and fibromyalgia. A summary of the types of pain children with these diseases often experience is found in Exhibit 7.2.

The actual incidence of children with chronic disease who experience significant pain varies with diagnosis. For example, Hirschfeld, Moss, Dragisic, Smith, and Pizzo (1996) found that 59% of their outpatients with AIDS suffered from significant pain, whereas Strafford et al. (1991) found that 100% of their pediatric patients with AIDS required pain intervention. One study of pediatric pain associated with cancer indicated that at least 25% of outpatients and 50% of inpatients suffered from treatment- or disease-related pain, with the majority of the pain being caused by treatment-related

EXHIBIT 7.2
Types of Pain Experienced by Children With Chronic Disease

AIDS	Cancer
Encephalopathy, medicine toxicity, neuropathies, pneumonia, esophagitis, diarrhea, infection, perforated bowel, spasticity, medicine toxicity	*Disease-related:* bone pain, headache, back pain caused by tumor infiltration of bones or soft tissue or compression of the central or peripheral nervous system *Treatment related:* mouth sores, neuropathy, phantom limb pain, infection, skin necrosis, gastritis

Cystic Fibrosis	Sickle Cell Disease
Headache, chest pain (pleuritic, rib fracture, pneumothorax), ulcer, gastritis, reflux, arthritis, back pain, limb pain	Vaso-occulusive episodes, extremity pain, abdominal pain

Juvenile Rheumatoid Arthritis	Fibromyalgia
Joint pain and stiffness	Persistent/pervasive musculoskeletal pain, headaches, irritable bowel symptoms

toxicity (Miser, Dothage, Wesley, & Miser, 1987). The presence of pain is also a defining feature of JRA (Jaworski, 1993) and juvenile primary fibromyalgia syndrome (Yunas, 1992). Although the statistics reported for pain experienced by children with chronic disease vary greatly, it is obvious that these children are at risk for suffering from multiorgan pain syndromes caused by the disease itself or the procedures and treatments required for illness management.

Finally, perhaps one of the most frequently investigated statistics is the incidence of inadequate pain treatment in children. Numerous studies indicate that medical personnel and parents underestimate, and consequently undertreat, the pain experiences of children (e.g., Bauchner, 1991; Cummings et al., 1996; Romsing, Moller-Sonnergaard, Hertel, & Rasmussen, 1996; Woodgate & Kristjanson, 1996). For example, sometimes children undergoing medical procedures such as lumbar punctures receive no analgesia, whereas adults receive local anesthetic for the same procedure (Bauchner, 1991). A summary of explanations suggested in the literature as to why children continue to receive inadequate pain management is found in Exhibit 7.3. Empirical validation of these factors is needed, however, before their usefulness in designing pain interventions for children can be appreciated.

EXHIBIT 7.3
Possible Reasons for the Inadequate Management of Pain in Children

Inaccurate pain assessment by adults	Belief that treatment should have been adequately effective despite child report of pain
Inadequate reassessment of pain control	
	Expectation that the child will necessarily experience some "discomfort"
Misconceptions about children's experience of pain (e.g., infants don't feel pain)	
	Minimal expectations of adults that pain can be effectively controlled
Standard approach to care versus individualized treatment	
	Cultural value judgment of parents and staff about pain and its treatment
Intermittent pain episodes are not observed by medical staff	
	Parental reluctance to "bother" medical staff for pain medication
Poor communication between medical staff, including delineation of responsibility for pain assessment and treatment	
	Inability of some children (e.g., infants) to effectively communicate pain
Expectation of daily reduction in medication despite evidence of pain	Child reluctance to report pain (e.g., doesn't want to appear weak; fear of injection used to administer pain medication)
Overestimation of the medication's benefits	
Misconceptions of drug safety (e.g., fear of dependence, tolerance, addiction)	

FACTORS CONTRIBUTING TO A CHILD'S PAIN EXPERIENCE

Several factors have been identified as potential contributors to a child's pain experience and consequently pain management. These factors include both the unique characteristics of the individual child, such as age, gender, temperament, and past experiences with pain, and environmental aspects associated with pain experiences, such as parental reactions. Such factors may be important to consider when assessing a child's pain management needs, as well as when developing an effective intervention. As mentioned in the introduction of this volume, cultural issues related to pain experiences are beginning to be studied. Despite much theoretical speculation about the effect of culture on pain, little empirical research has been reported that supports or refutes these ideas (B. A. Bernstein & Pachter, 1993).

Child Factors

Age and Gender

Age and gender have been investigated as two characteristics of the individual child that may contribute to the manner in which a child deals with pain. First, a child's age or developmental level may influence how a child reacts to a painful experience, as well as what types of coping strategies they use for pain management. Compared with older children, younger children often demonstrate greater overt behavioral distress, such as screaming and crying, and less physical control during painful medical procedures (Jacobsen et al., 1990; S. M. Jay, Elliott, Katz, & Siegel, 1987; Katz, Kellerman, & Siegel, 1980).

Some researchers have speculated that pain responses due to age differences may be influenced in part by social factors (Favaloro & Touzel, 1990; P. A. McGrath, 1993). Older children, especially adolescents, may suppress pain behaviors or underreport pain intensity to avoid looking socially incompetent or out of control (Favaloro & Touzel, 1990). LeBaron and Zeltzer (1984) reported, however, that when more subtle observations of children's pain responses are made, there were no significant differences in the number of behavioral reactions indicating distress in children and adolescents undergoing a bone marrow aspiration. Similarly, Carr, Lemanek, and Armstrong (1998) found no significant difference in the pain and fear reported by children younger and older than age 12 years old who underwent allergy skin testing.

In addition to influencing how a child copes with a painful procedure, age may also play a factor in chronic pain experiences. For example, Conner-Warren (1996) reported that older children with sickle cell disease reported greater levels of pain compared with younger children. It is difficult to determine, however, if the greater reports of pain were due the child's age, the increased severity of the disease, or most probably both factors. The results of these studies demonstrate the intricate relationship between age and a child's pain experience. In general, however, younger children may display more behavioral distress although their self-reports of pain may not differ from those of their older peers.

Gender has also been examined as a moderator of a child's pain experience. Some studies have shown that girls tend to demonstrate more behavioral distress during painful procedures (e.g., Hilgard & LeBaron, 1982; Katz et al., 1980) and report more postoperative pain (e.g., Favaloro & Touzel, 1990) than boys. Carr et al. (1998) also found that girls reported more pain associated with allergy skin testing than did the boys in the study. In contrast, Conner-Warren (1996) did not find any significant differences in the level of pain reported between boys and girls with sickle cell disease. Some of these discrepancies related to the effects of gender may be due to how pain is currently assessed. Available measures may be more sensitive to how girls typically express pain (e.g., crying, seeking emotional support) and may inaccurately evaluate the pain responses of boys.

Finally, age and gender have also been related to how many and what types of coping strategies a child uses to manage painful experiences. Hodgins and Lander (1997) reported that most of the 85 school-age children, ages 5–13, in their study used at least one coping strategy to deal with the pain of venipuncture. The most commonly used strategy was categorized as "direct efforts to maintain control," which included such behaviors as looking away, moving, talking, and controlling breathing. Younger children were found to both identify and use fewer coping strategies than older children. Younger children also used fewer cognitive strategies such as diversionary thinking than older children. Girls were found to use more coping strategies than boys, including more use of seeking support from an adult or a comforting toy. Overall, Hodgins and Lander reported that strategies described as behavioral (e.g., seeking information, breathing) were found to be more effective in helping these children cope with the pain of a venipuncture procedure compared with cognitive strategies (e.g., cognitive reappraisal, diversionary thinking).

In contrast, Curry and Russ (1985) found that school-age children ages 8–10 used more cognitive strategies such as positive restructuring (e.g., thinking good thoughts) than behavioral strategies for managing pain associated with dental procedures. Such differences reflect the fact that children use a variety of behavioral and cognitive strategies depending on the pain-related situation and may not demonstrate the stable use of one particular type of strategy (Curry & Russ, 1985; Gil, Wilson, & Edens, 1997). It appears that children may try different strategies until they find one that works.

The individual preferences of each child, as well as the instability of the preferred coping strategy, influence the type of preparation most appropriate for each child and further complicates the choice of pain management strategies. The reliable assessment of a child's coping strategies is difficult. At present, health care providers must rely on verbal reports of the parent's and child's past experiences and preferred coping strategies. Obviously, the younger the child, the less developed his or her verbal skills, so the less information that can be obtained regarding the child's coping styles. Nevertheless, age and gender factors should be considered when offering pain management interventions and also when assessing a child's level of pain or the effectiveness of an intervention. Because a child's preference for coping strategies may not be stable, consistent reassessment of the effectiveness of pain management techniques is required.

Temperament

Preliminary evidence suggests that a child's temperament may influence how he or she experiences pain. Aspects of a child's disposition that may be important for coping with a painful experience include the child's physiological responsiveness, behavioral adaptability and approaches to the painful situation, and threshold for the intensity of physiological and behavioral responses (Rudolph, Denning, & Weisz, 1995). For example, Lee and White-Traut (1996) found that children who were described as adaptable and positive displayed less distress during a venipuncture procedure than children labeled with "difficult" temperaments. The parents of the less-difficult children were more likely to prepare their children for a potentially painful procedure, suggesting that temperament may interact with parental factors that contribute to the pain experience as well. The authors concluded that temperament may play a modest role in a child's response to painful procedures and that assessing a child's temperament, including typical responses to pain, may be useful for those attempting to prepare a child for a procedure. Such questions are often a part of pain interviews with the parents and child, which are described in the "Assessment" section of this chapter.

Previous Experience With Pain

A child's previous experience with pain or painful procedures may also interplay with developmental characteristics to determine how a child will experience future pain. Children experience a wide range of painful experiences from scraped knees to broken bones. The intensity and duration of the sensory and emotional components of the painful experience are thought to influence how the child experiences his or her next pain-related event (P. A. McGrath, 1990). The relationship between past experience and how a child manages a more recent painful procedure, however, is complicated. For some children, such as those required to endure repeated bone marrow aspirations, past experience may do little to alleviate their distress about the procedure (S. M. Jay, Ozolins, Elliott, & Caldwell, 1983; Katz et al., 1980). Some studies have also shown that children with previous medical experience do not necessarily benefit as much as naive children from intervention strategies such as viewing a filmed peer model coping with the procedure (e.g., Faust & Melamed, 1984; Klorman, Hilpert, Michael, LaGana, & Sveen, 1980). Because of the potential influence past pain experiences may have on a child's current pain experience and receptiveness to intervention strategies, it is important to assess these experiences through child and parent interviews. Suggestions on how to conduct these assessments are discussed below in the section on "Pain Interviews."

Environmental Factors

One of the most important environmental factors that contributes to how children experience pain may be the response of their parents to the painful situation. Parents can have a direct and immediate impact on their child's response to pain during medical procedures, as well as to how the child responds to chronic pain. For example, Blount and colleagues found that when parents demonstrated behaviors such as reassuring, criticizing, or apologizing to their child during a painful medical procedure, the child's distress was greater than when parents engaged in other behaviors such as trying to distract the child (e.g., Blount et al., 1989; Blount, Sturges, & Powers, 1990).

A child's pain may also be moderated by their parents' reaction to chronic pain situations, such as those experienced with recurrent abdominal pain (RAP). Walker, Garber, and Greene (1993) reported that children with RAP perceived their parents to be more encouraging of illness or pain behavior than children who were well. The children with RAP reported receiving attention and special privileges when they displayed illness or pain-related behaviors. Thus, parents may encourage and maintain a child's expressions of pain by not only providing positive consequences but also by discouraging the child's use of appropriate coping strategies (Dunn-Geier, McGrath, Rourke, Latter, & D'Astous, 1986; Osborne, Hatcher, & Richtsmeier, 1989). Children with chronic pain also have higher incidences of family illness, providing more opportunities for modeling how to cope with pain (Walker et al., 1993). Such modeling may be detrimental to the child's pain experiences if the other family members do not cope effectively or if they receive positive reinforcement for their pain-related behaviors.

ASSESSMENT OF PAIN IN CHILDREN

Three main purposes for assessing a child's pain experience are to obtain information about the child's current level of distress or pain, to investigate factors that may affect the child's current and past pain experiences, and to monitor and document the effectiveness of pain management interventions. To effectively manage a child's pain, one must conduct a comprehensive assessment of the many components that affect the child's pain experience. Such assessments often involve interviewing the parent and child about factors that may affect the child's pain experience, including characteristics of the pain, pain-related perceptions, and environmental factors (P. A. McGrath, 1990; Varni, Thompson, & Hanson, 1987). In addition to such an interview, numerous measures are available to assist the child and caregivers in providing a quantification of pain based on child self-reports, adult reports of the child's pain, and physiological indices. A description of pain interviews and other assessment methods is provided below and is summarized in Exhibit 7.4. With the exception of the physiological measures, the instruments included are those that report acceptable psychometric properties, and most have been used in pain intervention studies. The tools included in this chapter are also feasible for use in clinical settings, with some scales specifically designed to facilitate their clinical utility (e.g., Schade, Joyce, Gerkensmeyer, & Keck, 1996).

EXHIBIT 7.4
Examples of Clinical Assessment Measures for Child Pain and Distress

Pain Interviews	Child's Report of Pain/Distress
Pain Experience History (Acute Pain Management Guideline Panel, 1992)	Poker chip tool (Hester, 1979)
	Faces (e.g., LeBaron & Zeltzer, 1984)
General Acute Pain Assessment Form (P. A. McGrath, 1990)	Oucher (Beyer & Aradine, 1986)
Children's Comprehensive Pain Questionnaire (P. A. McGrath, 1990)	Visual analog scales
	Line indicators
	Pain thermometer
Varni/Thompson Pediatric Pain Questionnaire (Varni, Thompson, & Hanson, 1987)	Pain diaries

Adult Reports of Child's Pain/ Distress	Physiological Measures
Riley Infant Pain Scale (Schade, Joyce, Gerkensmeyer, & Keck, 1996)	Pulse rate
	Respiration rate
	Cortisol and cortisone levels
Nursing Assessment of Pain Inventory (Stevens, 1990).	Beta-endorphin levels
	Palmar sweating
Likert scales	
Visual Analog Scale	

Pain Interviews

Interviews for Acute Pain

Before providing an intervention to address a child's acute or chronic pain, clinicians must obtain background information about a child's pain experiences and related factors that may affect pain management efforts. Children with acute pain management needs may come to the attention of the clinician when such children are required to experience repetitive acute pain such as that associated with bone marrow aspirations, venipunctures, or growth hormone injections. Table 7.1 illustrates brief interviews with the child and the parent that can be used to guide pain management for acute pain often associated with medical procedures.

P. A. McGrath (1990) offered a more comprehensive acute pain interview that is appropriate for both outpatient and inpatient evaluations. This structured interview provides a way of collecting general demographic information, information on hospital experiences, and typical pain experiences

TABLE 7.1
Pain Experience History for Acute Pain Management

Child Form	Parent Form
Tell me what pain is.	What word(s) does your child use in regard to pain?
Tell me about the hurt you have had before.	Describe the pain experiences your child has had before.
Do you tell others when you hurt? If yes, who?	Does your child tell you or others when he/she is hurting?
What do you do for yourself when you are hurting?	How do you know when your child is in pain?
What do you want others to do for you when you hurt?	How does your child usually react to pain?
What don't you want others to do for you when you hurt?	What do you do for your child when he/she is hurting?
What helps the most to take your hurt away?	What does your child do for himself/herself when he/she is hurting?
Is there anything special that you want me to know about you when you hurt? (If yes, have child describe)	What works best to decrease or take away your child's pain?
	Is there anything special that you would like me to know about your child and pain? (If yes, describe.)

Note. From *Acute Pain Management in Infants, Children, and Adolescents: Operative and Medical Procedures. Quick Reference Guide for Clinicians,* by the Acute Pain Management Guideline Panel (AHCPR Publication No. 92-0020), 1992, Rockville, MD: Agency for Health Care Policy and Research, Public Health Service, U.S. Department of Health and Human Services.

for children in the hospital such as finger pricks and dressing changes. The parents' perceptions of how their child typically reacts to various pain experiences are thoroughly assessed, along with their typical response to their child's pain or distress.

These interviews can assist the clinician in choosing the most suitable intervention for the patient and can facilitate communication about pain by allowing the clinician to use the child's language to describe pain experiences and the expected outcomes of intervention. For example, the clinician could tell the child, "You are going to feel a little boo-boo on your arm but if you blow these bubbles, the boo-boo will go away faster." The answers to interview questions can also alert clinicians to possible difficulties with cooperation on the part of the child or parent with recommended interventions.

Interviews for Recurrent or Chronic Pain

More extensive questioning may be needed to effectively assess and intervene with children who are experiencing recurrent or chronic pain.

These children may be referred to a clinician to supplement pharmacological pain interventions or when standard medical pain management has failed to bring the child sufficient relief. P. A. McGrath (1990) provided a structured interview that assesses pain history components relevant to recurrent and chronic pain experiences. This interview is designed to collect information about the child's sensory experience of the pain, past efforts at pain relief, and emotional and environmental factors that may impact the pain experience and treatment. It also includes affective facial scales and visual analog scales that are described later in this section.

Another interview tool for assessing recurrent and chronic pain is the Varni/Thompson Pediatric Pain Questionnaire (PPQ), which was developed and validated by Varni and his colleagues (Gragg et al., 1996; Varni et al., 1987). Similar to P. A. McGrath's (1990) interview, this questionnaire includes a structured parent and child interview to assess the child's pain history and subjective pain experiences, including sensory and affective aspects of pain. To assess the sensory experiences of pain, the clinician first asks the child to describe the pain, then shows the child a list of words that may assist the child in his or her descriptive efforts. The PPQ also asks questions about the family pain history as well as other socioenvironmental factors that may influence the child's pain experience. A body outline is included for the child to indicate the location and intensity of his or her pain using colors. In addition, a visual analog scale is provided to assist the child and parent in measuring pain intensity. The PPQ is a comprehensive instrument that combines both structured interview questions with methods for quantifying the child's pain.

P. A. McGrath (1987) offered some useful suggestions to clinicians for conducting interviews with children experiencing pain, such as recommending that the interview be completed in a relaxing setting where the child has some privacy. The child should be informed of the confidential nature of his or her answers. It may also be helpful to tell the child that the information is vital to the clinician's understanding of the child's pain and how best to help him or her manage it. If the child begins to appear distressed about a particular line of questioning, move on to less threatening questions. Finally, despite the structured format of some pain interviews, children should be allowed to elaborate on any questions that might be particularly relevant or important to them.

Child Reports of Pain

Numerous assessment methods are available to help children report their experience of pain to others. A description of some recommended self-report measures, including their descriptions for use and advantages and disadvantages, is found in Table 7.2.

TABLE 7.2
Pain as Impairment-Recommended Self-Report Measures in Children

Measure	Description	Indications for Use	Advantages	Disadvantages
Self-report measures	Child is asked about intensity, rhythm, and variations in pain	Adequate cognitive and communicative abilities	Simple and efficient Can be administered easily	Subject to bias (e.g., demand characteristics, inaccurate or selective memory)
Poker chip tool (Hester, 1979)	Child chooses 1 to 4 chips ("pieces of hurt")	4–8 years old	Correlates with overt behaviors in injections Adequate convergent validity Partial support for discriminate validity	May be childish for older children
Faces Scale (Bieri et al., 1990)	Faces indicating intensity were derived from children's drawings	6–8 years old	Strong agreement among children regarding pain severity of faces and consistency of intervals Adequate test–retest reliability	Validity studies not yet completed
Visual Analog Scale (VAS)	Vertical or horizontal line with verbal, facial, or numerical anchors on a continuum of pain intensity	5 years and older	Reliable and valid (e.g., child report correlates with behavioral measures and with parent, nurse, physician ratings) Versatile (can rate different dimensions—pain and affect on same scale)	Must understand proportionally Intervals on numerical scales may not be equal from a child's perspective

(continued)

TABLE 7.2 *(continued)*

Measure	Description	Indications for Use	Advantages	Disadvantages
Oucher Scale (Beyer & Wells, 1989)	Six photos of children's faces indicated intensity; 100-point corresponding vertical scale	3–12 years	Reliable; adequate content validity; correlates with other VAS scales Presentation of both pictorial and numerical scales is applicable for broader age range	See VAS
Pain diary	Numerical ratings are repeated, along with recording of other relevant information (e.g., time, activity, medication)	Older child/adolescent Measurement of chronic or recurrent pain (e.g., headache, limb pain, or cancer pain)	Adequate interrater reliability between parent and child Useful in determining patters of pain and in teaching self-management strategies (thereby providing a sense of mastery)	Requires commitment to record regularly and accurately Requires effort and prompting if moving from one situation to another (memory over time is rarely accurate)

Note. From "Assessment and Measurement of Pain in Children" (p. 99), by J. R. Mathews, P. J. McGrath, & H. Pigeon. In N. L. Schechter, C. B. Berde, & M. Yaster (Eds.). *Pain in Infants, Children, and Adolescents,* 1993, Baltimore: MD: Williams & Wilkins. Copyright 1993 by Williams & Wilkins. Reprinted with permission.

Pictorial Scales

Scales that use pictures or photographs depicting pain intensity are often used for younger children, whereas scales with numeric quantifications are used for older children. For example, Hester and her colleagues (Hester, 1979; Hester, Foster, & Kristensen, 1990) have developed the Poker Chip Tool to help young children express the amount of pain they feel associated with medical procedures such as immunizations (see Exhibit 7.5). This method has been used effectively with children ages 3–15 (Hester, 1979; Romsing et al., 1996). Four poker chips are used to quantify pain as "pieces" of hurt. Thus, one chip represents the least amount of pain a child is experiencing or has experienced, whereas four chips represent the worst pain the child could have. The number of chips chosen by the child can then be the focus of discussion and pain management efforts, both pharmacological and psychological.

Likert-type scales using children's faces depicting various levels of pain are also commonly used as a visual method for measuring pain and fear intensity in children. Two examples of such scales are the Faces (LeBaron & Zeltzer, 1984) and the Oucher (Beyer & Aradine, 1986, 1987). Facial scales typically consist of line drawings of unisex children expressing increasing levels of distress from neutral to intense pain. Children are typically asked to rate their pain before and after a procedure (e.g., LeBaron & Zeltzer, 1984; S. M. Jay, Elliott, Fitzgibbons, Woody, & Siegel, 1995). Similar scales with drawings depicting various levels of fear have also been used in addition to the pain scales (e.g., S. M. Jay et al., 1995; S. M. Jay, Elliott, Woody, & Siegel, 1991). As with most of the other measures, facial scales, including the Faces, have been used to assess pain related to medical procedures as well as to evaluate the effectiveness of pain management interventions

EXHIBIT 7.5
Poker Chip Tool

1. Place four poker chips horizontally in front of the child on a firm surface.
2. Point each chip one at a time and say "These are pieces of hurt."
3. Point to the chip on the child's left side and say "This is a little bit of hurt."
4. Move hands along chips and point to the fourth chip and say "And this is the most hurt you could ever have."
5. Ask the child "How many pieces of hurt do you have right now?"
6. Reiterate the child's level of hurt and discuss if needed (e.g., "So you have a little bit of hurt? What can make it feel better?")
7. Record the child's response on the appropriate charting if indicated.
8. Use child's responses to monitor and adapt pain management strategies.

Note. From "The Preoperational Child's Reaction to Immunization," by N. Hester, 1979, *Nursing Research, 28,* 250–256. Copyright 1979 by Lippincott Williams & Wilkins. Adapted with permission.

(L. L. Cohen, Blount, & Panopoulos, 1997; S. M. Jay et al., 1995; Pfefferbaum, Adams, & Aceves, 1990). The Faces scale has also been demonstrated to be a reliable instrument for assessing self-reported pain in Hispanic children (Pfefferbaum et al., 1990). A version of a facial scale used by McGrath and her colleagues (e.g. P. A. McGrath, 1990; P. A. McGrath, deVeber, & Hearn, 1985) is reproduced in Figure 7.1.

The Oucher scale (Beyer & Aradine, 1986, 1987) is another visual scale that has been used to measure pain intensity in children. This poster-like instrument comprises six photographs of a Caucasian child depicting various levels of pain on one side and a corresponding vertical number scale from 0 to 100 on the other side. The two different measurement systems on the same scale are provided to accommodate children who may want to use pictures or numbers to represent their pain (Beyer & Aradine, 1987). The actual photographs of children may also be more attractive and readily interpreted by young children than abstract or line drawings (Villarruel & Denyes, 1991). Similar to the other pictorial scales, the Oucher can be used to assess pain related to procedures or pain associated with recurrent or chronic illness. Alternative versions of the Oucher have also been validated for children of minority populations using photographs of Hispanic and African American children (Conner-Warren, 1996; Villarruel & Denyes, 1991).

Visual Analog Scales

Once a child can understand the concepts of order and numbering, other measures of pain may be useful as well. Variations of a visual analog

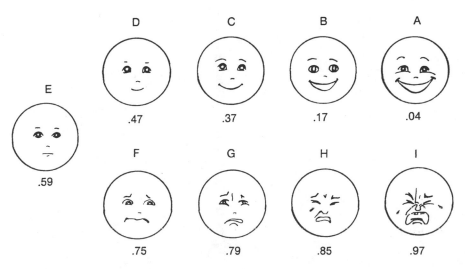

FIGURE 7.1. Example of a pain affect facial scale.

Note. From *Pain in Children: Nature, Assessment, and Treatment* (p. 76), by P. A. McGrath, 1990, New York: Guilford Press. Copyright 1990 by Guilford Press. Reprinted with permission.

scale are often used to help children quantify their pain for the adults involved in their care. Visual analog scales that have been used with children include simple horizontal or vertical line drawings with the increased length or height of the line indicating more severe pain. Some scales include written anchors to assist the child in interpreting the scale (e.g., no pain to severe pain), whereas others require the examiner to explain the scale using verbal anchors. The child makes a mark on the line where he or she interprets his or her current level of pain. Seymour, Simpson, and Charlton (1985) reported that a visual analog scaling line of 10 cm has the least amount of measurement error compared with lines that are 5 and 20 cm in length. Again, such scales have been used to obtain self-reports of procedure-related pain and recurrent or chronic pain. For example, Walco, Varni, and Ilowite (1992) asked children with juvenile rheumatoid arthritis, or JRA, to mark a visual analog scale in the morning and evening to indicate their intensity of pain. The children also marked the scale during acute pain episodes and after using cognitive–behavioral strategies to evaluate the effectiveness of these strategies.

Another visual analog scale used in pain research with children is the pain thermometer. An example of a pain thermometer is displayed in Figure 7.2.

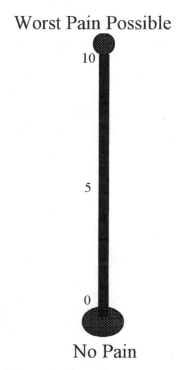

FIGURE 7.2. Example of a pain thermometer.

This method uses a picture of a vertical thermometer numbered from 0 to 10, with 0 indicating *no pain* and 10 portraying the *worst pain possible*. Children are required to indicate, typically by marking or coloring up the thermometer, "how much" hurt they experienced during a procedure. The pain thermometer can also be used for children who suffer from recurrent or chronic pain. As with the other visual analog scales, it is important to be sure that the child understands numerical concepts to use the pain thermometer accurately.

Pain Diaries

One of the most commonly used methods of assessing chronic or recurrent pain episodes is the use of a pain diary. Pain diaries may be most effective with children over the age of 8 years and are useful for monitoring fluctuations and trends in a child's pain experiences (Brown, 1996). An example of a pain diary is found in Exhibit 7.6. Typically, the child provides some type of quantitative rating for his or her pain, either by assigning a number to it or by using a visual analog scale. Relevant information, such as the time of the rating and concurrent activities, is also recorded. In addition, the child may be asked to record his or her use of pain management strategies, both pharmacological and nonpharmacological, and postintervention ratings. These ratings can be used to assist in monitoring treatment effectiveness.

As with most self-report measures, a child's self-report of pain has limitations. One may be the lack of credibility that adults give to such reports, especially if the child is not "behaving" like he or she is in pain (Cassidy & Walco, 1996). Despite a child's report of pain, medical personnel may rely on a parent's or their own assessment of pain based on their own criteria. Children are able, however, to accurately report their pain from approximately 4 to 5 years of age and should be given primary consideration when a pain assessment is made (Cassidy & Walco, 1996; P. A. McGrath, 1987).

Adult Reports of Child's Pain

The use of adult reports of the child's pain is another method of assessing a child's level of pain. The observations and perceptions of parents and nursing staff who have contact with the child are most often used. Adult reports may be particularly important for the preverbal child or for the child with disabilities that may preclude effective communication. Unfortunately, infants are particularly difficult to assess because of the inconsistent responses of their nervous system. For example, infants, especially those who are preterm, have variable physiological and behavioral responses to painful stimuli, demonstrate rapid changes in states of alertness, have a low threshold for stimulation, and show less physiological distinction between responses to innocuous stimuli, stress, and pain (Andrews & Fitzgerald, 1997).

EXHIBIT 7.6
Pain Diary

Date/ time started	Time ended	Type of pain	Location of pain	Intensity 1–10	What were you doing when it started?	What did you do to stop it?	Intensity 1–10 after trying to stop it

Health care providers and parents who are charged with managing a preverbal or nonverbal child's pain must typically rely on their observations of the child's behaviors, such as facial expressions, body movements, vocalizations, and responsiveness to touch. Consequently, the preverbal pain scales that have been developed generally include numeric rating scales to assist these adults in quantifying the child's level of such behaviors. Two examples of scales that have been used to assess infant pain in research studies are the Nursing Assessment of Pain Intensity (NAPI; Stevens, 1990) and the Riley Infant Pain Scale (RIPS; Joyce et al., 1994; Schade et al., 1996). The RIPS (Schade et al., 1996) was refined from a measure developed by Joyce et al. to provide health care providers with a practical and comprehensive measurement of pain intensity in pediatric patients. This scale requires the health care provider to rate the intensity of the behavior in each category, such as body movements, on a scale from 0 to 3, with 3 indicating greatest severity. A total pain intensity score is then calculated. Clinically, such a score would be used to monitor the effectiveness of pain management efforts such as medication for preverbal children following surgery or in pain as the result of a chronic disease state. Schade et al.'s study extended the reliability and validity data of these scales to children under the age of 1 month old and to children with cerebral palsy whose disabilities limit their ability to self-report. The NAPI provides similar information using a 0-to-3 scale and also includes rating of vocal responses. These types of measures may be most useful to the clinician who serves children in the hospital setting. Parents could also use such a measure to monitor medical and behavioral intervention effectiveness at home, reporting their findings to their clinician during outpatient appointments.

Parents and health care providers may also be asked to rate their perceptions of a child's pain using visual analog scales similar to those used by children. The scales for adults include horizontal or vertical lines with anchor points representing various levels of the behavior being measured, such as pain or fear (e.g., *no fear* or *most fear possible*). For example, Blount et al. (1992) used visual analog scales for parents to assess how much procedure-related fear and pain their child experienced, as well as to rate how much they were able to help their child during the procedure. A simple 5- or 7-point Likert scale is another way adults have been asked to rate a child's pain (e.g., Kazak et al., 1996; Manne et al., 1990). A caution should be noted about the use of parent report for assisting in the evaluation and treatment of pediatric pain. Although it is safe to assume that parents know their child better than a health care provider, it may also be true that the parents have never seen their child experiencing significant amounts of pain and thus may also have a difficult time accurately assessing it (Woodgate & Kristjanson, 1996).

Physiological Measures of Pain

When a child experiences a painful stimulus, measurable physiological changes occur. Although direct correlations cannot be made between physiological changes and a child's experience with pain, several physiological responses to pain, such as pulse rates, respiration rates, cortisol and beta-endorphin levels, and palmar sweating, continue to be the focus of research (P. A. McGrath, 1990). Some of these responses, such as pulse rates, cortisol levels, and sweating, have been found to increase when a child is in apparent distress related to a medical procedure (e.g., Johnston, Stevens, Yang, & Horton, 1995). Similar responses have also been found, however, when the child is involved in innocuous activities (e.g., being weighed, pretend procedures; Craig, Whitfield, Grunau, Linton, & Hadjistavropoulos, 1993). Thus, it is difficult to know whether changes in physiology are due to anxiety, distress, pain, or conditioned physiological responses (P. A. McGrath, 1990).

Despite the lack of clear evidence that physiological measures are accurate indicators of pain in children, some studies have used them as evidence of intervention outcomes. For example, S. M. Jay et al. (1987) reported that children involved in a cognitive–behavioral intervention had significantly lower pulse rates prior to a bone marrow aspiration, suggesting less distress, than children in a control group. Due to the lack of sensitivity and specificity of physiological measures, the current recommendation is that physiological measures only be used as adjunct assessment tools when evaluating pain in children (Acute Pain Management Guideline Panel, 1992).

INTERVENTIONS FOR PAIN MANAGEMENT

Interventions designed to assist children with pain management have included both pharmacological and nonpharmacological approaches. The simultaneous use of these approaches is often suggested as the most effective means of addressing pediatric pain (Kuttner, 1997; Leith & Weisman, 1997a), although unfortunately nonpharmacological strategies are sometimes requested only after pharmacological treatments fail. An overview of common pharmacological treatment options for children with pain is provided below. Because of the nature of this chapter, however, this review is brief and intended only to familiarize the reader with more frequently used options for medical intervention of pain in children. Nonpharmacological pain intervention strategies follow the discussion of pharmacological treatments. These include interventions for pain associated with medical procedures, with recurrent medical conditions, and with chronic diseases such as JRA.

Pharmacological Interventions

Procedure-Related (Acute) Pain

The information in this section is based on recommendations made in a clinical practice guideline developed by the Agency for Health Care Policy and Research and distributed by the U.S. Department of Health and Human Services for acute pain management in children (Acute Pain Management Guideline Panel, 1992). Although medical practices in individual medical facilities may differ, these guidelines provide basic information about standard, acceptable pharmacological interventions for children experiencing acute pain related to medical and operative procedures. The interested reader is also referred to Leith and Weisman (1997b) and Morton (1998) for more extensive reviews of common pharmacological interventions for children.

The usual initial step for addressing procedure-related pain is to provide the child with analgesics (e.g., acetaminophen, ibuprofen), local anesthetics (e.g., Lidocaine, EMLA cream), or both. These treatments are used to reduce pain associated with procedure preparation such as needle sticks or central venous access port punctures.

If a child is anxious, an oral or intravenous sedative or medication to reduce anxiety (e.g., anxiolytic) may also be provided to reduce anxiety and promote sedation. Such anxiety-relieving medications are generally not considered to be pain-relievers, however. Analgesic effects may be achieved by using oral, intravenous, or transmucosal opiods given in increments and titrated to an effective level. Finally, general anesthesia (e.g., nitrous oxide, ketamine) may also be used by trained personnel with appropriate monitoring mechanisms in place. Because of the possible negative impact of anxiety with an initial procedure, it is important to provide maximum pain and anxiety treatment at the time of the first procedure to decrease the development of anticipatory anxiety or increased resistance.

Postoperative pain is often managed using opiod and nonopiod analgesics. Opiods such as codeine and nonsterodial antiinflammatory drugs (NSAIDs) are used to manage pain associated with minor surgery, whereas regional or parenteral opiods are options for managing pain after major surgery. Patient-controlled analgesic (PCA) devices are also being investigated as a promising technology for acute pain control in the pediatric population. These devices, which have been used extensively with adults, allow the patient to control the delivery of analgesics, typically opiods such as morphine, at a rate that addresses their pain needs. Empirical investigations of PCA for procedure-related pain in children are few, however, and show mixed support for its effectiveness (Kotzer, Coy, & LeClaire, 1998; Tyler, 1990; Williams, 1996). Kotzer et al. suggested that patients and families may need more education addressing their fears about PCA, such as overdosing and addiction, before this method of drug administration will be consistently effective in the pediatric population.

Recurrent and Disease-State Pain

The pharmacological treatment of choice for pain associated with recurrent medical conditions and chronic disease states is often disease-specific. Some general statements can be made, however, regarding typical pain medications for such disorders. Pain is often managed using an analgesic "ladder," starting with nonopiod analgesics for mild pain, adding weak opiods for moderate pain, and then strong opiods for more severe pain (Miser, 1993).

Other issues such as dosing schedules (as needed or continuous), available routes of administration, and a long-term pain management plan are also considered when determining the appropriate choice of medication.

More specifically, NSAIDs have been suggested as a common, initial medical therapy for both hospital and home use for pain associated with cystic fibrosis (Ravilly, Robinson, Suresh, Wohl, & Berde, 1996) and JRA (Varni & Bernstein, 1991). JRA is also treated with antirheumatic drugs, such as oral or injectable gold and methotrexate, should initial drug therapies prove to be inadequate (Walco & Oberlander, 1993). These drugs often do not work beyond a certain dosage and have variable action, resulting in "breakthrough" pain, adding to the challenge of effective pharmacological management for patients with JRA.

Pain management strategies for children with cancer also include the use of analgesic ladders, which guide the physician in choosing the appropriate drug on the basis of the child's source of pain, available routes for administration, potential side effects, the child's level of pain, and environmental factors. These same strategies have also been recommended for treating pediatric pain associated with AIDS (Wishnie & Weisman, 1997). Pain management recommendations for these two diseases also support continuous administration of appropriate medications rather than use on an "as-needed" basis.

Opiods are often considered for children with chronic disease pain in addition to the use of nonopiod analgesics or after first-line therapies such as the NSAIDS fail (Ravilly et al., 1996; Wishnie & Weisman, 1997). Children with sickle cell disease, in particular, are often started on opiods as a first-line therapy at a very young age, depending on the severity of their pain (B. S. Shapiro, 1993).

The use of PCA has also been suggested as an effective pain management strategy for pediatric patients with chronic diseases such as sickle cell (Morton, 1998). Similar to the use of PCA for procedure-related pain, the effectiveness of PCA for chronic pain in pediatric patients has not been established. If children are experiencing intractable pain that is not being adequately managed by routine medications, the child may receive an opiod drug such as morphine through a spinal epidural.

Neuroleptics (tranquilizers) and antidepressants are also used as adjuvant medications for management of chronic pain (Leith & Weisman, 1997b; P. A. McGrath, 1990). These medications are often prescribed to assist patients with sleep, anxiety, and other factors that may negatively affect their pain.

A Comment About Opiod Drugs

The literature suggests that pain management in children may be less than effective, in part because of fears about dependence or addiction to pain medication, specifically opiods. Although opiod dependence requiring weaning may develop after prolonged treatment of at least 2 weeks (Shannon & Berde, 1989), addiction in children using opiods for analgesic purposes is considered to be uncommon (Acute Pain Management Guideline Panel, 1992; Cassidy & Walco, 1996; P. J. McGrath, 1996). Still, many physicians and parents are reluctant to use opiods to manage the child's pain. Their concern may stem from confusion about physiological dependence, resulting in increased drug tolerance, and psychological addiction.

P. J. McGrath (1996) recommended that physicians and parents be educated about the differences among dependence, tolerance, and addiction to facilitate the appropriate choice of analgesic medication to adequately alleviate the child's pain. Despite these controversies and misconceptions, there does seem to be a general agreement in the literature that opiod medications can be highly effective when managed properly and should not be withheld from children who need them for pain management.

Nonpharmacological Interventions

In general, the most well-researched, nonpharmacological intervention for pain management in children has been cognitive–behavioral therapy (CBT). CBT uses a wide variety of strategies to assist the child in developing and applying coping skills to manage pain and, when developmentally appropriate, to understand that thoughts and behavior can influence how pain is experienced (Keefe, 1996). CBT treatment strategies typically include breathing exercises, distraction, imagery, relaxation training, modeling, behavioral rehearsal, and reinforcement. Currently, support for the empirical validity of CBT varies across the type of pain being treated. Other nonpharmacological interventions such as hypnosis and biofeedback also have some support as valid pain treatments and are reviewed where applicable.

Pain Associated With Medical Procedures

The pain that children experience associated with medical procedures has been one of the most commonly researched topics in pediatric psychology. The majority of research has been done on pain associated with bone marrow aspirations and lumbar punctures, with less intervention research conducted on postoperative pain and pain associated with dental procedures or immunizations. Powers (1999) conducted a comprehensive review of intervention studies for procedure-related pain and found that CBT could be offered as a well-established treatment based on the Chambless criteria (Chambless et al., 1996; Task Force on Promotion and Dissemination of Psychological Procedures, 1995). The CBT components below are commonly used to address pain associated with medical procedures; they are followed by a discussion of other promising interventions for procedure-related

TABLE 7.3
Interventions for Addressing Procedure-Related Pain and Anxiety

	Before Procedure	During Procedure	After Procedure
Breathing Exercises	X	X	X
Party blower			
Paced counting			
Blowing bubbles			
Pretending to inflate or deflate a tire			
Distraction	X	X	X
Nonprocedural talk			
Humor			
Videotapes, games			
Bubbles			
Party blowers			
Interactive books			
Live music			
Imagery	X	X	X
Guided (enchanted forest)			
Relaxation training	X	X	X
Progressive muscle relaxation			
Filmed modeling	X		
Coping model			
Reinforcement	X	X	X
Stickers, toys, games, small trophies			
Rehearsal/Coaching	X		
Modeling, practice on doll, parent, psychologist, child			
Coaching to remind child to use strategies			
Hypnosis	X	X	X

pain, such as hypnosis. Table 7.3 provides information relevant to when each strategy may be used to help a child manage procedure-related pain.

Cognitive–Behavioral Therapy

Breathing exercises. Breathing exercises can actively divert a child's attention from the painful procedure. "Active" breathing may be elicited by having the child blow into a party blower during the procedure (e.g., Blount, Powers, Cotter, Swan, & Free, 1994) or by having the child count aloud while breathing (e.g., Kazak et al., 1996). Children can also be taught breathing exercises that use familiar experiences, such as pretending to pump up and deflate a tire (e.g., Jay, Elliott, Ozolins, Olson, & Pruitt, 1985) or pretending to blow on hot soup or blow bubbles to practice controlled breathing. Such strategies should be modeled and practiced before the procedure to increase the likelihood of their success in managing the child's pain.

Distraction. Distraction as a pain-management procedure refers to the patient, either alone or with the aid of a parent or clinician, engaging in a behavior that will "take his or her mind off" the painful procedure. While the child is being prepared for or is receiving the procedure, the parent or clinician talks with the child about nonprocedural topics or engages the child in video games, cartoons, bubbles, party blowers, or musical books (e.g., L. L. Cohen et al., 1997; Kazak et al., 1996). Other strategies have included directing the child to look for hidden objects in the procedure room (Elliott & Olson, 1983) or having the child look at an engaging poster while listening to a story through earphones (Stark et al., 1989). Many of these options are used because of their potential for surprise and interactive play, such as requiring the child to actively push buttons or search for objects on pages. Live music has also been suggested as an effective distraction technique for decreasing children's distress during procedures such as venipunctures and heel sticks, especially for infants (Malone, 1996).

Imagery. Imagery is a cognitive strategy that is used to encourage the child to cope effectively with the pain associated with the procedure instead of engaging in avoidance behaviors (S. M. Jay et al., 1987). Two types of imagery techniques, emotive and guided, are described in the intervention literature for procedure-related pain.

Emotive imagery, first described by Lazarus and Abramovitz (1962), involves having the child imagine scenarios that can elicit anxiety-inhibiting emotions such as pride or excitement. The most frequently reported emotive image that children undergoing medical procedures have been encouraged to develop is one that involves their favorite superhero. Typically, the clinician engages the child in discussions to determine his or her favorite hero image, then develops a story line incorporating the hero and the sensations of the medical experience (e.g., Jay et al., 1995; S. M. Jay et al., 1987). Children may be told that they are to go on a special mission for the hero that includes an act of bravery. The clinician then uses vivid detail of the visual, auditory, and kinesthetic experiences that accompany this mission and incorporates the physical sensations of the procedure into the image. For example, if the procedure involves pressure, the health care provider may describe how the child is trying to squeeze through a tight place in order to proceed with the mission. Such imagery techniques may require the parent or clinician to be present during the entire procedure to assist the child in developing and maintaining the story line. Older children, however, may be able to generate and practice their own images, especially for familiar, predictable procedures.

Another type of imagery strategy that has been used to help children cope with procedure-related pain is guided imagery (e.g., Elliott & Olson, 1983; Kazak et al., 1996). Guided imagery typically involves having the child imagine a relaxing scene and describing the elements and sensations of that scene to promote reduced anxiety and calmness during the procedure (Exhibit 7.7 describes elements that can be included in the image scenario). Common themes include sunny places, oceans or lakes, beaches, enchanted forests, caves, and amusement parks. For example, Elliott and Olson (1983) asked children undergoing painful treatments for burns to imagine they were floating in the ocean during hydrotherapy. Guided images can be used following the emotive strategies to facilitate relaxation after the child has experienced a sense of mastery over the situation. Similar to the emotive imagery, these techniques may require the assistance of a clinician or adult for younger children during the medical procedure. The image can also be tape recorded for the child to listen to during the procedure.

Relaxation training. Relaxation training has been used to assist with pain management in a wide variety of medical disorders. Such training is often offered as a way to help children identify their own bodily sensations associated with tension and learn how to relax. Typically, relaxation training involves deep-breathing strategies and the systematic tensing and relaxing of each separate muscle group in the body to facilitate patients' recognition of their bodily state. Age-appropriate analogies for the tensing and relaxing process can increase the appeal of these exercises. For example, the child can be told to pretend to squeeze a lemon in each hand as hard as he or she can for several seconds, then let it drop to the floor. A description of progressive muscle relaxation exercises appropriate for children is found in Appendix B.

EXHIBIT 7.7
Suggested Elements to Include in Guided Images

Element	Examples
Visual	Color of the water, trees, rocks, sky, plants; brightness; contrast; movement of the water, trees, animals
Auditory	Sound of the waves, animals, wind, child's deep breathing, soft music
Olfactory	Smell of the air, water, plants, flowers, trees
Kinesthetic	Feel of the ground, sun, wind, sand, rocks on child's feet, arms, hands, body; feel of child's deep breathing
Emotional	Peacefulness, calm, worry free, relaxed, happy, in control

Such relaxation training may be incorporated with the imagery techniques described above. The child may have to be coached to use these strategies appropriately during medical procedures because tensing may create more pain in some situations. Thus, these strategies may be most useful while the child is preparing for or recovering from the procedure. Similar to the imagery techniques, the steps of progressive muscle relaxation can also be recorded for the child to listen to and practice when needed.

Modeling. Modeling refers to the use of a person or an inanimate object, such as a doll, that a child can watch to see how medical procedures are conducted and how the model responds. Modeling can be an important strategy to include when a child's fears may be based on lack of information and when the behavior of the child (e.g., needing to lie still) is integral to the performance of the medical procedure (Dahlquist, 1992). The rationale behind using a peer model is that the child may be motivated to cope effectively or "master" the procedure as demonstrated by the model (S. M. Jay et al., 1985).

The type of modeling used most frequently to help children cope with painful medical procedures incorporates the use of a filmed peer model procedure (e.g., S. M. Jay et al., 1987, 1995). Jay and colleagues used a brief peer modeling film (11 to 12 minutes) as one component of their CBT intervention. The filmed peer model typically narrates the steps of the procedure, describes negative thoughts and feelings, demonstrates positive coping strategies such as positive self-talk, and ultimately copes effectively with the procedure.

Two factors that may be important when considering the use of modeling is the time available between the model exposure and the procedure, and a child's prior medical experience. Dahlquist (1992) suggested that modeling may not be the most effective strategy available to help children cope with a pending medical procedure if there is not sufficient time between viewing the model and participating in the procedure. For example, Faust and Melamed (1984) found that children who viewed a filmed model the same day as their surgery did not demonstrate any decrease in anxiety during the procedure. In comparison, children who saw the same film the night before the surgery demonstrated decreased self-reported anxiety and palmar sweating. Melamed and Siegel (1980) found, however, that children under the age of 7 years old might receive the most benefit from modeling if they view the video close to the time of the medical procedure. Thus, age seems to play a mediating role in the effect of the timing of the modeling and should be considered when using this strategy.

The effectiveness of this CBT component may be affected by a child's prior medical experience. For example, Melamed and Siegel (1980) found that children who had had prior operative procedures showed higher levels of emotion the night before surgery, regardless of whether or not they were shown a filmed model of the procedure. Other studies have also shown that filmed peer modeling was not effective in reducing procedure-related anxiety for children with previous medical experience and may, in fact, increase anxiety in such children (e.g., Faust & Melamed, 1984; Melamed, Dearborn, & Hermecz, 1983). The lack of therapeutic findings associated with peer modeling for children with previous medical experience may be due to the fact that the information provided by the model is not new or helpful in alleviating the child's anxieties about the procedure (Dahlquist, 1992). Thus, a child's prior medical experience may be important to consider when developing individualized strategies for pain management.

Positive reinforcement. Many different reinforcers or incentives have been used to elicit cooperation in children undergoing painful medical procedures. Stickers, small toys, trophies, and opportunities to play electronic games are some examples of rewards that have been offered to children for cooperating with procedures or for engaging in pain management techniques such as breathing exercises (Blount et al., 1994; S. M. Jay et al., 1995). Some researchers describe their rewards as incentives for the child's effort because the rewards are given to all children and are not contingent on their success with coping with the medical procedure.

Behavioral rehearsal and coaching. Many of the procedures described above are introduced and practiced using behavioral rehearsal before the procedure and coaching from a parent or clinician during the procedure. For example, Jay and colleagues (S. M. Jay et al., 1985, 1991, 1995) introduce several strategies to the child, such as breathing, reinforcement, and imagery, then have the child practice the procedure. The child may practice the procedure on a doll, the clinician, or parent while an adult coaches the recipient of the pretend procedure on the appropriate use of the intervention strategies. The actual medical equipment is used, if possible without potentially harmful components such as needles, and the child is guided in the step-by-step administration of the procedures. The pretend procedure is then "practiced" on the child while he or she is coached to use the pain management strategies. Behavioral rehearsal and coaching may be beneficial for children undergoing painful medical procedures by reducing medical fears associated with a lack of information, providing modeling, and role playing of effective coping strategies, thus desensitizing them to the components of the actual painful procedure (S. M. Jay et al., 1987).

Cognitive–Behavioral Therapy and Pharmacological Treatment

Studies have also investigated the benefits of CBT compared with the use of a pharmacological treatment to assist with pediatric pain management during painful medical procedures. S. M. Jay et al. (1987) found that CBT was more effective than Valium in decreasing the amount of behavioral distress and self-reported pain of children undergoing bone marrow aspirations. Another study by Jay and colleagues indicated that CBT was as effective as short-acting, general anesthesia for reducing self-reported pain and fear during bone marrow aspirations (S. M. Jay et al., 1995). CBT has also been found to be as efficacious as CBT plus oral Valium for reducing behavioral distress and self-reported pain and fear during bone marrow aspirations (S. M. Jay et al., 1991). Valium reportedly added very little if any beneficial effects to the CBT, but it may have interfered with the child's ability to successfully focus on the CBT strategies that were used. More research is clearly needed to further investigate this interesting finding of the possible interference of medication with a psychological intervention.

In a similar study, Kazak et al. (1996) found that children undergoing lumbar punctures and bone marrow aspirations who received CBT and medication for conscious sedation had less behavioral distress during the procedures compared with children who received medication only. Unfortunately, the CBT intervention used in this study was not adequately described, impeding any replications of these findings. Although these studies may demonstrate the effectiveness of CBT in comparison with pharmacological interventions, they are not included here to encourage the reduction or replacement of the use of medication treatments for children experiencing procedure-related pain. Such findings do support the usefulness of psychological interventions such as CBT as viable options for pediatric pain management.

Hypnosis for Procedure-Related Pain

Although hypnosis is not as well established as CBT as an intervention for procedure-related pain in children, it does show some promise as an additional pain management strategy. Hypnotic techniques often involve having the child visualize experiences, such as walking down stairs or a pathway to facilitate induction, followed by statements providing distraction from the pain. These distractors may also be incorporated with comments about the sensations associated with the procedure. For example, Kuttner (1988) used a child's favorite story of "Goldilocks and the Three Bears" to facilitate a hypnotic trance during a bone marrow aspiration. Kuttner (1988) incorporated procedural sensations into the story by telling the child: "and Goldilocks sat down to eat baby bear's porridge. It tasted so yummy and made her feel so comfortable, and now the poke is over and your back feels comfortable. But Goldilocks didn't stop eating" (p. 291).

Posthypnotic suggestions also may be incorporated into the scenario that facilitates relaxation after the procedure is over. For example, children may be told that when a nurse touches their shoulder later, they will feel as relaxed as they do during the trance. J. T. Smith, Barabasz, and Barabasz (1996) found that a child's receptiveness to being hypnotized may be an important factor in the success of hypnosis as a pain intervention strategy.

Smith et al. used the Stanford Hypnotic Clinical Scale for Children (Morgan & Hilgard, 1979) to estimate the child's hypnotizability. Children with low hypnotizability responded more positively to distraction techniques than to the hypnosis strategies used in this study. Further research in the area of hypnotizability may provide important information for determining the appropriateness of choosing hypnosis as an intervention strategy for a particular child. Appropriate training is required before a clinician can effectively and ethically attempt to hypnotize a child.

Summary

CBT has been demonstrated as an empirically supported intervention for assisting children in coping with the pain related to medical procedures such as immunizations, bone marrow aspirations, and lumbar punctures. One problem with the use of CBT may be the need for the clinician, specifically the psychologist, to be available to assist the child during every procedure to obtain successful results. Given the impracticality and cost of always having a therapist present, the training of medical staff such as nurses, parents, or both has been considered. Some studies demonstrate the effectiveness of training nurses or parents in CBT to assist the child with painful medical procedures (e.g., Blount et al., 1994; L. L. Cohen et al., 1997; Powers, Blount, Bachanas, Cotter, & Swan, 1993). The distress of parents may also be reduced if they are taught to effectively assist their child in managing painful experiences (L. L. Cohen et al., 1997).

Pain Associated With Recurrent Medical Conditions

Two recurrent medical conditions that have received the most attention in the pediatric pain literature are recurrent abdominal pain and headaches. Recurrent abdominal pain (RAP) is typically defined as sudden and intense abdominal pain occurring for three or more episodes over a 3-month period and resulting in impaired function such as missing school (Janicke & Finney, 1999). RAP typically has limited or no known physiological indications, with less than 5% of children diagnosed with RAP later being diagnosed with an organic medical condition (Walker, Garber, Van Slyke, & Greene, 1995). Despite the lack of verifiable organic etiology, however, RAP should always be considered real and can have a significant negative impact on a child's daily functioning.

Pediatric headache research has typically characterized headache pain as migraine or tension-type, although there is increasing recognition that headache pain most likely occurs on a continuum (Holden, Deichmann, & Levy, 1999; Rapoport & Sheftell, 1996). Similar to RAP, headaches can have a significant impact on children's functioning, limiting their school attendance and social involvement, and possibly increasing their risk for developing comorbid psychiatric disorders such as depression (Holden et al., 1999; Rapoport & Sheftell, 1996).

The most frequently investigated interventions designed to decrease pain associated with recurrent medical conditions, such as RAP and headaches, have been CBT and biofeedback. CBT, specifically the component of relaxation training, has the most support as an effective intervention for managing recurrent pain (Holden et al., 1999; Janicke & Finney, 1999). Biofeedback also shows promise as a pain management intervention for headaches, although its relative or additive effectiveness when compared with relaxation strategies appears to be minimal. A description of these strategies for use with recurrent pain conditions such as RAP and headaches is provided below.

Cognitive–Behavioral Therapy

The CBT component most commonly used for pain management with recurrent medical conditions has been relaxation training. Specific relaxation strategies typically include variations of progressive muscle relaxation and guided imagery as a means of self-"hypnosis." Relaxation strategies for children with recurrent pain are used not only to assist them with painful episodes but also to increase their ability to reduce socioenvironmental factors such as stress that may be influencing their pain experience.

These strategies are typically first presented to the child with an explanation of how negative events can affect his or her pain condition. The child is then introduced to the strategies, such as the steps of progressive muscle relaxation, and practices with the assistance of the therapist. The child is encouraged to practice his or her skills at home between appointments. This practice can be facilitated by giving the child an audiotape of the strategy to use at home or school. Adherence to practicing may also be facilitated by giving the child tangible rewards for completing the practice exercises. Finally, the child and therapist discuss how to integrate the child's newly acquired skills into his or her daily routine to both prevent and alleviate painful episodes. Relaxation therapies alone, and in combination with other interventions such as biofeedback, have been shown to be effective in reducing pediatric pain associated with recurrent medical conditions (e.g., Fentress, Masek, Mehegan, & Benson, 1986; D. G. Kohen, Olness, Colwell, & Heimel, 1984; P. J. McGrath et al., 1992). To increase the likelihood of generalization, some researchers have also investigated the effectiveness of training children with recurrent pain in nonclinical settings. The results of their efforts have been encouraging. For example, Larsson and Carlsson (1996) demonstrated that a school-based intervention using trained school nurses to teach progressive muscle relaxation to children with tension headaches was effective in reducing the children's headache pain. The nurses used audiotapes and a treatment manual to facilitate intervention fidelity. Other studies also support the feasibility and effectiveness of conducting group relaxation interventions in school settings to address pain associated with recurrent medical conditions such as headaches (e.g., Larsson, Daleflod, Hakansson, & Melin, 1987; Larsson & Melin, 1986).

There is also some support for the effectiveness of asking children, specifically adolescents, to teach themselves relaxation techniques without the presence of a therapist. For instance, Larsson et al. (1987) found that adolescents who taught themselves progressive muscle relaxation using information from audiotapes and a manual reduced their headache activity as much as adolescents who participated in a group, therapist-assisted relaxation intervention. Similar findings were also reported by McGrath et al. (1992), who also found that headache improvement obtained by adolescents using self-administered relaxation training was maintained through a 1-year follow-up.

More comprehensive CBT interventions have also been effective for managing recurrent pain in children. Two studies by Saunders and colleagues illustrate the use of a CBT intervention package with recurrent abdominal pain (Sanders et al., 1989; Sanders, Shepherd, Cleghorn, & Woolford, 1994). Their CBT strategies are summarized in Table 7.4.

The authors of these studies reported that the CBT strategies were effective in reducing self-reports of pain intensity, which were generally maintained at 6- and 12-month follow-up assessments. An important feature of these strategies is the incorporation of parent training in behavioral strategies as well. The recurrent nature of abdominal pain and headaches, as well as the significant contribution made by environmental factors in maintaining pain behaviors, supports the inclusion of parents in interventions for these disorders. These interventions were also conducted in a group format, suggesting a cost-effective means of providing treatment for recurrent pain disorders such as RAP. Finally, in an attempt to determine if a briefer intervention might be effective for treating pediatric headache pain, Barry and von Baeyer (1997) evaluated a two-session, comprehensive CBT intervention. Unlike the work of Sanders and colleagues, however, these authors found that this brief therapy was not effective in reducing the children's self-reports of headache pain. Thus, it appears that children must have adequate exposure to and practice with CBT strategies for these strategies to be effective in managing recurrent pain.

Biofeedback

Biofeedback also has been suggested as an effective strategy for reducing pain associated with recurrent medical conditions. Biofeedback is a strategy that involves the measurement and control of physiological functions not thought to be under the voluntary control of the individual (Kuttner, 1997). Biofeedback training attempts to teach the child to watch and

TABLE 7.4
Example of Group Cognitive–Behavioral Therapy for
Treating Recurrent Abdominal Pain

Session	Procedures
1	Explanations of child's pain behavior to parents; rationale for pain management procedures
2	Parents trained in differential reinforcement of well behavior with praise and token reinforcement to engage the child in competing responses and to avoid modeling sick behavior
3	Children taught coping skills using controlled breathing, distraction, and imagery
4	Children introduced to progressive muscle relaxation in addition to above strategies
5	Children introduced to more relaxation strategies (not specified) in addition to those in Session 4
6	Children introduced to positive self-talk strategies in addition to those taught in Sessions 4 and 5
7	Children practiced the skills they learned while distracted by parents and therapist and while walking
8	Children and parents engaged in problem-solving for potential future situations (also done in Sanders et al., 1989, during Session 6)

Note. Sessions 7 and 8 for Sanders et al. (1994) only.

From "Cognitive–Behavioral Treatment of Recurrent Nonspecific Abdominal Pain in Children: An Analysis of Generalization, Maintenance, and Side Effects," by M. R. Sanders, M. Rebgetz, M. Morrison, W. Bor, A. Gordon, M. Dadda, & R. Shepard, R., 1989, *Journal of Consulting and Clinical Psychology, 57,* 294–300; and "The Treatment of Recurrent Abdominal Pain in Children: A Controlled Comparison of Cognitive–Behavioral Family Intervention and Standard Pediatric Care," by M. R. Sanders, R. W. Shepherd, G. Cleghorn, & H. Woolford, H., 1994, *Journal of Consulting and Clinical Psychology, 62,* 306–314. Copyright 1989 and 1994 by the American Psychological Association. Adapted with permission of the author.

attenuate biological functions such as skin temperature and heart rate using specific equipment. Thermal biofeedback, which requires the monitoring of skin temperature on the basis of feedback from a thermistor held by the child, is the most common type of biofeedback used for recurrent pain management (Holden et al., 1999).

A review of behavioral intervention studies for pediatric headache pain indicated that thermal biofeedback alone and in combination with relaxation training was more effective than relaxation training alone or control conditions (Hermann, Kim, & Blanchard, 1995). A more recent review of intervention studies for pediatric headache also supports biofeedback as an effective intervention, although it is not as well established as relaxation strategies (Holden et al. 1999). The success of biofeedback training may be due to the immediate feedback that children can get about their bodies that may help them establish the connection between their thoughts and bodily responses of tension or relaxation (Collins, Kaslow, Doepke, Eckman, &

Johnson, 1998; P. A. McGrath, 1990). Attanasio et al. (1985) speculated that children may be less skeptical and more enthusiastic about their ability to control their biological functions than adults and thus may be more responsive to treatment.

Despite some evidence of effectiveness, the usefulness of biofeedback for recurrent pain is not consistently supported in the literature. Such lack of support may be based on research findings that demonstrate equal results using relaxation training and relaxation training plus biofeedback (e.g., Fentress et al., 1986). Thus, some authors suggest that although biofeedback can be effective for managing recurrent pain, it may not be needed in addition to relaxation training (M. L. McGrath & Masek, 1993). Given the additional equipment and training needs required of a clinician who wants to perform biofeedback, more evidence of the necessity of biofeedback is important. Of course, some simple biofeedback devices such as temperature-sensitive strips are available at a reasonable price for most consumers, offering at least one inexpensive option for the clinician and patient interested in pursuing biofeedback strategies (Kuttner, 1997).

Combined Treatments

Several studies have combined relaxation training, biofeedback, and other interventions to address recurrent pain in children. For example, K. D. Allen and Shriver (1998) combined thermal biofeedback with parent training in pain behavior management to effectively reduce the frequency of headaches experienced by their children. The parents met with the clinician at the end of the child's six biofeedback sessions for a discussion of how successfully they were implementing guidelines for managing their child's pain-related behavior. These guidelines provide the clinician with important issues to be discussed with parents of children with recurrent pain disorders. More research on the effectiveness of adding such parent training would be a welcome addition to the pain management literature.

Other combined treatment strategy interventions also have been effective in reducing recurrent pain. Finney and colleagues (Finney, Lemanek, Cataldo, Katz, & Fuqua, 1989) treated children ranging in age from about 6 to 13 years with RAP with some combination of five treatment components: self-monitoring, relaxation training, limited parental reinforcement for somatic complaints, dietary fiber, and routine activities. At follow-up, after an average of 2.5 office visits, 81% of the participants reported their pain symptoms were either improved or resolved.

Multicomponent psychological interventions have also been compared with pharmacological treatments for recurrent pain disorders. Sartory, Muller, Metsch, and Pothmann (1998) reported that children with migraines who received progressive muscle relaxation training and stress management strategies reported fewer and less intense headaches than children receiving biofeedback and stress management training or children receiving the prophylactic beta blocker metopolol. The positive reduction on headache frequency from the relaxation and stress management training was maintained at an 8-month follow-up. This study and the others reported in this section support the usefulness of psychological interventions as an effective option to add to the pharmacological agents available for treating recurrent pain in children.

Summary

The purpose of pain management interventions for recurrent medical conditions is to facilitate more effective coping skills in the child and to increase their independent, age-appropriate functioning. The use of relaxation strategies such as progressive muscle relaxation has been found to be effective in reducing pain associated with recurrent medical conditions such as RAP and headaches. There is also some evidence that these strategies can be effectively taught in both clinical and nonclinical settings such as the school. Biofeedback is also an effective strategy for managing recurrent headache pain, although evidence for biofeedback as a superior intervention when compared with relaxation training has not been demonstrated. Nevertheless, the technological appeal of biofeedback equipment and the availability of inexpensive, portable equipment such as temperature strips may enhance the likelihood that a child will practice the relaxation skills associated with biofeedback. Finally, interventions that combine numerous intervention strategies have also been effective in reducing recurrent pain in children. The clinician's choice of interventions may depend on the time available for intervention, access to groups of participants, and the preferences of the child and parents.

Pain Associated With Chronic Disease States

Many chronic disease states that affect children have pain associated with them. Diseases such as AIDS, cancer, sickle cell, and JRA have pain associated with their disease process, as well as a result of necessary medical treatments. A description of the types of pain children with these chronic illnesses experience was provided previously in Exhibit 7.2. Despite the prevalence of painful chronic diseases for children, very few intervention studies addressing the pain associated with the disease state or medical treatments have been conducted. One reason for the lack of such research in the area of childhood cancer specifically may be that children may experience less disease-related pain than procedure- or treatment-related pain (Miser, 1993). Consequently, many intervention studies can be found that address procedure-related pain for children with cancer, as discussed previously in this chapter. A recent review of intervention studies for pediatric disease-related pain found only six studies that included patients younger than age 18 (Walco, Sterling, Conte, & Engel, 1999). Clearly, this area of pain intervention research is not as well established as interventions for pain associated with medical procedures and recurrent medical conditions. Some strategies that do show promise for managing disease-related pain in children, however, include various components of cognitive–behavioral therapy, hypnosis, and biofeedback.

Cognitive–Behavioral Therapy

The CBT strategies that have been most frequently explored for managing disease-related pain in children have been controlled breathing, imagery, and progressive muscle relaxation. Such strategies are often used to assist children in distracting themselves from their painful experience (Walco et al., 1992). For example, Walco et al. taught children with JRA to use a combination of progressive muscle relaxation, controlled breathing accompanied by the instruction to say the word *relax* to themselves, and guided imagery similar to the techniques described for procedure-related pain. The guided imagery for these children also included suggestions to describe their pain as a concrete image or color, and to alter the image or color to a more relaxing state as they progressed through their image. Examples of such images included pain switches that could be turned off, needles to be removed, aversive colors to be transformed to more relaxing colors, and large colored areas to slowly shrink. The children were introduced to and practiced these strategies in the office for eight sessions and were also given audiotapes of the strategies to use at home. This package of CBT strategies was effective in reducing the self-reported pain intensity of the children, with reduced pain and improved adaptive functioning maintained at a 6- and a 12-month follow-up.

Other Strategies

Two other strategies that have been used to manage disease-related pain are hypnosis and biofeedback. Hypnosis has been suggested as a promising pain management intervention for disease-related pain in adults (e.g., Hilgard & LeBaron, 1982; Hornyak & Green, 2000; Peter, 1997) but is not currently supported as an empirically valid treatment for children. Small-sample studies of the benefits of hypnosis, however, suggest that this intervention may be worth continued investigation in the pediatric population (e.g. Dinges et al., 1997; LaClave & Blix, 1989; Olness, 1981). For example, Dinges et al. (1997) reported that teaching children and adolescents with sickle cell disease to use hypnosis during pain episodes helped to reduce the frequency of "bad days," nights of poor sleep because of pain, and the use of pain medication. Unfortunately, both the pain diary assessment tool and the intervention procedures were not described in enough detail to permit replication by the interested clinician. Hypnosis has been found to be effective in reducing emesis related to cancer treatments, suggesting an additional usefulness for this strategy for addressing treatment-related issues for children with cancer (Genuis, 1995).

Biofeedback, both alone and combined with CBT, has also been investigated as an intervention strategy for managing disease-related pain in children and adults. For example, preliminary findings from an intervention incorporating progressive muscle relaxation, electromyogram biofeedback, and thermal biofeedback suggested the effectiveness of such a treatment package for reducing pain associated with JRA (Lavigne, Ross, Berry, Hayford, & Pachman, 1992). Lavigne et al. also generated a treatment manual to accompany the six intervention sessions. More research on biofeedback and the other intervention strategies is needed and important as pain research moves beyond procedural pain to addressing the more complex issues of pain management.

Summary

Many childhood diseases are accompanied by pain as a result of the disease state or therapeutic treatments needed to manage the illness. Some components of CBT such as controlled breathing, progressive muscle relaxation, and guided imagery currently show the most promise for assisting children with their disease-related pain. Further investigations of hypnosis and biofeedback may add to the list of effective strategies available in the future. More research on interventions for disease-related pain is needed before any strategy can be considered empirically valid in this area. The effectiveness of pain management interventions should also be explored with other disease states, such as fibromyalgia and AIDS, which also have pain as a prominent characteristic of their presentation.

CONCLUSION

Many children are exposed to significant pain during their childhood because of medical procedures, recurrent medical conditions, or chronic disease. The effective management of pediatric pain has been investigated for more than 20 years, resulting in advances in pharmacological and nonpharmacological intervention strategies that have improved the quality of care received by children in pain. Unfortunately, there is still consistent evidence that pain is undertreated for children, especially for young children who are least able to communicate their pain management needs. Clinicians often receive referrals to address pain management issues when a child is having a difficult time with repetitive acute pain experiences necessary for medical treatment or when medical alternatives to recurrent or chronic pain are not sufficient.

Many assessment tools are available to assist health care providers evaluate a child's pain experience and to monitor the effectiveness of pain management efforts. Numerous interviews, adult observation tools, and self-report measures, including pain diaries, have demonstrated reliable and valid assessment of pediatric pain. Some efforts at developing culturally sensitive tools have also been demonstrated for children with African American and Hispanic heritage. As the United States continues to become more diverse, the development of such tools will be imperative. Furthermore, as our understanding of how children express pain grows, the assessment tools of the future may have to be sensitive to child characteristics such as age and gender as well.

Many interventions, both pharmacological and nonpharmacological, exist to assist children in managing their painful experiences. PCA devices are a promising venue for adequate medication delivery for children who may benefit from having some control over their own pain management. More patient, parent, and physician information on the safety of opiod drugs seems to be needed, however, before pediatric pain will be adequately managed. Regardless of how effective pharmacological agents are in treating a child's pain, the addition of nonpharmacological strategies will likely provide the most satisfactory care of children in pain. CBT has proved to be the most effective nonpharmacological strategy available for addressing procedure-related and recurrent pain. There is also some support for specific components of CBT, such as relaxation training, for addressing pain associated with recurrent and chronic medical conditions. Hypnosis and biofeedback are two other intervention strategies that have demonstrated some effectiveness in the management of procedure-related and recurrent pain, respectively. These two strategies are also being investigated as methods of pain management for pain related to chronic disease states.

The area of pain associated with chronic disease is perhaps the most in need of further research. The lack of psychological intervention studies in this area may be due to the obvious organic nature of the pain and thus a tendency to explore more pharmacological treatment options for pain management (S. M. Jay, Elliott, & Varni, 1986). As demonstrated with other areas of pain in children, however, the use of psychological interventions can have a substantial positive impact.

Finally, most pain research to date has focused on only a small aspect of the pain experiences of children, especially for children with recurrent and chronic diseases. In order for pain management efforts to be most successful, effective interventions may be needed to address other disease-related and environmental factors that contribute to a child's pain experience. McQuaid and Nassau (1999) provided a review of effective interventions for other disease-related symptoms besides pain that may have a negative impact on a child's chronic illness experience, including anticipatory nausea and vomiting associated with cancer treatments. Environmental interventions may also be needed to most effectively assist children with pain management. For example, preliminary studies show the effectiveness of training parents on how to respond to their child's pain behaviors (e.g., K. D. Allen & Shriver, 1998). Such studies broaden the scope of intervention to include the numerous factors that are often cited as significant contributors to the experience of pain.

In addition to increasing the availability of assessment tools to the health care provider, access to effective intervention information is also vital for successful pain management in children. Parents, nursing staff, and others who have consistent contact with children in pain can easily be trained to perform many of the strategies used in CBT. The communication and demonstration of effective interventions by health care providers to others who provide care to children in pain is imperative and most likely one of the few ways many health care providers may be exposed to nonpharmacological treatments for pediatric pain.

8

MANAGEMENT OF ADHERENCE TO PEDIATRIC MEDICAL REGIMENS

Traditionally, the extent to which a patient or a patient's parents follow the advice of medical professionals has been defined as *compliance*. Compliance with medical recommendations can mean keeping an appointment, taking a single pill, engaging in preventive care, altering one's lifestyle, or following a complex medical routine such as one required to manage diabetes. Clearly, compliance is a complex construct with numerous behavioral components (Delameter, 1993).

Recognizing that compliance can be a more complicated concept than traditional definitions indicate has led some researchers to search for conceptualizations that are more useful in clinical settings. The term *adherence* is now being used with more frequency as a means of describing the nature of a patient's response to a medical regimen. Current definitions recognize that adherence can occur on a continuum and that multiple factors in a person's daily life can influence health-related behaviors (Lutfey & Wishner, 1999; R. J. Thompson & Gustafson, 1996). Liptak (1996) added to the definition the responsibility of health care providers to offer patients understandable and feasible health management goals before they can expect patients to incorporate them into their routines. Such definitions recognize the importance of both the health care provider's and patient's contributions to the decision-making process and the success of the recommended medical care.

The term *adherence* is used in this chapter because of its broad-based conceptualization and focus on the patient, family, and health care providers as important contributors to the components and effectiveness of a medical regimen. Adherence issues often come to the attention of clinicians and other mental health professionals through referrals from physicians. For example, a primary-care physician may recognize that a child with a chronic illness, such as asthma, is exceptionally ill because of a lack of adherence to recommended inhaler treatments. Such a child may require the time and behavioral expertise that a clinician has been trained to provide. Major children's medical centers frequently have psychologists and social workers dedicated to specific medical subspecialties such as endocrinology and oncology to assist pediatric patients and their families in adequately performing the medical tasks necessary for optimal health. This chapter addresses how health care providers can improve patient and family adherence to medication regimens and to more complex treatment regimens often associated with chronic illness.

PREVALENCE

Given the variability in how adherence is defined and measured, reported prevalence rates also differ. In a review of pediatric adherence studies, Rapoff (1999) reported that medication nonadherence rates ranged from 5% to 85% for acute illness and from 4% to 98% for chronic illness. The most common statistic reported for pediatric adherence to medication and other components of medical regimens over the past 20 years, however, is a median rate of 50% (Dunbar-Jacob, Dunning, & Dwyer, 1993; Rapoff, 1999). This rate suggests little improvement in adherence rates over time despite increased interest and research.

CAUSES AND CORRELATES

The literature on pediatric adherence often lists a variety of factors thought to contribute to the patient's success in adhering to a medical regimen. Examples of such factors are provided in Exhibit 8.1.

The identification of such factors for a patient is meant to assist health care providers in recognizing potential barriers and strengths related to treatment adherence. Unfortunately, the ability to predict which patients may be nonadherent has been found to be quite limited (e.g., Mushlin & Appel, 1977). Thus, health care providers should be aware that although certain factors can alert them to patients who may require additional monitoring for potential nonadherence, the list is neither exhaustive nor predictive of all nonadherent patients. In fact, many of the factors included in Exhibit 8.1 are based on findings from case studies rather than from empirically based research (Lemanek, 1990). The complex nature of adherence, along with differences in the experimental methods of research in this area,

EXHIBIT 8.1
Factors That Influence Adherence to Medical Regimens

Illness Factors	Family Factors
Manifestations	Family supportiveness, coping skills
Level of disability	Level of dysfunction, conflict
Chronicity	Parental mental health, literacy

Treatment Factors	Health Care System Factors
Complexity	Patient satisfaction
Degree of required behavior change	Interpersonal style
Consequences of adherence	Accessibility, quality, continuity of care outcomes
Consequences of nonadherence	Finances
	Logistics (e.g., location of clinic)

Individual Characteristics	Social/Cultural Factors
Age	Social or peer pressure
Cognitive factors	Social stigma
Emotional functioning	Cultural beliefs, biases
General behavioral adherence	

may explain the lack of conclusive findings to date. Furthermore, these factors are rarely investigated with respect to intervention research (Rapoff, 1999). Thus, the ability to alter the influence of these factors through interventions has not been fully determined. Despite this limitation in the literature, however, a description of how the factors listed in Exhibit 8.1 may be related to intervention research is provided, when possible, in the "Intervention" section of this chapter.

ASSESSMENT

Numerous methods have been used to measure patient adherence to medical regimens. These methods, which are often categorized into direct and indirect measures, provide varying degrees of accuracy and objectivity with respect to adherence information. Given its complex nature, adherence is most accurately assessed by using multiple measures.

Direct Measures

Direct measures include analyzing samples of blood, urine, or saliva for the presence or concentration of a specific drug. Blood assays have also been used to infer adherence based on medical outcomes, such as blood glucose or hemoglobin A1c levels. Direct health outcomes such as weight loss or gain also have some usefulness in measuring adherence. Unfortunately, such measures may be a misleading means of assessment, because a one-to-one correspondence does not generally exist between adherence and outcome (Finney & Weist, 1988; Hays et al., 1994; S. B. Johnson et al., 1992). Thus, although it is tempting to assume that direct measures are "better" indices of adherence than indirect measures, they can be profoundly influenced by whether or not the patient is, in fact, on the correct treatment regimen. For example, a person with insulin-dependent (Type I) diabetes may have a high hemoglobin A1c level because of nonadherence to a treatment regimen or because an ineffective insulin regimen was being used at the time the blood glucose level was obtained. Despite such limitations, however, adherence is generally viewed as a key determinant in positive health outcomes for children with medical problems. Direct measures are typically obtained by the physician, but such information can be used by the clinician or mental health professional who is educated about the significance of such measures and their relationship to adherence.

Indirect Measures

Common indirect measures of adherence include counting pills, patient or parent self-reports, and health care professionals' estimates. Adherence also has been measured by such factors as patient knowledge and the demonstration of skills, such as insulin administration. These measures are less objective than direct measures but are also typically more practical for health care providers to use. Objectivity in self-reporting and parent reporting may be enhanced by nonjudgmental and specific questioning and by providing the family with a simple and explicit form to record important regimen data (Rapoff & Christophersen, 1982). An example of a Symptom Recording Sheet provided to the parents of a child with encopresis is described in chapter 5. This sheet provides parents with a way to record such daily regimen activities as the amount of daily fiber consumed, allowing the clinician to monitor adherence and progress. Further suggestions for assessment of adherence are found in the "Intervention" section of this chapter.

A Comment on General Behavioral Adherence

When attempting to improve a child's adherence to acute or chronic medical regimens, health care professionals must first assess the child's overall behavioral adherence and intervene if necessary. Children who are oppositional to nonmedical demands may understandably have difficulties adhering to treatment aspects that may be painful or limit their activities (Christophersen, 1994). Information about a child's level of overall adherence may be adequately assessed by parent interview and by obtaining information from parent and teacher behavior rating scales such as the Child Behavior Checklist (Achenbach & Edelbrock, 1983, 1986) or Behavior Assessment System for Children (Reynolds & Kamphaus, 1998). These measures have been discussed in more detail in chapter 1, on disruptive behavior disorders. Ideally, such information is obtained at the time of the child's medical diagnosis and before the child begins to demonstrate adherence or behavior problems related to the treatment regimen. Unfortunately, many children with adherence issues come to the attention of the clinician only after significant problems have been identified. If individual assessment information suggests that a patient demonstrating medical adherence problems also demonstrates more general behavior problems, intervention strategies for improving the child's general level of appropriate behavior should be implemented first, or at least in addition to efforts to improve medical adherence.

The specific adherence-related strategies described later in this chapter may also be useful for intervening with general behavior problems that are interfering with treatment. For example, Carton and Schweitzer (1996) used a token economy with a 10-year-old boy undergoing hemodialysis to successfully decrease negative behaviors, such as kicking or hitting the nurses, that were hindering his medical care. More detailed information about the assessment and treatment of general behavior problems can be found in chapter 1.

INTERVENTIONS

The availability of empirically supported interventions for improving adherence in the pediatric population is limited. Dunbar-Jacob et al. (1993) reviewed 91 studies on pediatric adherence and found that only 15 used experimental designs. The majority of studies provided only descriptive or correlational information about adherence. A more recent review by Rapoff (1999) found 34 intervention studies on adherence to acute and chronic illness regimens, suggesting an increased focus on intervention research in the last few years. On the basis of the current state of empirical interventions for adherence, the remainder of this chapter discusses the importance of providing accurate information as a first step for facilitating adherence and provides specific strategies for improving adherence to medication regimens and more complex treatment regimens. Suggestions for addressing family and social barriers to adherence are also offered.

Providing the Necessary Illness and Regimen Information

Health care providers need to communicate appropriate and understandable illness information and treatment recommendations if they expect pediatric patients and their families to follow regimen requirements. Although disease and treatment regimen information alone are not sufficient to guarantee adherence, many authors suggest that accurate information about disease or treatment regimens may have positive effects on adherence (Bender, Milgrom, Rand, & Ackerson, 1998; Jones, Jones, & Katz, 1989; Schoenberg, Mley, & Coward, 1998; Wysocki, 1997). In addition, effective communication can also be a vital part of patient satisfaction, which has been found to be a factor related to better adherence to medical regimens for pediatric patients (Auslander, Thompson, Dreitzer, & Santiago, 1997; Hazzard, Hutchinson, & Krawiecki, 1990; N. A. Smith, Seale, Ley, Shaw, & Bracs, 1986).

Although medical health care providers typically provide patients and families with necessary medical and regimen information to assist them in their health care, clinicians can assess the extent to which the information was understood and how well it is being adhered to by the patient. Frequent communication between health care providers is also essential to ensure that information is consistent and that adherence goals are compatible with the individual needs of the patient and family. Finally, discussions about the patient's medical condition and treatment need to be periodically repeated to determine if the patient or family needs updated information from the medical provider, as well as to assess any changes in the patient's or family's concerns about the treatment.

Medication is one area in particular that is subject to changing attitudes or concerns. Direct questions about patient or family concerns about medication, the frequency at which doses are forgotten, and any increased reluctance on the part of the patient to take the medication may be helpful in assessing current medication views (Stine, 1994). Several authors offer suggestions for providing patient information that are worth considering when attempting to improve patient adherence (Falvo, 1994; Ley, 1977; Rapoff & Christophersen, 1982; Stine, 1994; J. Thomas, 1994). These suggestions are summarized in Exhibit 8.2.

Developmentally Appropriate Information

Some individual characteristics of pediatric medical patients have been studied as potential contributors to regimen adherence and thus should be considered when providing illness and regimen information. For example, the influence of cognitive development has been included in many theories about adherence (Becker et al., 1979; Iannotti & Bush, 1993; Leventhal, 1993). Cognitive concepts such as perceptions of illness, self-efficacy, locus of control, and memory all have been suggested as potential factors affecting adherence in children. For example, children's memory for regimen instructions presented to them at a level beyond their comprehension ability is likely to be minimal and thus may interfere with adherence

EXHIBIT 8.2
Strategies for Providing Effective Patient Education

Building Rapport	Providing Information
■ Conduct interactions in a friendly, warm, and empathetic manner.	■ Avoid the use of medical jargon and technical wording.
■ Talk about nonmedical topics.	■ Use short sentences.
■ Engage patient in developmentally appropriate, personalized conversation.	■ Discuss the advantages and disadvantages of treatment.
■ Note important family events to ask about on return visits.	■ Be realistic about what the patient can and cannot expect as a result of treatment adherence.
	■ Inform patients of the likelihood of relapses.
	■ Repeat instructions, if necessary.
	■ Have parent or patient repeat instructions.
	■ Alert parents and patients when you are going to give an instruction (e.g., "now this is an important part of your care").
	■ Make advice specific and concrete.
	■ Tailor information and details to the individual (provide only the amount of detail necessary for a functional understanding; more details can be offered later as the patient becomes more adept at performing regimen tasks).

Assessing Patient and Family Adherence Characteristics	Problem Solving About Adherence Issues
■ Investigate preferred learning styles and learning problems (e.g., illiteracy) in parents and children.	■ Approach adherence problems with a supportive, nonjudgmental attitude.
■ Investigate emotional functioning and family stressors that may impact adherence.	■ Recognize how difficult adherence can be for families.
■ Ask about their understanding, worries, and expectations about the illness and treatment.	■ Assist family in identifying potential barriers to adherence.
■ If medication is involved, explore beliefs and concerns about medication.	■ Generate a list of solutions for the problem.
	■ Teach the family how to anticipate future problems and solutions.
	■ Focus on patient's personal best for adherence versus ideal care; gradually increase goals.
	■ Discuss the roles of each family member in carrying out the medical regimen.

efforts (Iannotti & Bush, 1993). Although more research is needed before specific cognitive factors can be offered as guidelines in providing appropriate information to children about their illness and treatment, suggestions are available for providing education according to a patient's developmental level (e.g., Falvo, 1994). For example, school-age children may learn tasks more effectively with hands-on examples. Adolescents should be asked about risk-taking behaviors and peer acceptance issues that may impact their adherence. Other suggestions can be found in Falvo (1994).

Written Educational Materials

Written handouts also may be used to supplement verbal instructions and increase patient understanding and recall, consequently improving adherence. Written materials have typically been used to describe medication regimens or other complex regimen components and have been shown to improve adherence (Colcher & Bass, 1972; Finney, Friman, Rapoff, & Christophersen, 1985; Maiman, Becker, Liptak, Nazarien, & Rounds, 1988). An example of an instructional handout on how to properly use an inhaler for asthma is provided in Figure 8.1. Of course, such handouts typically should be used to supplement the information and demonstration provided by the physician and not as the primary method of teaching a skill or regimen component.

Written instructions provided by clinicians can also be useful for providing supplemental information to patients and families about how to successfully implement treatment components, as well as how to carry out an intervention to improve adherence. For example, Blount, Dahlquist, Baer, and Wuori, (1984) demonstrated that children could be taught procedures to desensitize them to swallowing pills by progressing through a size hierarchy of nonmedicinal items (e.g., cake sprinkles, small hard candies). These procedures have been translated into a written handout for parents in our clinic to refer to when practicing at home (see Exhibit 8.3). Examples of written instructions about adherence interventions are found later in this chapter. These examples demonstrate the importance of using detailed instructions rather than general comments when providing written information about a treatment regimen or adherence intervention.

A Comment on Literacy

Literacy levels must be taken into consideration when providing patients and families with information about the patients' illness and medical regimen. Parents of pediatric patients who cannot read instructions, prescriptions, or informational material cannot follow the advice these written materials convey. Unfortunately, people may go to great extremes to hide their inability to read (Falvo, 1994; Stanley, 1999). Possible indicators of a person's poor reading ability may include using an X as a signature, asking to

STEPS FOR USING YOUR INHALER

Please demonstrate your inhaler technique at every visit.

1. Remove the cap and hold inhaler upright.
2. Shake the inhaler.
3. Tilt your head back slightly and breathe out slowly.
4. Position the inhaler in one of the following ways (A or B is optimal, but C is acceptable for those who have difficulty with A or B. C is required for breath-activated inhalers):

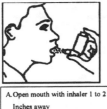	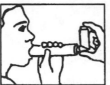	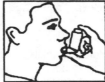	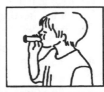
A. Open mouth with inhaler 1 to 2 Inches away	B. Use spacer/holding chamber (that is recommended especially for young children and for people using corticosteroids)	C. In the mouth. **Do not use for corticosteroids.**	D. NOTE: Inhaled dry powder capsules require a different inhalation technique. To use a dry powder inhaler, it is important to close the mouth tightly around the mouthpiece of the inhaler and to Inhale rapidly.

5. Press down on the inhaler to release medication as you start to breathe in slowly.
6. Breathe in slowly (3 to 5 seconds).
7. Hold your breath for 10 seconds to allow the medicine to reach deeply into your lungs.
8. Repeat puff as directed. Waiting 1 minute between puffs may permit second puff to penetrate your lungs better.
9. Spacers/holding chambers are useful for all patients. They are particularly recommended for young children and older adults and for use with inhaled corticosteroids.

Avoid common inhaler mistakes. Follow these inhaler tips:

- Breathe out *before* pressing your inhaler.
- Inhale *slowly.*
- Breathe in through your mouth, not your nose.
- Press down on your inhaler at the *start* of inhalation (or within the first second of inhalation). .
- Keep inhaling as you press down on inhaler.
- Press your inhaler only *once* while you are inhaling (one breath for each puff).
- Make sure you breathe in evenly and deeply.

NOTE: Other inhalers are becoming available in addition to those illustrated above. Different types of inhalers may require different techniques.

FIGURE 8.1. Asthma inhaler instruction sheet. From *Expert Panel Report 2: Guidelines for the Diagnosis and Management of Asthma* (NIH Publication No. 97-4051, p. 73), by National Asthma Education and Prevention Program, 1997, Washington, DC: National Institutes of Health.

fill out forms at home, and referring to items by visual cues (e.g., "the blue-labeled milk") instead of by the written label (Stanley, 1999). We often request that parents read aloud a few lines from written handouts to briefly assess their reading skills. It provides the opportunity to see if they can rely on the written instructions when necessary, but its purpose is probably never noticed by parents who take their reading ability for granted.

Most word-processing programs have a grade-level and readability tool that can help handout developers generate documents that are easy to read, typically defined as being at a 6th-grade reading level. For example,

EXHIBIT 8.3
Pill-Swallowing Handout for Parents

1. Model for your child the steps in swallowing a pill:
   A. Place pill on the back of your tongue.
   B. Keep the tongue flat.
   C. Take liquid in the mouth.
   D. Tilt the head backward slightly.
   E. Swallow.

2. Gradually increase the size of the pill in the following order:
   A. Oblong, multicolored sprinkle used for cake decoration.
   B. Spherical, silver cake decoration.
   C. Round, multicolored candy (0.3–0.7 cm diameter).
   D. Red licorice whip cut to 1-cm length.
   E. Capsule-shaped candy, multicolored, sold as "Tic Tacs" or "Dynamints."
   F. Normal-sized capsule: the child's actual pill.

Have your child practice swallowing each size piece of sprinkle or candy as many times as it takes for him or her to get accustomed to it. These procedures usually take about 45 minutes to 1 hour but may take you a little longer.

Note. From "A Brief, Effective Method for Teaching Children to Swallow Pills," by R. L. Blount, L. M. Dahlquist, R. A. Baer, and D. Wouri, 1984, *Behavior Therapy, 15,* p. 383. Copyright 1984 by Association for Advancement of Behavior Therapy. Adapted with permission of the publisher.

Microsoft Word (Version 7), under the "Spelling and Grammar" tab, provides a reading level for the text that is being examined. In this program, the reading level for this chapter is rated at the 12th grade. In contrast, the Chip System Treatment Manual (see Appendix A), which was written for parents, has a reading-level difficulty at the 7th grade. Some strategies for developing low literacy level materials are described in Exhibit 8.4.

Addressing Barriers to Medication Regimen Adherence

Interventions for improving adherence to medication regimens are some of the most commonly researched in the area of pediatric adherence. In fact, of the adherence studies reviewed by Rapoff (1999), all of the acute intervention studies targeted medication adherence, along with almost 50% of the chronic disease regimen adherence studies. In addition to the suggestion of written instructions mentioned previously, additional strategies for assisting parents and patients with their medication regimens are described below.

Increased Follow-Up

One strategy that has been found to be useful in assisting patients with medication adherence involves increased supervision of care from the health care provider. Some studies have found that increased monitoring of

EXHIBIT 8.4
Design Strategies for Developing Low-Literacy Materials

Language/Vocabulary	Content	Format
Use active voice.	Minimize the number of concepts presented.	Use high contrast between type and background color.
Use positive tones.	Try to limit to 1 concept per section per page.	Use color to create interest and emphasize points.
Use conversational style.	Concepts should be relevant to key instruction, not supplemental.	Use nonglossy paper.
Use a variety of sentence lengths, but emphasize short sentences.	Provide purpose of information and how it will affect the learner.	Use visual uses and illustrations.
Avoid use of slang.	Use advanced organizers (headings, purpose statements, titles).	Make illustrations simple and realistic (do not use cartoon style; simple line drawings are best).
Achieve desired readability level (< 6th grade).	Include practical information ("how-to" information).	Select simple font style, 12–14 point (large point helps for low vision, not low literacy).
Limit the number of polysyllabic words (> 3 syllables).	Make messages clear and break down into related sections.	Use upper- and lowercase letters.
Limit use of technical language.	Include frequent summaries and "how-to-use" information throughout.	Emphasize key points with use of underlines or bold print, not capitalization.
Define any technical language or words.		Arrange lists vertically and keep to fewer than 10 items.
		Allow for patient interaction and feedback.

Note. From "Low-Literacy Materials for Diabetes Nutrition Education," by K. Stanley, 1999, *Practical Diabetology, 15,* 36–44. Copyright 1999 by Rapaport Publishing. Adapted with permission.

patients may be an important component in improved adherence to regimen factors such as appointment keeping and taking medication (e.g., Casey, Rosen, Glowasky, & Ludwig, 1985; Eney & Goldstein, 1976). For example, Eney and Goldstein reported that when parents were told their child's level of asthma medication (theophylline) was going to be monitored using the child's blood serum or saliva, 42% of the children had serum levels in the therapeutic range, suggesting adherence to the medication regimen. In comparison, only 11% of children in a group that was not monitored had sufficient serum theophylline levels. Increased supervision also can be provided through telephone calls and home visits. The success of adherence intervention strategies also may be facilitated by increased follow-up or monitoring from the health care provider (Falvo, 1994; Rapoff, 1999; Rapoff & Christophersen, 1982). For example, the health care provider may call the patient or family a few days after an appointment to see if they have any questions on how to complete a self-monitoring sheet or to determine if the patient is being reinforced appropriately for adherence behaviors. Once again, communication between the health care providers is imperative for the success of adherence interventions. The clinician or mental health professional can often act as a liaison between the family and physician, communicating difficulties that may be able to be addressed before the next medical appointment. For example, blood sugar values for a child with diabetes could be faxed to the clinician by the school nurse as part of monitoring for the frequency of blood sugar checks. This information could then be forwarded to the child's endocrinologist to assist in evaluating the effectiveness of the insulin regimen.

Cues and Reinforcement

Behavioral strategies, such as providing cues to take medication and providing reinforcement for following a regimen, are also useful for promoting adherence. Similar to written instructions, these strategies typically are not used in isolation but are included as a component of a more comprehensive intervention. Thus, it is difficult to find empirical studies that validate these strategies separately. Cipes and Miraglia (1985) did demonstrate, however, that adherence to a daily fluoride mouth rinse was facilitated by having children use a calendar to remind and reward themselves for adherence by placing stickers on the calendar. Similarly, Cipes (1985) found that the self-management procedures described above were just as effective in facilitating adherence as parental reminding and parental reinforcement strategies for children using the fluoride mouth rinse. Thus, depending on the child, self-monitoring and parental management strategies can be suggested as means of encouraging adherence.

Token Economies and Contracting

The use of token economies and contracting that provides rewards to children for adherence to medication regimens have also been suggested as adherence-promoting strategies. These strategies typically involve giving the child tokens or points for demonstrating predefined adherence behaviors, which can later be exchanged for reinforcers. (See chapter 1 on disruptive behavior disorders for more information on token economies.) Although much of the research in this area has been conducted through the use of small sample sizes or single-subject design, there is some evidence of the effectiveness of token economies and contingency contracting for improving medication adherence behaviors in children. An example of a contingency contract that successfully increased medication use by children with thalassemia (Koch, Giardina, Ryan, MacQueen, & Hilgartner, 1993) is provided in Exhibit 8.5. Koch et al. also reported some evidence of adherence maintenance at 2-month follow-up.

Some authors report that the use of contingency contracting has not been as effective as other strategies, such as parental reinforcement or self-reinforcement (Cipes & Miraglia, 1985). The authors speculated that some of the families in their study may not have understood or liked the contracting concept, thus pointing to the importance of using socially acceptable intervention strategies that are adaptable to individual ability levels.

Comprehensive Strategies

Because of the complex nature of adherence issues, it is understandable that effective interventions may be those that combine numerous strategies. Typical comprehensive interventions include a combination of written instructions, increased monitoring from health care providers, and behavioral interventions such as self-monitoring or token economies (e.g., da Costa, Rapoff, Lemanek, & Goldstein, 1997; Finney et al., 1985; N. A. Smith, Seale, Ley, Mellis, & Shaw, 1994). For example, a comprehensive intervention for asthma medication adherence, which included written instructions, tailoring the regimen to the patient's routines, and increased supervision by the physician, resulted in improved adherence for families who had a child with asthma when compared with children who received standard clinic care (N. A. Smith et al., 1986, 1994). As with any intervention, the success of a comprehensive strategy will most likely require input from the patient, parents, and physicians to ensure acceptability and feasibility for implementation. Such interventions may also have to be frequently revised as the family determines which components are most helpful and which components are too difficult to complete.

EXHIBIT 8.5
Examples of Contract Components to Enhance Adherence
to a Medication Regimen

Goals	Rewards for Meeting Goals
Set as a goal the number of empty medication vials you would like to return, based on your current use.	Star on chart
	Stamp in pocket "credit card"
Renegotiate goal every 2 weeks on the basis of the performance during the prior 2 weeks.	Surprise gift for purchase with stars and credits at the end of each 2-week period
	10 credits redeemable for $20 gift

Note. From "Behavioral Contracting to Improve Adherence in Patients With Thalassemia," by Koch et al., 1993, *Journal of Pediatric Nursing, 8,* 106–111. Copyright 1993 by W. B. Sanders. Adapted with permission.

Addressing Barriers to Complex Treatment Regimen Adherence

The medical interventions necessary to control the effects of an illness such as diabetes, asthma, or juvenile arthritis may involve a complex interplay of diet, exercise, and medication, necessitating complex lifestyle changes that may be difficult to implement. Unfortunately, both the chronicity of a child's illness and the complexity of the treatment regimen have been suggested as factors related to poor adherence (Daviss et al., 1995; Haynes, Taylor, & Sackett, 1979; Jacobson et al., 1990; Kovacs, Goldston, Obrosky, & Iyanger, 1992). Because of the complexity of some treatment regimens, adherence often varies within the regimen itself (Kurtz, 1990; Van Sciver, D'Angelo, Rappaport, & Woolf, 1995). For example, children with diabetes may adhere closely to necessary emergent treatment, such as eating when they experience low blood sugar, but be less adherent to preventive or daily requirements of their regimen, such as following suggestions for foot care and regular exercise.

The interventions available to assist children in adhering to complex treatment regimens are similar to those described for medication adherence. Due to the often overwhelming nature of the regimen requirements, however, more complex and comprehensive interventions are needed to facilitate successful adherence. It is especially important to remember that the patient's and parents' motivation and cooperation may be the key to intervention success (Falvo, 1994). Thus, interventions that target specifically defined behaviors and socially valid behavior change goals (Finney & Weist, 1988) are more likely to be successful than those that take a less patient-relevant focus. In fact, several authors suggest that tailoring the patient's regimen to the patient's individual needs and schedules, including simplifying or reducing the number of treatment components, is important for facilitating adherence (Falvo, 1994; Rapoff & Christophersen, 1982; J. Thomas, 1994).

Reminders and Reinforcement

Similar to the methods used to facilitate medication adherence, reinforcement can be used to encourage adherence to specific parts of complex regimens. Figure 8.2 provides an example of a reinforcement and reminder strategy to help children with diabetes properly rotate their injection sites. This simple strategy has the child draw a favorite figure, mark potential injection sites with an X, and place stickers on each injection site on the figure to represent the site they chose on their own body. For example, if the child chose to get an injection in her arm, she would place a sticker on the corresponding arm of the figure as a visual reward and reminder of where she got the injection. Rewards are provided for having stickers on all of the indicated sites, and a new chart is developed once each site is "full." This strat-

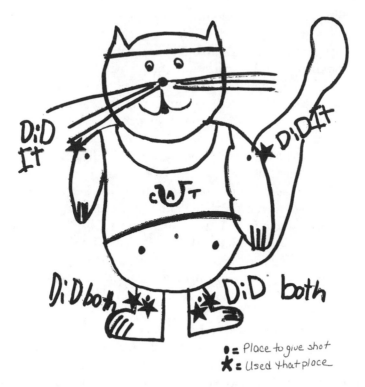

FIGURE 8.2. Visual motivation chart for rotating insulin injection sites.

egy allows children with diabetes to be reminded to rotate their injection sites and also to be reinforced for adhering to this important component of their treatment regimen.

Token Economies and Contracting

Token economies have been successfully used with children following both complex medical regimens, such as those required to manage diabetes (Lowe & Lutzker, 1979) and arthritis (Rapoff, Lindsley, & Christophersen, 1984), and for more acute regimens required to treat urinary tract infections, otitis media, and dental hygiene problems. Token economies and contracting that provide tokens or privileges for completing individual components of a regimen provide parents with a more effective and reinforcing means of encouraging adherence than the use of constant verbal reminders. For example, Rapoff et al. instructed parents in the use of a token economy to improve the adherence of a 7-year-old girl with juvenile rheumatoid arthritis.

She earned tokens for putting on wrist splints before being asked to do so by her parents, for keeping splints on, for taking medication, for taking a morning bath, and for performing morning and evening exercises. Medication, splint wearing, and body positioning adherence were all significantly improved at follow-up 10 weeks later. These results were replicated in a second study of a 14-year-old boy with juvenile rheumatoid arthritis (Rapoff, Purviance, & Lindsley, 1988). Medication compliance for this boy more than doubled with the implementation of a token economy. Improvements in clinical outcomes, defined as active joints determined by the rheumatologist and parental ratings of juvenile rheumatoid arthritis symptoms, were noted by the end of the study.

Lowe and Lutzker (1979) demonstrated the effectiveness of using a token economy for getting a child with Type I diabetes to perform his daily foot care and other tasks. The opportunity to earn tokens for performing a finger stick, testing blood properly, calculating diet points, and calmly taking insulin shots resulted in an improvement in the child's adherence to his medical regimen. A point system that rewarded 10 children with hemophilia for participating in exercise therapy resulted in average adherence rates of 94% during the intervention, compared with an average of 55% during baseline (Greenan-Fowler, Powell, & Varni, 1987). Once the reinforcement system was removed, there was some decrease in adherence over the 9-month follow-up period, with rates averaging from 66% to 84%. Finally, Wysocki, Green, and Huxtable (1989) used contingency contracting to enhance the self-monitoring of blood glucose (SMBG) completed by adolescents with diabetes. Wysocki et al. found that contracting resulted in maintenance of SMBG, whereas a control group demonstrated a sharp decline on this task. As mentioned previously, one limitation of token economy and contracting intervention studies is the almost exclusive use of single-subject designs (e.g., Greenan-Fowler et al., 1987; Rapoff et al., 1984; Schafer, Glasgow, & McCaul, 1982) with fewer studies using a group design (e.g., Wysocki et al., 1989). Nevertheless, token economies and contracting strategies do show some promise as effective interventions for helping children adhere to complex treatment regimens.

Comprehensive Strategies

Despite the obvious challenges presented to families that are trying to manage complex treatment regimens, most intervention studies focus only on a limited number of treatment components with a minimal number of intervention strategies. A meta-analysis of 153 studies on adherence conducted by Roter et al. (1998) indicated that comprehensive interventions comprising more than one strategy, such as those focusing on education, behavior change, and increased support, were more effective than individual strategies for improving adherence in adults and children. Most of the studies that address complex treatment regimens combine educational and behavioral intervention strategies (e.g., Epstein et al., 1981; Gross, 1983; Lowe & Lutzker, 1979). For example, Epstein et al. (1981) found improved adherence to urine testing in children with diabetes by using a combination of parent educational training and contingency contracting with the parents and children.

Child-Related Barriers for Complex Treatment Regimen Adherence

Each child may have individual characteristics independent of his or her medical condition that may present barriers to adherence to a complex treatment regimen. For example, a child's emotional functioning may negatively affect adherence by limiting his or her ability to adjust to and cope with the demands of chronic illness and related care. The impact of emotional distress and psychiatric illness on medical adherence, however, has been difficult to establish. Some studies show that disorders such as anxiety and depression correlate with poor adherence in chronically ill children whose treatment involves complex regimens (e.g., Brownbridge & Fielding, 1994; Jacobson et al., 1990). Similarly, Liss, Waller, Kennard, Capra, and Stephens (1998) suggested that children with Type I diabetes who are nonadherent to such a degree that hospitalization is required demonstrate more psychiatric disorders than children with Type I diabetes who do not require hospitalization. Other studies, however, do not report strong support for such findings (e.g., Bender et al., 1998; Daviss et al., 1995). Such discrepancies may be due to methodological differences in how the child's psychopathology was measured. Thus, further evaluation and treatment may be required for patients with attention, learning, or psychiatric problems. The impact of such disorders on children's ability to manage and adhere to their medical treatment, as well as on their quality of life and functioning in such other areas as school, should be considered when designing interventions to promote adherence.

Addressing Family Barriers to Adherence

Families play an important role in helping children adhere to a medical regimen. Thus, several characteristics of families and their interactions have been investigated as contributing factors to adherence. For example, just as children may have preexisting learning or mental health problems that may negatively impact their adherence behaviors, personal characteristics of the child's parents may also influence medical regimen adherence. For example, depression in parents of children with chronic illness has been correlated with poorer patient adherence (Brownridge & Fielding, 1994). Thus, referring parents to clinicians who specialize in adult disorders may be needed to ultimately facilitate the adherence and health of the pediatric patient. As mentioned previously, an evaluation of a parent's literacy level may also need to be conducted to determine the most appropriate approach to providing adherence-promoting strategies.

Other factors such as family cohesiveness, support, and empathy for illness issues have been positively associated with a high rate of adherence to complex medical regimens (e.g., Hauser et al., 1990; Liss et al., 1998). Family coping skills have also been related to adherence, with families that balance the needs of the child with the needs of the family demonstrating better adherence (Patterson, Budd, Goetz, & Warwick, 1993). However, family conflict, often defined as emotionally charged, minimally empathetic, confrontive, and negative parent–child interactions, has been associated with poor adherence (e.g., Bender et al., 1998; Bobrow, AvRuskin, & Siller, 1985; Hauser et al., 1990; Liss et al., 1998).

Unfortunately, only a few studies have investigated the impact of adherence interventions on such family relationship factors as those described above. One study by Gross, Magalnick, and Richardson (1985) demonstrated that families that participated in a self-management training program had greater adherence with a diabetes regimen and less family conflict compared with families in a control group. The self-management training consisted of teaching the children and parents common behavior management techniques (e.g., reinforcement, shaping, and contracting) to modify each other's behavior. For example, children praised their parents for positive comments, and parents provided reinforcement for their child for modifying problematic care-related behavior. This intervention demonstrates that the patient, parent, or both can be targeted as the focus of behavioral change strategies, depending on the needs and strengths of the family. In another study, families with children who were newly diagnosed with diabetes were provided with support from a family with more experience with diabetes in addition to diabetes education from a multidisciplinary team (Galatzer, Amir, Gil, Karp, & Laron, 1982). Galatzer et al. reported that the families receiving intervention demonstrated significantly better adherence and improved family relationships when compared with families that did not receive the intervention. Finally, an innovative study by Satin, La-Greca, Zigo, and Skyler (1989) that incorporated multifamily education with parent simulation of diabetes care tasks found that adolescents with diabetes enrolled in the intervention group demonstrated a significant improvement in their glycosylated hemoglobin, a commonly used indicator of an individual's metabolic control. No significant changes were reported for family functioning, however.

Addressing Social Barriers to Adherence

Social and cultural factors can also affect the patient's and family's adherence. Many aspects of treatment regimens for children with chronic illness can create difficulties for families in social situations, such as adhering to a dietary plan for diabetes management. Thus, peer and social pressure must be realized as a potential factor that may influence a child's adherence efforts (Delamater, 1993; Delamater, Smith, Kurtz, & White, 1988; A. M. Thomas, Peterson, & Goldstein, 1997). Such factors may be particularly relevant for adolescents, who are typically found to be less adherent with complex medical regimens than younger children (e.g., S. B. Johnson et al., 1992; Ricker, Delamater, & Hsu, 1998; A. M. Thomas et al., 1997). Differences in adherence across childhood and adolescence may be due, in part, to social pressure as well as to changes in parental supervision and the increasing responsibilities children have as they age (Gudas, Koocher, & Wypij, 1991; Iannotti & Bush, 1993).

The social stigma of an illness or its treatment requirements also may have a negative impact on adherence. For example, children who have to leave class to take stimulant medication for the treatment of attention deficit hyperactivity disorder may fail to do so in order to avoid being teased or being different from their peers. Media misinformation often perpetuates or magnifies problems with adherence by creating public anxiety about treatments that involve medication (Stine, 1994).

Peer Interventions

Although peers may have an influential role in pediatric adherence, especially for adolescents, few intervention studies have incorporated peers. The studies that are available, however, show that such interventions are promising for influencing pediatric adherence. For example, one study found that the use of peer counseling resulted in greater adherence to the use of oral contraceptives for adolescents when compared with nurse counseling (M. S. Jay, DuRant, Shoffitt, Linder, & Litt, 1984). Although this study did not address adherence to a regimen related to acute or chronic illness, it is one of the few studies available that investigates the influence of peers on the health behavior of adolescents.

Some preliminary studies on peer-group interventions designed to improve a patient's social problem-solving skills in situations that create adherence problems are showing promise. Kaplan, Chadwick, and Schimmel (1985) provided a social learning intervention that included role playing to help adolescents with diabetes identify difficult social situations and develop responses. When compared with a control group of adolescents who were presented with medical information about diabetes, the social learning group was reported to show better adherence, as demonstrated by the outcome measure of glycosylated hemoglobin. Schlundt et al. (1996) used groups of adolescents with diabetes to help develop a tool for assessing problematic dietary situations. Although Schlundt et al. did not evaluate the effects of such problem-solving efforts on adherence behaviors, their

EXHIBIT 8.6
Possible Solutions for Dealing With Problematic Mealtimes for Children With Diabetes

- Follow meal plan without any compromise.
- Plan ahead to limit potential problems with tempting mealtimes.
- Distract yourself during tempting mealtimes (e.g., talk with friends).
- Discuss problematic mealtimes with the person who created the situation.
- Substitute a healthy food choice for an inappropriate one.
- Eat only a small amount of an inappropriate food choice.
- Compensate for not following meal plan by adjusting insulin intake.
- Compensate for not following meal plan by adjusting exercise level.
- Compensate for not following meal plan at one meal by adjusting later meals.
- Make no attempt to follow the meal plan.

Note. From "Assessing and Overcoming Situational Obstacles to Dietary Adherence in Adolescents With IDDM," by D. G. Schlundt et al., 1996, *Journal of Adolescent Health, 19,* 282–288. Copyright 1996 by The Society for Adolescent Medicine. Adapted with permission.

preliminary findings indicated that adolescents can demonstrate effective problem-solving in role-played social situations that often present difficulties for dietary adherence. Examples of possible solutions based on this study are presented in Exhibit 8.6. Such a list could be used as a source of discussion with patients during an office visit or group intervention to introduce them to problem solving and recognizing solutions and consequences.

CONCLUSION

Children who have acute and chronic illness are frequent users of the health care system. A visit to a physician often results in a recommendation to follow a medication regimen or to alter some aspect of the child's daily life. Despite more than two decades of research, however, we as health care providers and researchers are unable to consistently help children and families adhere to the treatment regimens recommended to keep them well or to improve the quality of their lives. Unfortunately, as so aptly stated by Liptak (1996), "no matter how technologically advanced treatments become, they can only be as effective as compliance with their use" (p. 128).

Some interventions do show promise, however, for improving adherence rates for children who are coping with the demands of acute and chronic illness. One of the most effective ways of increasing the success of an adherence intervention may be to use a combination of strategies. Such comprehensive interventions can be individualized to incorporate parent and patient learning styles, skills, and needs to develop the most effective adherence intervention possible. For example, a patient whose parents cannot read may benefit from intervention strategies that focus more on concrete, behavioral strategies and supportive efforts than those that emphasize written educational materials.

Comprehensive interventions also may be better able to affect outcomes beyond the traditional direct and indirect measures of adherence that have been studied. After reviewing more than 100 studies on adherence, Roter et al. (1998) suggested that adherence research needs to be broader based in terms of outcome measures. For example, D. Baum and Creer (1986) found that although an educational intervention with tangible reinforcers did not enhance adherence among children with asthma, the children were more likely to try to manage their asthma (e.g., avoiding precipitants) compared with children who were asked only to monitor their asthma treatment and attacks. Thus, the intervention may have given the children important prerequisite skills to self-manage their asthma that could affect their ability to adhere to future medical recommendations.

As intervention research and clinical practice continues, strategies that focus on the multidimensional reality of adherence, are adaptable to the individual needs of patients and families, and are supported by health care providers have a greater chance of being effective. Of course, such strategies also must be useful for addressing the long-term and ever-changing adherence issues for families and patients faced with increasing responsibility for their own health care. Clinicians and other mental health professionals can be very useful in this pursuit by assisting families and physicians in developing and monitoring interventions that can have a positive and lasting effect on their adherence efforts.

APPENDIX A

The Home Chip System:
A Treatment Manual

For Children Ages 3 to 7

The Home Chip System was developed for use by parents who have children with behavior problems. The procedures in this system have been used with preschool-age children, in families with one to six children, with parents whose education ranged from less than high school to postgraduate studies, and with income levels ranging from poverty to upper-income professional, and with families from a variety of ethnic and racial backgrounds, including Caucasian, African American, Hispanic, and Asian American.

This system has been used with a range of problem behaviors from minor, everyday difficulties, such as getting children to bed at night and getting them to keep their rooms neat, to moderate problems, such as hitting, temper tantrums, hyperactivity, and talking back. The system has not been evaluated with such severe behavior problems as substance abuse.

This program requires dedicated and highly motivated parents who are willing to put forth the effort necessary to teach their children more appropriate ways of behaving. The program also requires that the children be supervised by someone most of the day. We train parents to be teachers. The parents cannot teach their children if they are not with them. Whether ad-

---

ministered by the parents, a nanny, or an alternative caregiver, the program requires that the children be supervised.

The Home Chip System is designed to provide a maximum amount of instruction and feedback to your child through you, the caregiver. Instruction, feedback, and consequences are the tools you will use to train your child in new desirable behaviors, to eliminate already present undesirable behaviors, or both. The system's effectiveness in changing behaviors will depend on your thoroughness. It will not operate by itself. Its success will depend on the degree to which you actively observe and reward or punish the behaviors you see your child demonstrate.

It has been more than 30 years since the Home Chip System was first introduced in the literature (Christophersen, Arnold, Hill, & Quilitch, 1972), and many professionals are still recommending its use. The most notable is probably Russell Barkley, PhD, who is an expert in the treatment of attention deficit hyperactivity disorder. He included an earlier version of the Chip System as an Appendix in his 1980 book and recommended the use of a Chip System in his 1998 book (see Barkley & Benton, 1998) on strategies for dealing with a defiant child.

HOW THE HOME CHIP SYSTEM WORKS

The Home Chip System is based on two simple, yet thoroughly effective, principles:

1. Behavior that is immediately followed by a good, rewarding consequence continues to occur.
2. Behavior that is followed by an unrewarding or punishing consequence ceases to occur or will occur less often.

Poker Chips

Like money, poker chips themselves have no value. Chips must be given meaning or value to become effective. It is only through their power to purchase necessary and enjoyable goods or activities that they gain meaning and become useful. They must always be available for you, the caregiver, to give and take. However, poker chips serve as rewards or punishments *only when they immediately follow your child's behavior*.

Making Chips Powerful

For chips to be used as an effective consequence for behavior, earning chips (like earning money) must be rewarding for your child; your child must feel like he or she has indeed gained something. Losing chips (like losing money) must be unpleasant or punishing for your child; your child must feel like he or she has lost something.

Chips will become meaningful for your child as he or she uses them to buy the "privileges" of having or doing something that the child desires. Privileges are items or activities, usually available in your home or community, that your child enjoys and can purchase with chips.

Earning Privileges

Privileges can be anything your child likes to do. For example, snacks, playing with friends, playing with toys or games, and shopping with Mom all might be considered privileges by some children. The privilege to have snacks, for instance, permits your child to have snacks when they are available and he or she has paid for them (given you some poker chips). Snacks might be available in the afternoon or before bed. You should decide what constitutes a snack (e.g., one scoop of ice cream, two cookies, or one can of soda) and the times they are available. For chips to be of value, *your child must be required to spend them for his or her privileges*. Thus, if snacks are on the privilege list, your child should not get a snack unless he or she spends his or her chips to purchase one. Privileges must be available as often as possible when your child has the chips. Again, unless the chips are worth something that cannot be purchased without them, they will not be an effective tool in changing your child's behavior.

Starting a Chip System

If you have more than one child in your home, the procedures can be implemented for each of them. It is better to start the chip system with all of your children at the same time rather than start with only the child you are the most concerned about. In this way, the children will be able to learn from each other. Just remember to individualize the behaviors that earn and lose chips on the basis of each child's strengths and weaknesses.

Prior to starting a Chip System, you must decide what behaviors you would like to have your child continue to do, such as making the bed or brushing his or her teeth, and what behaviors you would like to encourage your child to begin doing.

Sit down with your child and make a list of behaviors that you and your child think are positive and suitable for earning chips. It is important to be very specific when choosing behaviors. For example, "clean your room" might not be as clear to your child as providing chips for each of the individual steps involved in cleaning a room. For example, if you instructed your child to pick up the clothes on the floor, give your child chips for picking up the clothes. If you instructed your child to pick up the toys, give him or her chips for picking up the toys. Specifying the steps involved will probably do a much better job than if you just ask you child to clean the room.

The following examples represent behaviors that can earn chips. Fill in behaviors that apply in your home.

Behaviors That Earn Chips

Making bed
Picking up clothes in bedroom
Picking up toys in bedroom
Brushing teeth
Getting dressed on time
Saying please and thank you

_____

_____

Next, you have to agree on how many chips your child will earn each time a household chore has been successfully completed. If you are using this system with more than one child in your family, the point value of similar items on each list should be equal. For example, if "making bed" is on two of your children's lists, it should be worth two chips for both children.

Making bed	+ 2
Picking up clothes in bedroom	+ 2
Picking up toys in bedroom	+ 2
Brushing teeth	+ 2
Getting dressed on time	+ 2
Saying please and thank you	+ 2

_____

_____

One mistake parents usually make is paying their children only for chores. Parents need to find a number of different social skills to pay chips for as well. Please think about a variety of social behaviors that you consider important. Again, it is important to be specific when choosing these behaviors. Some examples are provided below, along with space to add your own.

Social Behaviors That Earn Chips

Sharing with brother	+ 4
Taking verbal feedback without arguing	+ 4
Practicing going to "time-out"	+ 4
Verbalizing a coping strategy	+ 4
Doing homework (per 15 minutes)	+ 8

_____

_____

Each of these behaviors, if completed, results in a chip gain. If not completed, they result in a chip loss. For example, if your child brushed his or her teeth, two chips would be gained. If your child failed to brush his or her teeth, two chips would be lost. *It is more important to give chips than it is to take chips away.* Such behaviors as "helping" or "playing quietly" only earn chips. These are behaviors that are worthwhile to add to your list and to reward consistently, because they are the types of behaviors you would like to see more of every day.

Privileges and Their Value

The privileges listed on your home chip system are privileges your child can "buy" if he or she has the right number of chips. However, the list may change. You will need to be aware of what your child is doing for fun so you can add those activities to the list as necessary. Most of the activities children naturally do in their spare time are things they enjoy. Thus, these activities can be viewed as privileges and can be added to the list of privileges. Some examples are as follows:

Privilege	Cost, in Chips (number of chips)
Watching television	5 chips per 1/2 hour
Playing outside	5 chips
Snacks	5 per snack
Going to friend's	10 chips
Riding bike	5 chips

Behaviors That Lose Chips	Number of Chips Lost
Throwing things	−2
Jumping on furniture	−2
Talking back	−2
Tantrums	−3
Coming downstairs after bedtime	−2
Interrupting	−4
Running in the house	−2
_____	
_____	
_____	

Behaviors that lose chips are behaviors you would like your child to stop doing. For this system to be effective, you *must* take the chips away *immediately* every time one of these behaviors occurs. As mentioned with the behaviors above, it is important to be specific about these behaviors as well. Probably the most frequent behavior that children lose chips for is stalling. So, if you ask your son to pick up his coat and he does not respond within 5 seconds, ask him to give you 4 chips for stalling.

Extra Jobs That Earn Privileges

Setting the table	Sweeping the porch
Picking up trash in yard	Dusting
Wiping off kitchen table	Folding wash cloths

Your child is capable of doing many small jobs around the house. It is important that your child share the responsibilities of the house. This is also an excellent time for you to interact with and to teach your child. A list of jobs, made by you in advance, will provide a chance for your child to earn chips when he or she needs to or when he or she wants to help. Such a list could be attached to the front of your refrigerator with a piece of tape or magnets.

HOW TO GIVE CHIPS AND TAKE THEM AWAY

Both giving and taking away chips should be as pleasant as possible. Here are several things you and your child need to do whenever there is a chip exchange.

Rules for Parents

When giving chips, remember to:

1. Be near your child and able to touch him or her (not 20 feet or two rooms away).
2. Look at your child and smile.
3. Use a pleasant voice.
4. Make sure your child is facing you and looking at you. Praise your child by saying something like, "Hey that's great. You're really doing a nice job. That's really helping me."
5. Reward your child with chips and say, "Here's two chips for helping me with the dishes."
6. Describe the appropriate behavior for your child so your child knows exactly what behavior he or she is being praised and rewarded for.
7. Hug your child occasionally—kids love it!
8. Have your child acknowledge you by saying something like, "Thanks, Mom" or "OK."

When demonstrating to parents and children how to give chips in the office, we always hold the chips between our thumb and first finger and tell the child that he or she has just earned two chips, for example, for picking up his or her jacket. As soon as the child places his or her thumb and fingers on the chips, makes eye contact, and says, "thank you," we release the chips to the child.

Children should have some place to keep their chips. This can be a Tupperware bowl, a "fanny pack," or simply a ceramic bowl from your kitchen. To discourage children from taking each other's chips, use a different color for each child. Also, make certain that you do not have any extra chips somewhere in your home. Children seem to know exactly where to find extra chips if they are anywhere in the home.

228   *APPENDIX A*

When taking away chips, remember to:

1. Be near your child and able to touch him or her.
2. Look at your child and smile.
3. Use a pleasant voice. Your child should not be able to tell by the tone of your voice or your facial expression whether you are going to give or take away chips.
4. Make sure your child is facing you and looking at you.
5. In a calm manner, explain what was inappropriate (see section on instruction).
6. Be sympathetic by saying something like, "I know it's hard to lose chips, but that's the rule."
7. Tell the child how much the chip fine costs.
8. Make sure your child gets the chips appropriately (see next section).
9. Prompting the appropriate responses is sometimes necessary by saying, for example, "Come on, give me a smile. That's right."
10. If a chip loss is taken well by your child, give him or her back one-half of the chip fine, and say, "You took off the chips so well, I'm going to give you back half of the chip fine!" For example, if the fine were two chips, your child would immediately earn one chip back simply by being cooperative when he or she gave you the two chips.
11. If your child is too mad or upset to give you the chips, don't forget the issue. Place your child in time-out (to cool off) and take the chips out of your child's chip container while he or she is in time-out.

Rules for Children

When getting chips, children should:

1. Be facing their parents, looking at them, and smiling.
2. Place their thumb and first finger on the chips and acknowledge receiving the chips by saying, "OK," "Thanks," or something else in a pleasant voice.
3. Put the chips in the specified container. (Any chips left lying around are returned to the bank.)

When losing chips, children should:

1. Face their parents, look at them, and smile (not frown).
2. Acknowledge the chip loss with, "OK," "All right," "I'll get the chips," or something else in a pleasant voice. (Children must keep looking at the parent and be pleasant.)

3. Give the chips to their parents in a pleasant manner. Most parents find that the exchange works best if they ask their child to "count out the chips." So, for a six-chip fine, children count the chips, one by one, as they place them in their mother's hand.

PRACTICE GIVING AND TAKING AWAY CHIPS

Once on the chip system, families frequently encounter instances in which a child has done something to earn chips but has not done it very well. This is an excellent time to teach your child how to do it correctly by having him or her practice doing it correctly. Practicing can be done with both chores and social behaviors.

Practicing With Maintenance Behaviors

When teaching your child how to do a new job correctly or when giving him or her feedback on a job poorly done, practice is essential. For example, if your child is doing the dishes but, when you check, he or she is not doing them correctly, the following rules will help you teach your child the correct way.

Practicing With Dish Washing

Dish Washing Example	Parent Rule
"You're really working steadily and the table looks really clean. Thanks."	Praise a related behavior.
"But it looks like you haven't gotten all the food off the plates."	Describe fully the inappropriate or inadequate behavior.
"It's important that all the dishes are clean with no food left on the plates."	Describe the appropriate behavior.
"Because germs can grow on the dishes, and besides, the next time you use the plate you will want it to be clean."	Give a reason for the appropriate behavior.
"Do you understand?"	Request acknowledgment.
"When food is stuck, a good way to get it off is to use the scraper instead or the cloth—like this."	Model: Show child how to do it.

Dish Washing Example	Parent Rule
"Now you try it."	Practice.
"Great, you're doing a much better job of getting them clean now."	Praise or feedback.
"When you get done, come get me and you will get your chips, plus two for practicing so nicely. You're really doing a good job now."	Praise and reward.

Practicing With Social Behaviors

If your child becomes unpleasant and talks back when he or she loses points, the following rules will be useful to teach your child the appropriate response.

Talking Back Example	Parent Rule
"You came quickly when I called and I really appreciate that."	Praise a related behavior.
"But the rule is that you don't back-talk after a chip loss. I'll have to take off two more chips for talking back."	Describe fully the inappropriate or inadequate behavior.
"Remember, you're supposed to look at me, be pleasant, and say "OK, Dad" in a nice tone of voice."	Describe the appropriate behavior.
"This way we'll get along better at home and it will help you take criticism better at school."	Give a reason for the appropriate behavior.
"Do you understand what you're supposed to do?"	Request acknowledgment.
"Say it pleasantly and give me a big smile—like this" (parent says "OK" and smiles).	Model: Show child how to do it.
"Now you try it."	Practice.
"That's right, you're looking at me with a pleasant facial expression."	Praise or feedback.
"Great, that's how it's done. You practiced very well. You can have a chip back."	Praise and reward.

WHEN TO PRACTICE

The best time to practice any behavior is during a pleasant time of the day, preferably when your child has not done anything wrong. A great time to practice is when your child needs more chips to purchase an item or activity he or she wants. This teaches your child—under pleasant circumstances—how to respond to important situations. Prompting and practicing correct responses, however, are still important after a rule violation or a poorly done job has occurred.

When there has not been a rule violation, practice using make-believe violations and a make-believe time-out. For example, if your child says he or she needs a job to earn some chips, tell your child you will give him or her five chips if he or she will do a good pretend time-out. If your child says, "OK," direct him or her to go to time-out. When your child has completed the pretend time-out, give your child the five chips and tell him or her what a good job he or she did. This is a good way for your child to earn chips at the same time that he or she practices important social behaviors.

You may also practice taking off chips. For example,

Mother: Jim, let's practice how you're supposed to take a chip loss and you can earn two chips.

Jimmy: OK.

Mother: Jim, would you please take two chips off for throwing the ball in the house? Remember the rule is that balls can only be thrown outdoors.

Jimmy: Sure, Mom (with pleasant facial expression and tone of voice).

Mother: That was great! If you can remember to do that the next time you lose chips, I'll give you back half of the chips you lost.

Jimmy: Gee, thanks, Mom.

Mother: Let me give you your chips back because we were just practicing, and I'll give you 4 chips for practicing so well.

CHECKING JOBS

Checking jobs, whether daily or extra work, is a vital aspect of the chip system. It not only helps you teach your child the right way to do things, but it also provides a good opportunity for you to interact with your child in an appropriate way. The rules that apply to practice situations also apply to checking jobs. If the job was done correctly the first time, you need not go through all the steps. Instead, make sure you specifically praise the things done well and give chips.

GIVING CHIPS FOR JOBS COMPLETED WELL

The number of chips given for a job should be decided beforehand; that way, you can reward with extra chips a job done especially well and take away chips for a job performed poorly. All jobs, however, must be done as specified—a poorly done job is not acceptable and must be done again. For this reason, it is good to define how a job is done, then write the description down on the job list so you can look at it whenever a question comes up.

If your child asks you to check the table and all of the steps have been done correctly the first time, praise your child and give him or her the full chip value. If the job was not done correctly, however, go through the practice components and tell your child that if he or she corrects the faulty job components, he or she can get back half the chips that were possible. Be sympathetic but firm. Encourage your child to do it right this time so he or she can get the full number of chips. If, when checked again, the job still is not done correctly, it is probably not because the child does not know how. Place the child in time-out (without loss of privileges). After the time-out is completed, ask your child, again, to do the steps that were not done right. Be sure to practice each time before asking the child to repeat the job (see section on the time-out procedure).

If, after the time-out, your child cooperates and corrects the job, give chips for correcting the job. If your child will not cooperate, place him or her in time-out again. Most children will do what is required of them rather than sit in time-out. The first couple of times they may choose to go to time-out several times in a row—as a test to see if you really intend to follow through. Once in a while, a child will test both you and the rules. Don't give in to such tests, as it may only make it harder to convince your child that your rules are an important part of your family's functioning.

MONITORING YOUR CHILD: THE 10-MINUTE RULE

It is important that you be aware of what your child is doing. Periodic checks should be made so you can reward (give chips and praise) such appropriate behavior as playing quietly or working on a job, and punish (take away chips) such inappropriate behavior as fighting, stalling, or getting into things. You do not have to check every 10 minutes on the dot. However, the checks should be done at intervals somewhere between 5 and 20 minutes. This rule should not be used to harass your child. When you go to see what your child's doing, you do not need to interrogate him or her. Instead, look at your child's behavior and either praise and give chips or take some chips away and give him or her feedback. If your child is quietly engaged in a privilege, such as playing with a game in his or her room with the door closed, you do not need to open the door every 10 minutes to see what your child is doing.

PUNISHMENT: WHEN CHIPS DON'T WORK

The use of brief time-outs, when you do not interact with your child in any way until she has calmed down, can be used at two different times: when your child refuses to do a job or a chore and when your child is out of chips.

Time-out means the temporary revoking of all privileges and social interaction. Traditionally, this has been done by having the child stand in the corner or go to his or her room. We have changed this somewhat to include places where children can see what they are missing by being in time-out. The time-out place should be a dull, but not a scary, place (no closets or dark places!). The best places are a living-room chair, a kitchen chair, or a front step if the child is outside.

The child should be directed to time-out with no more than three or four words. For example, "Time out, stalling," or "Time out, talking back." No further words should be exchanged until your child has calmed down.

There is no such thing as a time-out within a time-out. Once you have directed your child to a time-out, you should not say another word until he or she has calmed down—regardless of what he or she does. Time-outs should be used when your child has lost as many or more chips than he or she has gained. This may occur at any time during the day. In other words, when your child has no chips, he or she must go to time-out.

First, practice time-outs when your child is not upset so it will be easier for him or her when a time-out actually happens. For example, during a nonemotional time of the day, especially if your child has told you he or she needs chips to gain access to an activity he or she wants, your child can earn chips for practicing time-out.

TIME-OUT PROCEDURE

If your child has either refused to do a job or has run out of chips, you need to direct him or her to time-out. To institute a time-out:

Briefly explain to your child that he or she has lost all of the chips and is in time-out.

1. Do not interact with your child until your child is calm. If your child is really upset, he or she may get very obnoxious, including yelling, calling you names, or telling you that you can't make him or her do a time-out if he or she doesn't want to.

2. When the initial stay in time-out is completed, your child then has the choice either to earn some chips or to stay in time-out. Many children choose to stay in time-out, hoping you will give in and let them do what they want to. Don't give in. Just let the time-out last as long as the child wants it do. It is far better to have a couple of long time-outs (even 30 to 45 minutes!) than to have your child think he or she doesn't have to follow your rules. Remember, the time-out is not a substitute for doing the work.

3. Your child must work until he or she has earned at least five chips and may then go about his or her business. That means your child will have to complete some assigned jobs or your child will have to ask you for a job that he or she can do to earn some chips.

Rules for Children in Time-Out

1. While a child is in time-out, no chips are earned or lost.
2. If undesirable behavior occurs while the child is in time-out, ignore it.
3. Social interaction is forbidden during time-out. Instruct other family members to observe this rule and fine the other children each time they interact with anyone in time-out. If the other children are not on the chip system, separate them from the child who is in time-out.
4. Ignore all inappropriate behavior that may follow placement of your child in time-out.
5. As soon as your child is quiet for 2 to 3 *seconds*, tell him or her the time-out is over. Do not remind your child why he or she went to time-out. Do not ask your child why he or she went to time-out. If you're using time-outs to help a child to learn how to calm down, you can't nag him or her after each time-out.
6. Children of all ages should be started out with these very brief time-outs.
7. As your child learns to calm down when he or she is in time-out, gradually increase the amount of time between calming down and the end of the time-out.
8. It is critical that your child learns to associate calming down with a time-out.
9. Later, after your child can readily calm down in time-out, you can begin using time-out with your child when he or she is angry or frustrated, and you won't need the chip system anymore.

Example of a Time-Out

The following conversation is an example of when time-out should be used:

Father: Susie, you were really good about getting home on time, but you forgot to hang up your coat. Remember, the rule is that we all hang up our coats as soon as we get home. Would you give me four chips and then hang your coat up, please?

Susie: I don't want to do it right now.

Father: I know it's hard sometimes, but we all have to follow the rules. That's back-talk. Remember, you're supposed to say "OK Dad," and then go do it. Why don't you give me four more chips for back-talk and we'll try it again.

Susie: I'm not going to give you any chips.

Father: Right now, you're a little upset so you'll have to go to time-out and cool off. [As soon as Susie is quiet, the father can continue.] You're really being quiet, that's great. You're out of time-out now.
[Susie would then be asked to return the four chips to the bank. As soon as she relinquishes the four chips nicely, she'll be given two of the four back because she took them off so nicely. Then, the father would ask her again.]

Father: Susie, would you please hang up your coat for me?

HELPFUL HINTS FOR PARENTS

1. *Nothing good is free*. For chips to be powerful and useful as consequences for behavior, it is absolutely necessary that all privileges be purchased with chips.
2. *If it bugs you, it's worth improving*. If your child does something that annoys you, it probably annoys other adults too. Explain this to your child, set a chip consequence, fine this behavior, and reward a more appropriate one. Thus, any behavior that bothers you should probably be modified. You should define it, instruct your child about the appropriate behavior, and provide feedback.
3. *Baby-sitters*. Have a baby-sitter you can call on short notice. There will undoubtedly be a time before a family outing when one of your children has no chips to pay for the outing. Since it is not fair to make the rest of the family stay home, you will need someone to stay with your child or somewhere to take him or her. If you allow your child to participate in a privilege he or she cannot purchase, you are weakening the whole system.

4. *Don't be discouraged when a behavior doesn't change overnight.* Change will happen more quickly if you are consistent with both taking away chips and giving chips. Frequent practice can also be helpful for changing behavior.
5. *Don't be impatient.* Keep in mind that your child has, on the average, 70 more years to live. A couple of months teaching him or her some critical skills does not seem like such a big deal when you put it in this perspective.
6. *Be prepared.* Prepare your child for the right response before you tell the child what he or she did wrong. Example: "Tommy, I'm going to tell you something that might make you a little angry, but if you keep looking at me, stay pleasant, and take it well, you'll earn an extra five chips." Try it—it works.
7. *Be sympathetic.* When chip fines are given, remember you can express your sympathy with your child's unfortunate situation at the same time that you stay firm in applying the chip fine. Reassure the child who is receiving a lot of chip fines that when you take away chips it does not mean you are mad; it only means he or she is behaving in a manner unacceptable to you.
8. *Refrain from all nagging.* Don't use unenforceable threats, warnings, emotional pleading, or anger as methods of changing behavior; data indicate these do not work. Also, nagging, tantrums, and anger by a parent make life very unpleasant for the whole family. Firm but unemotional, even sympathetic, feedback works best.
9. *Chips and praise should go together.* Chips are not powerful just because they are chips. They must be made to be powerful. *That's the secret to making your chip system work.* To make chips powerful, they must be the *only* way the child can get his or her privileges. When you give chips, also give praise. And, if it is worth a few words of praise, it couldn't hurt to give a few chips.

PHASING OUT THE CHIP SYSTEM

The prime criterion used for deciding when to phase out the chip system should be your child's overall behavior. Your child doesn't need to be "perfect" before the chips are taken out. Rather, when your child's behavior has been satisfactory to you over a period of a month, and he or she has clearly learned self-quieting skills, it is a good time to begin phasing out the chips.

If it is obvious that you phased out the chips too soon, you can always reinstitute them as soon as necessary. To reinstitute the chips, just pick a job that your child completes when asked and give your child the correct number of chips for doing the job when asked.

TRIAL DAYS

While you are still using the chips on a daily basis, initiate trial days off the chip system. The following steps should be followed for any trial day.

1. Explain to your child that you would like to try a day off the chip system.
2. Stress that if things go well, you'll have another trial day the next day, too.
3. Explain that the child must follow the rules just as if he or she were on the chip system.
4. Explain what will happen if the rules are not followed: You will be using time-out for any misbehavior. If time-out is used more than two times for the same behavior, the next day cannot be a trial day. The chips may be started again at any time during any day.
5. Prompting the right response from your child can be very effective in obtaining or regaining cooperation, as the following example shows:
   Mother: Michael, I'm going to give you 4 chips for helping me bring in the groceries. You remember, don't you, that you would have earned twice as many chips if you had carried in the groceries without being asked first?
   Michael: Yes, I understand. Thanks, Mom.

It is important for parents to remember that not all trial days are successful; it may take some time before the chips can be completely phased out. Chips can always be used again, whether it has been 1 day off the system or 4 weeks. After your child once knows how you want him or her to behave, it is up to you to follow through when a rule is broken.

CONCLUSION

When your child is on the chip system, breaking a rule should result in a chip loss. When your child is off the system, breaking a rule should result in time-out. If these procedures are not followed by you, your child will not follow the rules. Praise for desirable behavior is also a must, whether you are on or off the system. If being good does not have a reward (attention, praise, or extra privileges), the desired behavior will not occur as often. When phasing out the chip system, all the procedures for practicing, checking jobs, and time-out should still be followed consistently with praise rather than chips.

The implementation of a chip system provides the necessary structure so parents and children interact in predictable ways with predictable consequences. Over time, parents learn to provide appropriate consequences in a matter-of-fact, consistent, unemotional manner. Children learn how to earn the privileges they desire and to avoid the behaviors that prevent them from earning those privileges. In this way, the chip system can make your family's time together more satisfying and enjoyable.

APPENDIX B

Progressive Muscle Relaxation Exercises

NAME: _____

Week of: _____

Practice for 2 weeks, 15–20 minutes, twice a day.
Check off the positions you practice (or have someone help you).

	Mon	Tues	Weds	Thurs	Fri	Sat	Sun
Relaxing Position							
Tense/Relax:							
Toes							
Legs							
Stomach							
Back							
Shoulders							
Arms							
Jaw							
Nose							
Eyes							
Forehead							
Relaxing Position							

STEPS FOR PROGRESSIVE MUSCLE RELAXATION

Present the following rationale using developmentally appropriate language.

Whenever you feel tense, nervous, upset, or in pain, the muscles in your body can get tight. But when you are having fun and are relaxed, your muscles are relaxed too and feel loose. Today, I am going to teach you how to feel when your muscles are tight and loose. That way when you notice that they are tight, you can relax them. After you practice tensing and relaxing for awhile, you will be able to tell all by yourself when you are tense, and you will be able to make your muscles relax. That can help you be less nervous or feel less pain.

First, you will start in a relaxed position with the breathing we have practiced before, then you will learn how to slowly tense and relax your muscle groups until you feel relaxed from your toes to your head. To get really good at relaxing you will have to practice! Let's start with practicing twice a day. You can practice others times of the day too when you really need to. Find a quiet place to practice and plan for at least 15 minutes so you have enough time. You can practice before school, before bed time, after dinner, or whenever you feel pain or tension.

Do you have any questions?

1. *Starting Out Relaxed*
   Get in a relaxed position in the chair with your feet flat on the floor, arms at your side or hands in your lap. Let yourself sink into the chair and close your eyes. Now start to practice your deep breathing. When you feel as relaxed as you can be, raise your finger for me so I know.

2. *Toes*
   We are going to start by relaxing your toes. I want you to pretend that you are barefoot and standing in the mud. Now take your toes and squish them deep into the mud for 5 seconds. OK, now relax your toes. Try it again, hold for 5 seconds. This time relax your toes a little more slowly.

3. *Legs*
   Now you are going to relax your legs. I want you to lift your legs straight out in front of you and hold them there and don't let them drop. Pretend like your mom is vacuuming underneath your feet and you have to hold your legs up out of the way. Hold for 5 seconds. OK, now let them drop like they are too heavy to hold up anymore. Try it again. This time drop your legs down very slowly and feel the difference between tense and relaxed.

4. *Stomach*

Now your whole lower body should feel relaxing. Take a few deep, relaxing breaths before we move on to your stomach. Tighten your stomach as tight as you can. Try to make it feel like your belly button is touching your spine. Hold it for 5 seconds. Now relax it. Try it again and this time relax a little more slowly.

5. *Back*

Moving on to your back. I want you to move a little bit forward in your chair. Now bring your arms up like you are holding on to the chains of a swing. Now bring your elbows back and try to get them to meet behind your back. Feel how tense your shoulders and back are? Hold it that way for 5 seconds. Now move your hands back and let them drop into your lap. Try it again.

6. *Shoulders*

Time to move onto your shoulders. I want you to stretch your arms way up over your head like a cat might do. Keep your arms up there and spread out your fingers and hold it for 5 seconds. OK, now let your arms drop back into your lap. Arms up again, feel how tight your back and shoulders feel? Hold for 5 seconds, now drop them way down. Feel how relaxed your shoulders and back feel now.

7. *Arms*

Pretend like you have half a lemon in each hand. First I want you to squeeze those lemons as hard as you can for 5 seconds. Pretend like you are squeezing all of the juice out. OK, now let the lemons drop to the floor as you relax your arms. Try it again.

8. *Jaw*

Now it is time to move onto your face muscles. First we are going to practice relaxing your jaw. I want you to smile as big as you can. Make the corners of your lips touch your ears. Hold for 5 seconds. Now let your smile relax back to normal. Big stretchy smile again, hold it. Now relax. Wiggle your mouth around a little to make sure it is relaxed.

9. *Nose*

Let's move up your face to your nose. First, I want you to pretend that you have a fly on your nose and wiggle your nose around to try to get rid of it. Keep moving your nose from side to side for 5 seconds. Now stop and relax like the fly is gone. Try it again.

10. *Eyes*

Now I want you to close your eyes very tightly like you are watching a scary movie and don't want to see the scary part. Feel how tight it is above and below your eye. Hold that for 5 seconds. Now relax your eyes slowly and open them if you want to. Try it again and relax nice and slowly.

11. *Forehead*

This will be our last muscle group to tense and relax. I want you to wrinkle up your forehead like you are really surprised at something. Pull your eyebrows up into your hair. Feel how tense the top of your head is right now. Hold it for 5 seconds. Now relax it. Feel how your eyebrows spread back into a re-laxing place. Now try it again.

12. *Ending Up Relaxed*

To finish up, I want you to sit quietly in your chair with your eyes closed. Start with your toes and feel how relaxed your body is. Your toes, legs, stomach, back, arms, shoulders, and face all feel very relaxed. Take a few minutes to practice your deep breathing and think about how relaxed you feel so you can remember it when you practice at home. If you want to, you can say the word *relax* as you breath out. When you are ready you can open your eyes.

REFERENCES

Achenbach, T. M. (1991). *Manual for the Child Behavior Checklist: 4–18 and 1991 profile*. Burlington: University of Vermont, Department of Psychiatry.

Achenbach, T. M. (1994). *Manual for the Child Behavior Checklist: 2–3 and 1994 profile*. Burlington: University of Vermont, Department of Psychiatry.

Achenbach, T. M., & Edelbrock, C. (1983). *Manual for the Child Behavior Checklist and Revised Child Behavior Profile*. Burlington: University of Vermont, Department of Psychiatry.

Achenbach, T. M., & Edelbrock, C. (1986). *Manual for the Teacher's Report Form and Teacher Version of the Child Behavior Profile*. Burlington: University of Vermont, Department of Psychiatry.

Achenbach, T. M., & Edelbrock, C. (1988). *Manual for the Child Behavior Checklist and Revised Child Behavior Profile*. Burlington: University of Vermont, Department of Psychiatry.

Achenbach, T. M., & McConaughy, S. H. (1996). Relations between *DSM–IV* and empirically based assessment. *School Psychology Review, 25*, 329–341.

Acute Pain Management Guideline Panel. (1992). *Acute pain management: Operative or medical procedures and trauma. Clinical practice guideline* (AHCPR Publication No. 92-0032). Rockville, MD: Agency for Health Care Policy and Research, Public Health Service, U.S. Department of Health and Human Services.

Adair, R., Bauchner, H., Philipp, B., Levenson, S., & Zuckerman, B. (1991). Night waking during infancy: Role of parental presence at bedtime. *Pediatrics, 87*, 500–504.

Adair, R., Zuckerman, B., Bauchner, H., Philipp, B., & Levenson, S. (1992). Reducing night waking in infancy: A primary care intervention. *Pediatrics, 89*, 585–588.

Adams, L. A., & Rickert, V. I. (1989). Reducing bedtime tantrums: Comparison between positive routines and graduated extinction. *Pediatrics, 84*, 756–761.

Ahmann, P. A., Waltonen, S. J., Olson, K. A., Theye, F. W., van Erem, A. J., & LaPlant, R. J. (1993). Placebo-controlled evaluation of Ritalin side effects. *Pediatrics, 91*, 1101–1106.

Allen, J. S., Jr., Tarnowski, K. J., Simonian, S. J., Elliott, D., & Drabman, R. S. (1991). The generalization map revisited: Assessment of generalized treatment effects in child and adolescent behavior therapy. *Behavior Therapy, 22*, 393–405.

Allen, K. D., & Shriver, M. D. (1998). Role of parent-mediated pain behavior management strategies in biofeedback treatment of childhood migraines. *Behavior Therapy, 29*, 477–490.

Allen, K. W. (1996). Chronic nailbiting: A controlled comparison of competing response and mild aversion treatments. *Behavior Research and Therapy, 34*, 269–272.

American Academy of Child and Adolescent Psychiatry. (1997a). Practice parameters for the assessment and treatment of children, adolescents, and adults with attention-deficit/hyperactivity disorder. *Journal of the American Academy of Child and Adolescent Psychiatry, 36*(Suppl.), 85S–121S.

American Academy of Child and Adolescent Psychiatry. (1997b). Practice parameters for the assessment and treatment of children and adolescents with anxiety disorders. *Journal of the American Academy of Child and Adolescent Psychiatry, 36*(Suppl.), 69S–84S.

American Academy of Pediatrics. (2000). Clinical practice guideline: Diagnosis and evaluation of the child with attention-deficit/hyperactivity disorder. *Pediatrics, 105,* 1158–1170.

American Psychiatric Association. (1987). *Diagnostic and statistical manual of mental disorders* (3rd ed., Rev.) Washington, DC: Author.

American Psychiatric Association. (1994). *Diagnostic and statistical manual of mental disorders* (4th ed.). Washington, DC: Author.

Anastopoulos, A. D., Barkley, R. A., & Shelton, T. L. (1996). Family-based treatment: Psychosocial intervention for children and adolescents with attention deficit hyperactivity disorder. In E. D. Hibbs & P. S. Jensen (Eds.), *Psychosocial treatments for child and adolescent disorders: Empirically based strategies for clinical practice* (pp. 267–284). Washington, DC: American Psychological Association.

Anastopoulos, A. D., DuPaul, G. J., & Barkley, R. A. (1992). Stimulant medication and parent training therapies for attention deficit-hyperactivity disorder. *Journal of Learning Disabilities, 24,* 210–218.

Anders, T. F. (1979). Night-waking in infants during the first year of life. *Pediatrics, 63,* 860–864.

Anders, T. F. (1982). Neurophysiological studies of sleep in infants and children. *Journal of Child Psychology and Psychiatry and Allied Disciplines, 23,* 75–83.

Anders, T. F., Halpern, L. F., & Hua, J. (1992). Sleeping through the night: A developmental perspective. *Pediatrics, 90,* 554–560.

Andrews, K., & Fitzgerald, M. (1997). Biological barriers to paediatric pain management. *Clinical Journal of Pain, 13,* 138–143.

Ankjaer, J. A., & Sejr, T. E. (1994). Costs of the treatment of enuresis nocturna: Health economic consequences of alternative methods in the treatment of enuresis nocturna. *Ugeskr-Laeger, 156,* 4355–4360.

Aponte, H. J., & Van Deusen, J. M. (1981). Structural family therapy. In A. S. Gurman & D. P. Kniskern (Eds.), *Handbook of family therapy* (pp. 310–360). New York: Bruner/Mazel.

Arndorfer, R. E., Allen, K. D., & Aljazireh, L. (1999). Behavioral health needs in pediatric medicine and the acceptability of behavioral solutions: Implications for behavioral psychologists. *Behavior Therapy, 30,* 137–148.

Attanasio, V., Andrasik, F., Burke, E. J., Blake, D. D., Kabela, E., & McCarran, M. S. (1985). Clinical issues in utilizing biofeedback with children. *Clinical Biofeedback and Health, 8,* 134–141.

Auslander, W. F., Thompson, S. J., Dreitzer, D., & Santiago, J. V. (1997). Mothers' satisfaction with medical care: Perceptions of racism, family stress, and medical outcomes in children with diabetes. *Health and Social Work, 22,* 190–199.

Azrin, N. H., & Foxx, R. M. (1974). *Toilet training in less than a day.* New York: Simon & Schuster.

Azrin, N. H., & Nunn, R. G. (1973). Habit reversal: A method of eliminating nervous habits and tics. *Behaviour Research and Therapy, 11,* 619–628.

Azrin, N. H., & Nunn, R. G. (1977). *Habit control in a day.* New York: Simon & Schuster.

Azrin, N. H., Nunn, R. G., & Frantz, S. E. (1980). Treatment of hair pulling (trichotillomania): A comparative study of habit reversal and negative practice training. *Journal of Behavior Therapy and Experimental Psychiatry, 11,* 13–20.

Azrin, N. H., Nunn, R. G., & Frantz-Renshaw, S. E. (1982). Habit reversal vs. negative practice treatment of self-destructive oral habits (biting, chewing, or licking of the lips, cheeks, tongue, or palate). *Journal of Behavior Therapy and Experimental Psychiatry, 13,* 49–54.

Azrin, N. H., & Peterson, A. L. (1990). Treatment of Tourette syndrome by habit reversal: A waiting-list control group comparison. *Behavior Therapy, 21,* 305–318.

Azrin, N. H., Sneed, T. J., & Foxx, R. M. (1974). Dry-bed training: Rapid elimination of childhood enuresis. *Behaviour Research and Therapy, 12,* 147–156.

Baker, S. S., Liptak, G. S., Colletti, R. B., Croffie, J. M., DiLorenzo, C., Ector, W., & Nurko, S. (1999). Constipation in infants and children: Evaluation and treatment. *Journal of Pediatric Gastroenterology and Nutrition, 29,* 612–626.

Banerjee, S., Srivastav, A., & Palan, B. M. (1993). Hypnosis and self-hypnosis in the management of nocturnal enuresis: A comparative study with imipramine therapy. *American Journal of Clinical Hypnosis, 36,* 113–119.

Baren, M., & Swanson, J. M. (1996). How not to diagnosis ADHD. *Contemporary Pediatrics, 13,* 53–64.

Barkley, R. A. (1981). *Hyperactive children: A handbook for diagnosis and treatment.* New York: Guilford Press.

Barkley, R. A. (1987). *Defiant children: A clinician's manual for parent training.* New York: Guilford Press.

Barkley, R. A., & Benton, C. M. (1998). *Your defiant child: 8 steps to better behavior.* New York: Guilford Press.

Barkley, R. A., & Grodzinsky, G. M. (1994). Are tests of frontal lobe functions useful in the diagnosis of attention deficit disorders? *Clinical Neuropsychologist, 8,* 121–139.

Barkley, R. A., Guevremont, A. D., Anastopoulos, A. D., & Fletcher, K. E. (1992). A comparison of three family therapy programs for treating family conflicts in adolescents with attention-deficit hyperactivity disorder. *Journal of Consulting and Clinical Psychology, 60,* 450–462.

Barkley, R. A., McMurray, M. B., Edelbrock, C. S., & Robbins, K. (1990). Side effects of methylphenidate in children with attention deficit hyperactivity disorder: A systemic, placebo-controlled evaluation. *Pediatrics, 86*, 184–192.

Barnard, J. D., Christophersen, E. R., & Wolf, M. M. (1977). Teaching children appropriate shopping behavior through parent training in the supermarket setting. *Journal of Applied Behavior Analysis, 10*, 49–59.

Barr, R. G., Levine, M. D., Wilkinson, R. H., & Mulvihill, D. (1979). Chronic and occult stool retention: A clinical tool for its evaluation in school-aged children. *Clinical Pediatrics, 18*, 674–686.

Barrett, P. M. (1995a). *Group coping koala workbook.* Unpublished manuscript, School of Applied Psychology, Griffith University, Queensland, Australia.

Barrett, P. M. (1995b). *Group family anxiety management workbook.* Unpublished manuscript, School of Applied Psychology, Griffith University, Australia.

Barrett, P. M. (1998). Evaluation of cognitive–behavioral group treatment for childhood anxiety disorders. *Journal of Clinical Child Psychology, 27*, 459–468.

Barrett, P. M., Dadds, M. R., & Holland, D. E. (1994). *The coping koala: Prevention manual.* Unpublished manuscript, University of Queensland, Queensland, Australia.

Barrett, P. M., Dadds, M. R., & Rapee, R. M. (1996). Family treatment of childhood anxiety: A controlled study. *Journal of Consulting and Clinical Psychology, 64*, 333–342.

Barry, J., & von Baeyer, C. L. (1997). Brief cognitive–behavioral group treatment for children's headache. *Clinical Journal of Pain, 13*, 215–220.

Bauchner, H. (1991). Procedures, pain, and parents. *Pediatrics, 87*, 563–565.

Baum, C. G. (1989). Conduct disorders. In T. H. Ollendick & M. Hersen (Eds.), *Handbook of child psychopathology* (2nd ed., pp. 171–196). New York: Plenum.

Baum, D., & Creer, T. L. (1986). Medication compliance in children with asthma. *Journal of Asthma, 23*, 49–59.

Becker, M. H., Maiman, L. A., Kirscht, J. P., Haefner, D. P., Drachman, R. H., & Taylor, D. W. (1979). Patient perceptions and compliance: Recent studies of the health belief model. In R. B. Haynes, D. W. Taylor, & D. L. Sackett (Eds.), *Compliance in health care* (pp. 78–109). Baltimore: Johns Hopkins University Press.

Bell-Dolan, D. J., Last, C. G., & Strauss, C. C. (1990). Symptoms of anxiety disorders in normal children. *Journal of the American Academy of Child and Adolescent Psychiatry, 29*, 759–765.

Bellman, M. (1966). Studies on encopresis [Special supplement]. *Acta Paediatrica Scandanavica, 170*.

Bender, B., Milgrom, H., Rand, C., & Ackerson, L. (1998). Psychological factors associated with medication nonadherence in asthmatic children. *Journal of Asthma, 35*, 347–353.

Benton, A. L., & Hamsher, K. (1978). *Multilingual aphasia examination* (Revised manual). Iowa City: University of Iowa Press.

Bergin, A., Wranch, H. R., Brown, J., Carson, K., & Singer, H. S. (1998). Relaxation therapy in Tourette syndrome: A pilot study. *Pediatric Neurology, 18,* 136–142.

Bernstein, B. A., & Pachter, L. M. (1993). Cultural considerations in children's pain. In N. L. Schechter, C. B. Berde, & M. Yaster (Eds.), *Pain in infants, children, and adolescents* (pp. 113–122). Baltimore: Williams & Wilkins.

Bernstein, G. A., Warren, S. L., Massie, E. D., & Thuras, P. D. (1999). Family dimensions in anxious-depressed school refusers. *Journal of Anxiety Disorders, 13,* 513–528.

Beyer, J. E., & Aradine, C. R. (1986). Content validity of an instrument to measure young children's perceptions of the intensity of their pain. *Journal of Pediatric Nursing, 1,* 386–395.

Beyer, J. E., & Aradine, C. R. (1987). Patterns of pediatric pain intensity: A methodological investigation of a self-report scale. *Clinical Journal of Pain, 3,* 130–141.

Beyer, J. E., & Wells, N. (1989). The assessment of pain in children. *Pediatric Clinics of North America, 36,* 837–854.

Biederman, J., Faraone, S. V., Doyle, A., Lehman, B. K., Kraus, I., Perrin, J., & Tsuang, M. T. (1993). Convergence of the Child Behavior Checklist with structured interview-based psychiatric diagnoses of ADHD children with and without comorbidity. *Journal of Child Psychology and Psychiatry, 34,* 1241–1251.

Biederman, J., Faraone, S. V., Milberger, S., Jetton, J. G., Chen, L., Mich, E., Greene, R. S., & Russell, R. L. (1996). Is childhood oppositional defiant disorder a precursor to adolescent conduct disorder? Findings from a four-year follow-up study of children with ADHD. *Journal of the American Academy of Child and Adolescent Psychiatry, 35,* 1193–1204.

Biederman, J., Rosenbaum, J. F., Bolduc-Murphy, E. A., Faraone, S. V., Chaloff, J., Hirshfeld, D. B., & Kagan, J. (1993). A 3-year follow-up of children with and without behavioral inhibition. *Journal of the American Academy of Child and Adolescent Psychiatry, 32,* 814–821.

Bieri, D., Reeve, R. A., Champion, G. D., Addicoat, L., & Ziegler, J. B. (1990). The Faces Pain Scale for the self-assessment of the severity of pain experienced by children: Development, initial validation, and preliminary investigation for ratio scale properties. *Pain, 41,* 139–150.

Binderglas, P. M. (1975). The enuretic child. *Journal of Family Practice, 5,* 375–380.

Birmaher, B., Brent, D. A., Chiappetta, L., Bridge, J., Monga, S., & Baugher, M. (1999). Psychometric properties of the screen for child anxiety related emotional disorders (SCARED): A replication study. *Journal of the American Academy of Child and Adolescent Psychiatry, 38,* 1230–1236.

Birmaher, B., Khetarpal, B., Brent, S., Cully, D., Balach, L., Laufman, J., & Neer, S. M. (1997). The screen for child anxiety related emotional disorders (SCARED): Scale construction and psychometric characteristics. *Journal of the American Academy of Child and Adolescent Psychiatry, 36,* 545–553.

Blader, J. C., Koplewicz, H. S., Abikoff, H., & Foley, C. (1997). Sleep problems of elementary school children: A community survey. *Archives of Pediatric and Adolescent Medicine, 151,* 473–480.

Blount, R. L., Bachanas, P. J., Powers, S. W., Cotter, M. C., Franklin, A., Chaplin, W., Mayfield, J., Henderson, M., & Blount, S. D. (1992). Training children to cope and parents to coach them during routine immunizations: Effects on child, parent, and staff behaviors. *Behavior Therapy, 23,* 689–705.

Blount, R. L., Corbin, S. M., Sturges, J. W., Wolfe, V. V., Prater, J. M., & James, L. D. (1989). The relationship between adults' behavior and child coping and distress during BMA/LP procedures: A sequential analysis. *Behavior Therapy, 20,* 585–601.

Blount, R. L., Dahlquist, L. M., Baer, R. A., & Wuori, D. (1984). A brief, effective method for teaching children to swallow pills. *Behavior Therapy, 15,* 381–387.

Blount, R. L., Powers, S. W., Cotter, M. W., Swan, S., & Free, K. (1994). Training pediatric oncology patients to cope and their parents to coach them during BMA/LP procedures. *Behavior Modification, 18,* 6–31.

Blount, R. L., Sturges, J. W., & Powers, S. W. (1990). Analysis of child and adult behavioral variations by phase of medical procedure. *Behavior Therapy, 21,* 33–48.

Blum, N. J., & Carey, W. B. (1996). Sleep problems among infants and young children. *Pediatrics in Review, 17,* 87–92.

Bobrow, E. S., AvRuskin, T. W., & Siller, J. (1985). Mother–daughter interaction and adherence to diabetes regimens. *Diabetes Care, 8,* 146–151.

Brody, J. E. (1992, January 29). Personal health: Silence on fecal incontinence is harmful; from 1 to 2 percent of children over 4 have the problem. *New York Times,* p. B8.

Broughton, R. J. (1968). Sleep disorders: Disorders of arousal? *Science, 159,* 1070–1078.

Brown, R. T. (1996). Introduction to a special series on pain: Refuting clinical folklore. *Children's Health Care, 25,* 237–251.

Brownbridge, G., & Fielding, D. M. (1994). Psychosocial adjustment and adherence to dialysis treatment regimens. *Pediatric Nephrology, 8,* 744–749.

Bruun, R. D., & Budman, C. L. (1996). Risperidone as a treatment for Tourette's syndrome. *Journal of Clinical Psychiatry, 57,* 29–31.

Bushell, D., Jr. (1978). An engineering approach to the elementary classroom: The behavior analysis follow through project. In A. C. Catania & T. A. Brigham (Eds.), *Handbook of applied behavior analysis: Social and instructional processes* (pp. 525–563). New York: Irvington.

Campbell, S. B. (1995). Behavior problems in preschool children: A review of recent research. *Journal of Child Psychology and Psychiatry, 36,* 113–149.

Campbell, S. B., & Ewing, L. J. (1990). Follow-up of hard-to-manage preschoolers: Adjustment at age 9 and predictors of continuing symptoms. *Journal of Child Psychology and Psychiatry, 31,* 871–889.

Canadian Task Force on the Periodic Health Examination. (1979). The periodic health examination. *Canadian Medical Association Journal, 121,* 1194–1254.

Cantwell. D. P. (1989a). Conduct disorder. In H. I. Kaplan & B. J. Sadock (Eds.), *Comprehensive textbook of psychiatry* (5th ed., pp. 1821–1828). Baltimore: Williams & Wilkins.

Cantwell, D. P. (1989b). Oppositional defiant disorder. In H. I. Kaplan & B. J. Sadock (Eds.), *Comprehensive textbook of psychiatry* (5th ed., pp. 1842–1845). Baltimore: Williams & Wilkins.

Cantwell, D. P. (1996). Attention deficit disorder: A review of the past 10 years. *Journal of the American Academy of Child and Adolescent Psychiatry, 35,* 978–987.

Carr, T. D., Lemanek, K. L., & Armstrong, F. D. (1998). Pain and fear ratings: Clinical implications of age and gender differences. *Journal of Pain and Symptom Management, 15,* 305–313.

Carton, J., & Schweitzer, J. B. (1996). Use of a token economy to increase compliance during hemodialysis. *Journal of Applied Behavior Analysis, 29,* 111–113.

Casey, R., Rosen, B., Glowasky, A., & Ludwig, S. (1985). An intervention to improve follow-up of patients with otitis media. *Clinical Pediatrics, 24,* 149–152.

Cassidy, R. C., & Walco, G. A. (1996). Pediatric pain: Ethical issues and ethical management. *Children's Health Care, 25,* 253–264.

Castellanos, D., & Hunter, T. (1999). Anxiety disorders in children and adolescents. *Southern Medical Journal, 92,* 946–954.

Cavior, N., & Deutsch, A. (1975). Systematic desensitization to reduce dream-induced anxiety. *Journal of Nervous and Mental Disease, 161,* 433–435.

Cendron, M. (1999). Primary nocturnal enuresis: Current concepts. *American Family Physician, 57,* 1205–1218.

Chambless, D. L., Sanderson, W. C., Shoham, V., Johnson, S. B., Pope, K., Crits-Christoph, P., Baker, M., Johnson, B., Woody, S. R., Sue, S., Beutler, L., Williams, D., & McCurry, S. (1996). Update on empirically validated therapies. *Clinical Psychologist, 49,* 5–15.

Chappell, P. B., McSwiggan-Hardin, M. T., Scahill, L., Rubenstein, M., Walker, D. E., Cohen, D. J., & Leckman, J. F. (1994). Videotape tic counts in the assessment of Tourette's syndrome: Stability, reliability, and validity. *Journal of the American Academy of Child and Adolescent Psychiatry, 33,* 386–393.

Christophersen, E. R. (1983). Methodological issues in behavioral and developmental pediatrics. In M. D. Levine, W. B. Carey, A. C. Crocker, & R. T. Gross (Eds.), *Developmental–behavioral pediatrics* (pp. 1197–1209). Philadelphia: Saunders.

Christophersen, E. R. (1991). Toileting problems in children. *Pediatric Annals, 20,* 240–244.

Christophersen, E. R. (1994). *Pediatric compliance: A guide for the primary care physician.* New York: Plenum.

Christophersen, E. R. (1998a). *Beyond discipline: Parenting that lasts a lifetime* (2nd ed.). Shawnee Mission, KS: Overland Press.

Christophersen, E. R. (1998b). *Little people: Guidelines for commonsense child rearing* (4th. ed.). Shawnee Mission, KS: Overland Press.

Christophersen, E. R., Arnold, C. M., Hill, D. W., & Quilitch, H. R. (1972). The home point system: Token reinforcement procedures for application by parents of children with behavior problems. *Journal of Applied Behavior Analysis, 5,* 485–497.

Christophersen, E. R., Barnard, J. D., & Barnard, S. R. (1981). The family training program manual: The home chip system. In R. A. Barkley (Ed.), *Hyperactive children: A handbook for diagnosis and treatment* (pp. 437–448). New York: Guilford Press.

Christophersen, E. R., Cataldo, M. F., Russo, D. C., & Varni, J. W. (1984). Behavioral pediatrics: Establishing and maintaining a program of training, research, and clinical service. *The Behavior Therapist, 7,* 43–46.

Christophersen, E. R., & Purvis, P. C. (2001). Toileting problems in children. In C. E. Walker & M. C. Roberts (Eds.), *The handbook of clinical child psychology* (3rd ed., pp. 453–469). New York: Wiley.

Cipes, M. H. (1985). Self-management versus parental involvement to increase children's compliance with home fluoride mouthrinsing. *Pediatric Dentistry, 7,* 111–118.

Cipes, M. H., & Miraglia, M. (1985). Monitoring versus contingency contracting to increase children's compliance with home fluoride mouthrinsing. *Pediatric Dentistry, 7,* 198–204.

Clark, J. H., Russell, G. J., Fitzgerald, J. F., & Nagamori, K. E. (1987). Serum beta-carotene, retinol, and alpha-tocopherol levels during mineral oil therapy for constipation. *American Journal of Diseases of Childhood, 141,* 1210–1212.

Clark, L. A., Watson, D., & Reynolds, S. (1995). Diagnosis and classification of psychopathology: Challenges to the current system and future directions. *Annual Review of Psychology, 46,* 121–153.

Clay, R. A. (1998). State boards consider Rx recommendations. *APA Monitor, 29,* 5.

Cobham, V. E., Dadds, M. R., & Spence, S. H. (1998). The role of parental anxiety in the treatment of childhood anxiety. *Journal of Consulting and Clinical Psychology, 66,* 893–905.

Cohen, H. A., Barzilai, A., & Lahat, E. (1999). Hypnotherapy: An effective treatment modality for trichotillomania. *Acta Paediatrica, 88,* 407–410.

Cohen, L. L., Blount, R. L., & Panopoulos, G. (1997). Nurse coaching and cartoon distraction: An effective and practical intervention to reduce child, parent, and nurse distress during immunizations. *Journal of Pediatric Psychology, 22,* 355–370.

Cohen, M. W. (1975). Enuresis. *Pediatric Clinics of North America, 22,* 545–560.

Colcher, I. S., & Bass, J. W. (1972). Penicillin treatment of streptococcal pharyngitis: A comparison of schedules and the role of specific counseling. *Journal of the American Medical Association, 222,* 657–659.

Coleman, J., Wolkind, S., & Ashley, L. (1977). Symptoms of behaviour disturbance and adjustment to school. *Journal of Child Psychology and Psychiatry, 18,* 201–209.

Collins, M., Kaslow, N., Doepke, K., Eckman, J., & Johnson, M. (1998). Psychosocial interventions for children and adolescents with sickle cell disease. *Journal of Black Psychology, 24,* 432–454.

Conners, C. K. (1969). A teacher rating scale for use in drug studies with children. *American Journal of Psychiatry, 126*, 884–888.

Conners, C. K. (1995). *Conners' continuous performance test.* New York: Multi Health Systems, Inc.

Conner-Warren, R. L. (1996). Pain intensity and home management of children with sickle cell disease. *Issues in Comprehensive Pediatric Nursing, 19*, 183–195.

Connor, D. F., Barkley, R. A., & Davis, J. T. (2000). A pilot study of methylphenidate, clonidine, or the combination in ADHD comorbid with aggressive oppositional defiant or conduct disorder. *Clinical Pediatrics, 39*, 15–25.

Costello, A. J., Edelbrock, C. S., Dulcan, M. K., Kalas, R., & Klaric, S. H. (1984). *Development and testing of the NIMH diagnostic interview schedule for children on a clinical population: Final report* (Contract RFP-DB-81-0027). Rockville, MD: Center for Epidemiological Studies, National Institute of Mental Health.

Costello, E. J., & Angold, A. (1995). Epidemiology. In J. S. March (Ed.), *Anxiety disorders in children and adolescents* (pp. 109–124). New York: Guilford Press.

Costello, E. J., Angold, A., Burns, B. J., Stangl, D. K., Tweed, D. L., Erkanli, A., & Worthman, C. M. (1996). The great smoky mountains study of youth: Goals, design, methods, and the prevalence of *DSM–III–R* disorders. *Archives of General Psychiatry, 53*, 1129–1136.

Cox, D. J., Sutphen, J., Borowitz, S., Kovatchev, B., & Ling, W. (1998). Contribution of behavior therapy and biofeedback to laxative therapy in the treatment of pediatric encopresis. *Annals of Behavioral Medicine, 20*, 70–75.

Coyle, J. T. (2000). Psychotropic drug use in very young children. *Journal of the American Medical Association, 283*, 1059–1060.

Craig, K. D., Whitfield, M. F., Grunau, R. V., Linton, L., & Hadjistavropoulos, H. D. (1993). Pain in the preterm neonate: Behavioural and physiological indices. *Pain, 52*, 287–299.

Crowther, J. K., Bond, L. A., & Rolf, J. E. (1981). The incidence, prevalence and severity of behavior disorders among preschool-age children in day care. *Journal of Abnormal Child Psychology, 9*, 23–42.

Cummings, E. A., Reid, G. J., Finley, A., McGrath, P. J., & Ritchie, J. A. (1996). Prevalence and source of pain in pediatric inpatients. *Pain, 68*, 25–31.

Curry, S. L., & Russ, S. W. (1985). Identifying coping strategies in children. *Journal of Clinical Child Psychology, 14*, 61–69.

Curtis, A. C., & Ballmer, R. S. (1939). The prevention of carotene absorption by liquid petroleum. *Journal of the American Medical Association, 113*, 1785–1788.

da Costa, I. G., Rapoff, M. A., Lemanek, K., & Goldstein, G. L. (1997). Improving adherence to medication regimens for children with asthma and its effect on clinical outcome. *Journal of Applied Behavior Analysis, 30*, 687–691.

Dadds, M. R., Holland, D. E., Barrett, P. M., Laurens, K. R., & Spence, S. H. (1997). Prevention and early intervention for anxiety disorders: A controlled trial. *Journal of Consulting and Clinical Psychology, 65*, 627–635.

Dadds, M. R., Holland, D. E., Laurens, K. R., Mullins, M., Barrett, P. M., & Spence, S. H. (1999). Early intervention and prevention of anxiety disorders in children: Results at 2-year follow-up. *Journal of Consulting and Clinical Psychology,* *67,* 145–150.

Dahlquist, L. M. (1992). Coping with aversive medical treatments. In A. M. La-Greca, L. J. Siegel, J. L. Wallander, & C. E. Walker (Eds.), *Stress and coping in child health* (pp. 345–376). New York: Guilford Press.

Davidson, M. (1958). Constipation and fecal incontinence. *Pediatric Clinics of North America, 5,* 749–757.

Davidson, M., Kugler, M. M., & Bauer, C. H. (1963). Diagnosis and management in children with severe and protracted constipation and obstipation. *Journal of Pediatrics, 62,* 261–275.

Daviss, W. B., Coon, H., Whitehead, P., Ryan, K., Burkley, M., & McMahon, W. (1995). Predicting diabetic control from competence, adherence, adjustment, and psychopathology. *Journal of the American Academy of Child and Adolescent Psychiatry, 34,* 1629–1635.

De Jong, P. J., Andrea, H., & Muris, P. (1997). Spider phobia in children: Disgust and fear before and after treatment. *Behavior Research and Therapy, 35,* 559–562.

Delamater, A. M. (1993). Compliance interventions for children with diabetes and other chronic diseases. In N. A. Krasnegor, L. Epstein, S. B. Johnson, & S. J. Yaffe (Eds.), *Developmental aspects of health compliance behavior* (pp. 335–354). Hillsdale, NJ: Erlbaum.

Delamater, A. M., Smith, J. A., Kurtz, S. M., & White, N. H. (1988). Dietary skills and adherence in children with insulin-dependent diabetes mellitus. *Diabetes Educator, 14,* 33–36.

Determining reasonable expectations: A multi-disciplinary roundtable discussion on special problems in toilet training. (1990). Durham: Duke University Medical Center, Office of Continuing Medical Education.

Dinges, D. F., Whitehouse, W. G., Orne, E. C., Bloom, P. B., Carlin, M. M., Bauer, N. K., Gillen, K. A., Shapiro, B. S., Ohene-Frempong, K., Dampier, C., & Orne, M. T. (1997). Self-hypnosis training as an adjunctive treatment in the management of pain associated with sickle cell disease. *International Journal of Clinical and Experimental Hypnosis, 45,* 417–432.

Doleys, D. M., Ciminero, A. R., Tollison, J. W., Williams, D. L., & Wells, K. C. (1977). Dry-bed training and retention control training: A comparison. *Behavior Therapy, 8,* 541–548.

Drabman, R. S., & Jarvie, G. (1977). Counseling parents of children with behavior problems: The use of extinction and time-out techniques. *Pediatrics, 59,* 78–85.

Dunbar-Jacob, J., Dunning, E. J., & Dwyer, K. (1993). Compliance research in pediatric and adolescent populations: Two decades of research. In N. A. Krasnegor, L. Epstein, S. B. Johnson, & S. J. Yaffe (Eds.), *Developmental aspects of health compliance behavior* (pp. 29–51). Hillsdale, NJ: Erlbaum.

Dunn-Geier, B. J., McGrath, P. J., Rourke, B. P., Latter, J., & D'Astous, J. (1986). Adolescent chronic pain: The ability to cope. *Pain, 26,* 23–32.

DuPaul, G. J., Anastopoulos, A. D., Shelton, T. L., Guevremont, D. C., & Metevia, L. (1992). Multimethod assessment of attention-deficit hyperactivity disorder:

The diagnostic utility of clinic-based tests. *Journal of Clinical Child Psychology*, *21*, 394–402.

Edwards, K. J., & Christophersen, E. R. (1993). Automated data acquisition through time-lapse videotape recording. *Journal of Applied Behavior Analysis*, *26*, 503–504.

Edwards, K. J., & Christophersen, E. R. (1994). Treating common sleep problems of young children. *Journal of Developmental and Behavioral Pediatrics*, *15*, 207–213.

Eifert, G. H., Schulte, D., Zvolensky, M. J., Lejuez, C. W., & Lau, A. W. (1997). Manualized behavior therapy: Merits and challenges. *Behavior Therapy*, *28*, 499–509.

Eisen, A. R., & Kearney, C. A. (1995). *Practitioner's guide to the treatment of fear and anxiety in children and adolescents*. Northvale, NJ: Aronson.

Elliott, C. H., & Olson, R. A. (1983). The management of children's distress in response to painful medical treatment for burn injuries. *Behavioral Research and Therapy*, *21*, 675–683.

Eney, R. D., & Goldstein, E. O. (1976). Compliance of chronic asthmatics with oral administration of theophylline as measured by serum and salivary levels. *Pediatrics*, *57*, 513–517.

Epstein, L. H., Beck, S., Figueroa, J., Farkas, G., Kazdin, A. E., Daneman, D., & Becker, D. (1981). The effects of targeting improvements in urine glucose on metabolic control in children with insulin dependent diabetes. *Journal of Applied Behavior Analysis*, *14*, 365–375.

Erenberg, G. (1999). Tics. In R. A. Dershewitz (Ed.), *Ambulatory pediatric care* (3rd ed., pp. 806–809). Philadelphia: Lippincott-Raven.

Evidence-Based Working Group. (1992). Evidence-based medicine: A new approach to teaching the practice of medicine. *Journal of the American Medical Association*, *268*, 2420–2425.

Eyberg, S. M. (1985). Behavioral assessment: Advancing methodology in pediatric psychology. *Journal of Pediatric Psychology*, *10*, 123–139.

Eyberg, S. M., Edwards, D., Boggs, S. R., & Foote, R. (1998). Maintaining the treatment effects of parental training: The role of booster sessions and other maintenance strategies. *Clinical Psychology: Science and Practice*, *5*, 544–554.

Falvo, D. R. (1994). *Effective patient education: A guide to increased compliance* (2nd ed.). Gaithersburg, MD: Aspen.

Farrington, D. P. (1991). Childhood aggression and adult violence: Early precursors and later-life outcomes. In D. J. Pepler & K. H. Rubin (Eds.), *The development and treatment of childhood aggression* (pp. 189–197). Hillsdale, NJ: Erlbaum.

Faust, J., & Melamed, B. G. (1984). Influence of arousal, previous experience, and age on surgery preparation of same day surgery and in hospital pediatric patients. *Journal of Consulting and Clinical Psychology*, *52*, 359–365.

Favaloro, R., & Touzel, B. (1990). A comparison of adolescents' and nurses' postoperative pain ratings and perceptions. *Pediatric Nursing*, *16*, 414–424.

Fentress, D. W., Masek, B. J., Mehegan, J. E., & Benson, H. (1986). Biofeedback and relaxation-response training in the treatment of pediatric migraine. *Developmental Medicine and Child Neurology, 28,* 139–146.

Ferber, R. (1985). *Solve your child's sleep problems.* New York: Simon & Schuster.

Ferber, R. (1986). Sleepless child. In C. Guilleminault (Ed.), *Sleep and its disorders in children* (pp. 141–163). New York: Raven.

Ferber, R. (1987). Sleeplessness, night awakenings, and night crying in the infant and toddler. *Pediatrics in Review, 9,* 1–14.

Findling, R. L., McNamara, N. K., Branicky, L. A., Schluchter, M. D., Lemon, E., & Blumer, J. L. (2000). A double-blind pilot study of risperidone in the treatment of conduct disorder. *Journal of the American Academy of Child and Adolescent Psychiatry, 39,* 509–516.

Finley, G. A., McGrath, P. J., Forward, S. P., McNeill, G., & Fitzgerald, P. (1996). Parents' management of children's pain following "minor" surgery. *Pain, 64,* 83–87.

Finney, J. W., Friman, P. C., Rapoff, M. A., & Christophersen, E. R. (1985). Improving compliance with antibiotic regimens for otitis media: Randomized clinical trial in a pediatric clinic. *American Journal of Diseases of Children, 139,* 89–95.

Finney, J. W., Lemanek, K. L., Cataldo, M. F., Katz, H. P., & Fuqua R. W. (1989). Pediatric psychology in primary health care: Brief targeted therapy for recurrent abdominal pain. *Behavior Therapy, 20,* 283–291.

Finney, J. W., Rapoff, M. A., Hall, C. L., & Christophersen, E. R. (1983). Replication and social validation of habit reversal treatment for tics. *Behavior Therapy, 14,* 116–126.

Finney, J. W., & Weist, M. D. (1988). Medical compliance with pediatric regimens: Matching health behavior and health outcome. *Wellness Perspectives, 2,* 17–20.

Fisher, C., Kahn, E., Edwards, A., & Davis, D. M. (1973). A psychophysiological study of nightmares and night terrors: The suppression of Stage 4 night terrors with diazepam. *Archives of General Psychiatry, 28,* 252–259.

Fleischman, M. J. (1981). A replication of Patterson's "Intervention for boys with conduct problems." *Journal of Consulting and Clinical Psychology, 49,* 342–251.

Forbes, G. B. (1998). Clinical utility of the Test of Variables of Attention (TOVA) in the diagnosis of attention-deficit/hyperactivity disorder. *Journal of Clinical Psychology, 54,* 461–476.

Forehand, R. L., & Long, N. (1996). *Parenting the strong-willed child.* Chicago: Contemporary Books.

Forehand, R. L., & McMahon, R. J. (1981). *Helping the noncompliant child: A clinician's guide to parent training.* New York: Guilford Press.

Forsythe, W. I., & Butler, R. J. (1989). Fifty years of enuretic alarms. *Archives of Diseases in Childhood, 64,* 879–885.

Fox, J. E., & Houston, B. K. (1983). Distinguishing between cognitive and somatic trait and somatic state anxiety in children. *Journal of Personality and Social Psychology, 45,* 862–870.

France, K. G., Blampied, N. M., & Wilkinson, P. (1991). Treatment of infant sleep disturbance by trimeprazine in combination with extinction. *Journal of Developmental and Behavioral Pediatrics, 12*, 308–314.

France, K. G., & Hudson, S. M. (1990). Behavior management of infant sleep disturbance. *Journal of Applied Behavior Analysis, 23*, 91–98.

Frank, N. C., Spirito, A., Stark, L., & Owens-Stively, J. (1997). The use of scheduled awakenings to eliminate childhood sleepwalking. *Journal of Pediatric Psychology, 22*, 345–353.

Friedman, A. G., & Ollendick, T. H. (1989). Treatment programs for severe nighttime fears: A methodological note. *Journal of Behavior Therapy and Experimental Psychiatry, 20*, 171–178.

Friman, P. C., Barone, V. J., & Christophersen, E. R. (1986). Aversive taste treatment of finger and thumb sucking. *Pediatrics, 78*, 174–176.

Friman, P. C., Handwerk, M. L., Swearer, S. M., McGinnis, J. C., & Warzak, W. J. (1998). Do children with primary enuresis have clinically significant behavior problems? *Archives of Pediatric and Adolescent Medicine, 152*, 537–539.

Friman, P. C., & Hove, G. (1987). Apparent covariation between child habit disorders: Effects of successful treatment for thumb sucking on untargeted chronic hair pulling. *Journal of Applied Behavior Analysis, 20*, 309–314.

Friman, P. C., & Leibowitz, J. M. (1990). An effective and acceptable treatment alternative for chronic thumb- and finger-sucking. *Journal of Pediatric Psychology, 15*, 57–65.

Friman, P. C., Mathews, J. R., Finney, J. W., Christophersen, E. R., & Leibowitz, M. (1988). Do encopretic children have clinically significant behavior problems? *Pediatrics, 82*, 407–409.

Gabel, S., Hegedus, A. M., Wald, A., Chandra, R., & Chiponis, D. (1986). Prevalence of behavior problems and mental health utilization among encopretic children: Implications for behavioral pediatrics. *Journal of Developmental and Behavioral Pediatrics, 7*, 293–297.

Galatzer, A., Amir, S., Gil, R., & Karp, M., & Laron, Z. (1982). Crisis intervention program in newly diagnosed diabetic children. *Diabetes Care, 5*, 414–419.

Genuis, M. L. (1995). The use of hypnosis in helping cancer patients control anxiety, pain, and emesis: A review of recent empirical studies. *American Journal of Clinical Hypnosis, 37*, 316–325.

Giebehain, J. E., & O'Dell, S. L. (1984). Evaluation of a parent-training manual for reducing children's fear of the dark. *Journal of Applied Behavior Analysis, 17*, 121–125.

Gil, K. M., Wilson, J. J., & Edens, J. L. (1997). The stability of pain coping strategies in young children, adolescents, and adults with sickle cell disease over an 18-month period. *Clinical Journal of Pain, 13*, 110–115.

Glick, B. S., Schulman, D., & Turecki, S. (1971). Diazepam (Valium) treatment in childhood sleep disorders: A preliminary investigation. *Diseases of the Nervous System, 32*, 565–566.

Gold, D. M., Levine, J., Weinstein, T. A., Kessler, B. H., & Pettei, M. J. (1999). Frequency of digital rectal examination in children with chronic constipation. *Archives of Pediatric and Adolescent Medicine, 153*, 377–379.

Goldman, L. S., Genel, M., Bezman, R. J., & Slanetz, P. J. (1998). Diagnosis and treatment of attention-deficit/hyperactivity disorder in children and adolescents. *Journal of the American Medical Association, 279*, 1100–1107.

Goodman, W. K., Price, L. H., Rasmussen, S. A., Mazure, C., Delgado, P., Heninger, G. R., & Charney, D. S. (1989). The Yale–Brown Obsessive–Compulsive Scale: II. Validity. *Archives of General Psychiatry, 46*, 1012–1016.

Goodman, W. K., Rasmussen, S. A., Riddle, M. A., Price, L. H., & Rapoport, J. L. (1986). *Children's Yale–Brown Obsessive–Compulsive Scale* (CY-BOCS). Gainesville, FL: University of Florida, Department of Psychiatry.

Gordon, M. (1983). *The Gordon Diagnostic System*. DeWitt, NY: Gordon Systems.

Goyette, C. H., Conners, C. K., & Ulrich, R. F. (1978). Normative data on revised Conners parent and teacher rating scales. *Journal of Abnormal Child Psychology, 6*, 221–236.

Gragg, R. A., Rapoff, M. A., Danovsky, M. B., Lindsley, C. B., Varni, J. W., Waldron, S. A., & Bernstein, B. H. (1996). Assessing chronic musculoskeletal pain associated with rheumatic disease: Further validation of the pediatric pain questionnaire. *Journal of Pediatric Psychology, 21*, 237–250.

Graziano, A. M., & Mooney, K. C. (1980). Family self-control instruction for children's nighttime fear reduction. *Journal of Consulting and Clinical Psychology, 48*, 206–213.

Graziano, A. M., & Mooney, K. C. (1982). Behavioral treatment of "nightfears" in children: Maintenance of improvements at 2 1/2- to 3-year follow-up. *Journal of Consulting and Clinical Psychology, 50*, 598–599.

Green, W. H. (1989). Stereotypy and habit disorder. In H. I. Kaplan & B. J. Sadock (Eds.), *Comprehensive textbook of psychiatry* (5th ed., pp. 1903–1909). Baltimore: William & Wilkins.

Greenan-Fowler, E., Powell, C., & Varni, J. (1987). Behavioral treatment of adherence to therapeutic exercise by children with hemophilia. *Archives of Physical Medicine and Rehabilitation, 68*, 846–849.

Greenhill, L. L., Pine, D., March, J., Birmaher, B., & Riddle, M. (1998). Assessment issues in treatment research of pediatric anxiety disorders: What is working, what is not working, what is missing, and what needs improvement. *Psychopharmocology Bulletin, 34*, 155–164.

Gross, A. M. (1982). Self-management training and medication compliance in children with diabetes. *Child and Family Behavior Therapy, 4*, 47–55.

Gross, A. M., Magalnick, L. J., & Richardson, P. (1985). Self-management training with families of insulin-dependent diabetic children: A controlled long-term investigation. *Child and Family Behavior Therapy, 7*, 35–50.

Gudas, L. L., Koocher, G. P., & Wypij, D. (1991). Perceptions of medical compliance in children and adolescents with cystic fibrosis. *Developmental and Behavioral Pediatrics, 12*, 236–242.

Hall, C. C. I. (1997). Cultural malpractice: The growing obsolescence of psychology with the changing U.S. population. *American Psychologist, 52,* 642–651.

Harcherik, D. F., Leckman, J. F., Detlor, J., & Cohen, D. J. (1984). A new instrument for clinical studies of Tourette's syndrome. *Journal of the American Academy of Child and Adolescent Psychiatry, 23,* 153–160.

Hauser, S. T., Jacobson, A. M., Lavori, P., Wolfsdorf, J. I., Herskowitz, R. D., Milley, J. E., & Bliss, R. (1990). Adherence among children and adolescents with insulin-dependent diabetes mellitus over a four-year longitudinal follow-up: II. Immediate and long-term linkages with family milieu. *Journal of Pediatric Psychology, 15,* 527–542.

Haynes, R. B., Taylor, D. W., & Sackett, D. L. (1979). *Compliance in health care.* Baltimore: Johns Hopkins University Press.

Hays, R. D., Kravitz, R. L., Mazel, R. M., Sherbourne, C. D., DiMatteo, M. R., Rogers, W. H., & Greenfield, S. (1994). The impact of patient adherence on health outcomes for patients with chronic disease in the medical outcomes study. *Journal of Behavioral Medicine, 17,* 347–360.

Hazzard, A., Hutchinson, S. J., & Krawiecki, N. (1990). Factors related to adherence to medication regimens in pediatric seizure patients. *Journal of Pediatric Psychology, 15,* 543–555.

Heard, P. M., Dadds, M., & Conrad, P. (1992). Assessment and treatment of simple phobias in children: Effects on family and marital relationships. *Behaviour Change, 9,* 73–82.

Heaton, R. K. (1981). *A manual for the Wisconsin Card Sorting Test.* Lutz, FL: Psychological Assessment Resources.

Hermann, C., Kim, M., & Blanchard, E. B. (1995). Behavioral and prophylactic pharmacological intervention studies of pediatric migraine: An exploratory meta-analysis. *Pain, 60,* 239–256.

Hester, N. K. (1979). The preoperational child's reaction to immunization. *Nursing Research, 28,* 250–255.

Hester, N., Foster, R., & Kristensen, K. (1990). Measurement of pain in children: Generalizability and validity of the pain ladder and the poker chip tool. In D. C. Tyler & E. J. Krane (Eds.), *Advances in pain research and therapy* (Vol. 15, pp. 79–84). New York: Raven.

Hibbs, E. D., Clarke, G., Hechtman, L., Abikoff, H. B., Greenhill, L. L., & Jensen, P. S. (1997). Treatment guideline development. *Psychopharamacology Bulletin, 33,* 619–629.

Hibbs, E. D., & Jensen, P. S. (1996). Attention deficit hyperactivity disorder: Introduction. In E. D. Hibbs & P. S. Jensen (Eds.), *Psychosocial treatments for child and adolescent disorders: Empirically based strategies for clinical practice* (pp. 263–266). Washington, DC: American Psychological Association.

Hilgard, J., & LeBaron, S. (1982). Relief of anxiety and pain in children and adolescents with cancer: Quantitative measures and clinical observations. *International Journal of Clinical and Experimental Hypnosis, 30,* 417–442.

Hirschfeld, S., Moss, H., Dragisic, K., Smith, W., & Pizzo, P. A. (1996). Pain in pediatric human immunodeficiency virus infection: Incidence and characteristics in a single-institution pilot study. *Pediatrics, 98,* 449–452.

Hirshfeld, D. R., Rosenbaum, J. F., Biederman, J., Bolduc, E. A., Faraone, S. V., Snidman, N., Reznick, J. S., & Kagan, J. (1992). Stable behavioral inhibition and its association with anxiety disorder. *Journal of the American Academy of Child and Adolescent Psychiatry, 31*(1), 103–110.

Hjalmas, K. (1992). Functional daytime incontinence: Definitions and epidemiology. *Scandinavian Journal of Urology and Nephrology, 141,* 39–44.

Hoder, E. L., & Cohen, D. J. (1992). Repetitive behavioral patterns of childhood. In M. D. Levine, W. B. Carey, & A. C. Crocker (Eds.), *Developmental-behavioral pediatrics* (2nd ed.). Philadelphia: Saunders.

Hodgins, M. J., & Lander, J. (1997). Children's coping with venipuncture. *Journal of Pain and Symptom Management, 13,* 274–285.

Holden, E. W., Deichmann, M. M., & Levy, J. D. (1999). Empirically supported treatments in pediatric psychology: Recurrent pediatric headache. *Journal of Pediatric Psychology, 24,* 91–109.

Hornyak, L. M., & Green, J. P. (2000). *Healing from within.* Washington, DC: American Psychological Association.

Houts, A. C. (1996). Behavioral treatment of enuresis. *Clinical Psychologist, 49,* 5–6.

Houts, A. C., Berman, J. S., & Abramson, H. (1994). Effectiveness of psychological and pharmacological treatments for nocturnal enuresis. *Journal of Consulting and Clinical Psychology, 62,* 737–745.

Houts, A. C., Liebert, R. M., & Padawer, W. (1983). A delivery system for the treatment of primary enuresis. *Journal of Abnormal Child Psychology, 11,* 513–519.

Houts, A. C., Mellon, M. W., & Whelan, J. P. (1988). Use of dietary fiber and stimulus control to treat retentive encopresis: A multiple-baseline investigation. *Journal of Pediatric Psychology, 13,* 435–445.

Hudziak, J. J., Helzer, J. E., Wetzel, W. W., Kessel, K. B., McGee, B., Janca, A., & Przybeck, T. (1993). The use of the *DSM–III–R* Checklist for initial diagnostic assessments. *Comprehensive Psychiatry, 34,* 375–383.

Hufford, M. R. (2000). Empirically supported treatments and comorbid psychopathology: Spelunking Plato's cave. *Professional Psychology: Research and Practice, 31,* 96–99.

Hurley, R. M. (1990). Enuresis: The difference between night and day. *Pediatrics in Review, 12,* 167–170.

Iancu, I., Weizman, A., Kindler, S., Sasson, Y., & Zohar, J. (1996). Serotonergic drugs in trichotillomania: Treatment results in 12 patients. *Journal of Nervous and Mental Disease, 184,* 641–644.

Iannotti, R. J., & Bush, P. J. (1993). Toward a developmental theory of compliance. In N. A. Krasnegor, L. Epstein, S. B. Johnson, & S. J. Yaffe (Eds.), *Developmental aspects of health compliance behavior* (pp. 59–76). Hillsdale, NJ: Erlbaum.

Ingebo, K. B., & Heyman, M. B. (1988). Polyethylene glycol-electrolyte solution for intestinal clearance in children with refractory encopresis. *American Journal of Diseases of Children, 142*, 340–342.

Iwamasa, G. Y., & Orsillo, S. M (1997). Individualizing treatment manuals as a challenge for the next generation. *Behavior Therapy, 28*, 511–515.

Jacobsen, P. B., Manne, S. L., Gorfinkle, K., Schorr, O., Rapkin, B., & Redd, W. H. (1990). Analysis of child and parent behavior during painful medical procedures. *Health Psychology, 9*, 559–576.

Jacobson, A. M., Hauser, S. T., Lavori, P., Wolfsdorf, J. I., Herskowitz, R. D., Milley, J. E., Bliss, R., Gelfand, E., Wertlieb, D., & Stein, J. (1990). Adherence among children and adolescents with insulin-dependent diabetes mellitus over a four-year longitudinal follow-up: I. The influence of patient coping and adjustment. *Journal of Pediatric Psychology, 15*, 511–526.

Janicke, D. M., & Finney, J. W. (1999). Empirically supported treatments in pediatric psychology: Recurrent abdominal pain. *Journal of Pediatric Psychology, 24*, 115–127.

Jaspers, J. P. C. (1996). The diagnosis and psychopharmacological treatment of trichotillomania: A review. *Pharmacopsychiatry, 29*, 115–120.

Jaworski, T. M. (1993). Juvenile rheumatoid arthritis: Pain-related and psychosocial aspects and their relevance for assessment and treatment. *Arthritis Care and Research, 6*, 187–196.

Jay, M. S., DuRant, R. H., Shoffitt, T., Linder, C. W., & Litt, I. F. (1984). Effect of peer counselors on adolescent compliance in use of oral contraceptives. *Pediatrics, 73*, 126–131.

Jay, S. M., Elliott, C. H., Fitzgibbons, I., Woody, P., & Siegel, S. (1995). A comparative study of cognitive behavior therapy versus general anesthesia for painful medical procedures in children. *Pain, 62*, 3–9.

Jay, S. M., Elliott, C. H., Katz, E., & Siegel, S. E. (1987). Cognitive–behavioral and pharmacologic interventions for children's distress during painful medical procedures. *Journal of Consulting and Clinical Psychology, 55*, 860–865.

Jay, S. M., Elliott, C. H., Ozolins, M., Olson, R. A., & Pruitt, S. D. (1985). Behavioral management of children's distress during painful medical procedures. *Behavioral Research and Therapy, 23*, 513–520.

Jay, S. M., Elliott, C. H., & Varni, J. W. (1986). Acute and chronic pain in adults and children with cancer. *Journal of Consulting and Clinical Psychology, 54*, 601–607.

Jay, S. M., Elliott, C. H., Woody, P. D., & Siegel, S. (1991). An investigation of cognitive–behavior therapy combined with oral valium for children undergoing painful medical procedures. *Health Psychology, 101*, 317–322.

Jay, S. M., Ozolins, M., Elliott, C. H., & Caldwell, S. (1983). Assessment of children's distress during painful medical procedures. *Health Psychology, 2*, 133–147.

Jenkins, S., Bax, M., & Hart, H. (1980). Behavior problems in preschool children. *Journal of Child Psychology and Psychiatry, 21*, 5–18.

Jensen, P. S., Kettle, L., Roper, M. R., Sloan, M. T., Dulcan, M. K., Hoven, C., Hector, P. H., Bird, H. R., Bauermeister, J. J., & Payne, J. D. (1999). Are stimulants overprescribed? Treatment of ADHD in four U.S. communities. *Journal of the American Academy of Child and Adolescent Psychiatry, 38,* 797–804.

Jensen, P. S., Salzberg, A. D., Richters, J. E., & Watanabe, H. K. (1993). Scales, diagnoses, and child psychopathology: I. CBCL and DISC relationships. *Journal of the American Academy of Child and Adolescent Psychiatry, 32,* 397–406.

Johnson, C. M., Bradley-Johnson, S., & Stack, J. M. (1981). Decreasing the frequency of infants' nocturnal crying with the use of scheduled awakenings. *Family Practice Research Journal, 1,* 98–104.

Johnson, S. B., Kelly, M., Henretta, J. C., Cunningham, W. R., Tomer, A., & Silverstein, J. H. (1992). A longitudinal analysis of adherence and health status in childhood diabetes. *Journal of Pediatric Psychology, 17,* 537–553.

Johnston, C. C., Abbott, F. V., Gray-Donald, I., & Jeans, M. E. (1992). A survey of pain in hospitalized patients aged 4–14 years. *Clinical Journal of Pain, 8,* 154–163.

Johnston, C. C., Stevens, B. J., Yang, F., & Horton, L. (1995). Differential response to pain by very premature neonates. *Pain, 61,* 471–479.

Jones, S. L., Jones, P. K., & Katz, J. (1989). A nursing intervention to increase compliance in otitis media patients. *Applied Nursing Research, 2,* 68–73.

Joyce, B. A., Schade, J. G., Keck, J. F., Gerkensmeyer, J., Raftery, T., Moser, S., & Huster, G. (1994). Reliability and validity of preverbal pain assessment tools. *Issues in Comprehensive Pediatric Nursing, 17,* 121–135.

Kagan, J. (1966). Reflection-impulsivity: The generality and dynamics of conceptual tempo. *Journal of Abnormal Psychology, 71,* 17–24.

Kahn, A., Mozin, M. J., Rebuffat, E., Sottiaux, M., & Muller, M. F. (1989). Milk intolerance in children with persistent sleeplessness: A prospective double-blind crossover evaluation. *Pediatrics, 84,* 595–602.

Kahn, A., Rebuffat, E., Blum, D., Casimir, G., Duchateau, J., Mozin, M. J., & Jost, R. (1987). Difficulty in initiating and maintaining sleep associated with cow's milk allergy in infants. *Sleep, 10,* 116–121.

Kales, J. D., Soldatos, C. R., & Caldwell, A. B. (1980). Nightmares: Clinical characteristics and personality patterns. *American Journal of Psychiatry, 137,* 1197–2001.

Kaplan, R. M., Chadwick, B. A., & Schimmel, L. E. (1985). Social learning intervention to promote metabolic control in Type I diabetes mellitus: Pilot experiment results. *Diabetes Care, 8,* 152–155.

Kataria, S., Swanson, M. S., & Trevathon, G. E. (1987). Persistence of sleep disturbances in preschool children. *Journal of Pediatrics, 110,* 642–646.

Katz, E. R., Kellerman, J., & Siegel, S. E. (1980). Behavioral distress in children with cancer undergoing medical procedures: Developmental considerations. *Journal of Consulting and Clinical Psychology, 48,* 356–365.

Kaufman, A. S., & Kaufman, N. L. (1983). *Kaufman Assessment Battery for Children—Interpretive manual.* Circle Pines, MN: American Guidance Service.

Kazak, A. E., Penati, B., Boyer, B. A., Himelstein, B., Brophy, P., Waibel, M. K., Blackall, G. F., Daller, R., & Johnson, K. (1996). A randomized controlled prospective outcome study of a psychological and pharmacological intervention protocol for procedural distress in pediatric leukemia. *Journal of Pediatric Psychology, 21*, 615–631.

Kazdin, A. E. (1977). *The token economy: A review and evaluation.* New York: Plenum.

Kazdin, A. E. (1982). The token economy: A decade later. *Journal of Applied Behavior Analysis, 15*, 431–445.

Kazdin, A. E. (1985). *Treatment of antisocial behavior in children and adolescents.* Homewood, IL: Dorsey.

Kazdin, A. E. (1995). *Conduct disorder in childhood and adolescence* (2nd ed.). Newbury Park, CA: Sage.

Kazdin, A. E. (1996). Problem solving and parent management in treating aggressive and antisocial behavior. In E. D. Hibbs & P. S. Jensen (Eds.), *Psychosocial treatments for child and adolescent disorders: Empirically based strategies for clinical practice* (pp. 377–408). Washington, DC: American Psychological Association.

Kazdin, A. E., Bass, D., Ayers, W. A., & Rodgers, A. (1990). Empirical and clinical focus of child and adolescent psychotherapy outcome research. *Journal of Consulting and Clinical Psychology, 58*, 729–740.

Kazdin, A. E., Bass, D., Siegel, T., & Thomas, C. (1989). Cognitive–behavioral therapy and relationship therapy in the treatment of children referred for antisocial behavior. *Journal of Consulting and Clinical Psychology, 57*, 522–535.

Kazdin, A. E., Siegel, T. C., & Bass, D. (1992). Cognitive problem-solving skills training and parent management training in the treatment of antisocial behavior in children. *Journal of Consulting and Clinical Psychology, 60*, 733–747.

Kazdin, A. E., & Wassell, G. (2000). Therapeutic changes in children, parents, and families resulting from treatment of children with conduct problems. *Journal of American Academy of Child and Adolescent Psychiatry, 39*, 414–420.

Kazdin, A. E., & Weisz, J. R. (1998). Identifying and developing empirically supported child and adolescent treatments. *Journal of Consulting and Clinical Psychology, 66*, 19–36.

Kearney, C. A., & Silverman, W. K. (1998). A critical review of pharmacotherapy for youth with anxiety disorders: Things are not as they seem. *Journal of Anxiety Disorders, 12*, 83–102.

Keefe, F. J. (1996). Cognitive behavioral therapy for managing pain. *Clinical Psychologist, 49*, 4–5.

Kellerman, J. (1979). Behavioral treatment of night terrors in a child with acute leukemia. *Journal of Nervous and Mental Disease, 167*, 182–185.

Kellerman, J. (1980). Rapid treatment of nocturnal anxiety in children. *Journal of Behavior Therapy and Experimental Psychiatry, 11*, 9–11.

Kemph, J. P., DeVane, C. L., Levin, G. M., Jarecke, R., & Miller, R. L. (1993). Treatment of aggressive children with clonidine: Results of an open pilot study.

Journal of the American Academy of Child and Adolescent Psychiatry, 32, 577–581.

Kendall, P. C. (1990). *Coping cat workbook.* (Available from P. C. Kendall, Department of Psychology, Temple University, Philadelphia, PA 19122)

Kendall, P. C. (1992). *Coping cat workbook.* Ardmore, PA: Workbook Publishing.

Kendall, P. C. (1994). Treating anxiety disorders in children: Results of a randomized clinical trial. *Journal of Consulting and Clinical Psychology, 62*, 100–110.

Kendall, P. C. (2000). *Cognitive–behavioral therapy for anxious children therapist manual, 2nd edition.* Ardmore, PA: Workbook Publishing.

Kendall, P. C., & Braswell, L. (1985). *Cognitive–behavioral therapy for impulsive children.* New York: Guilford Press.

Kendall, P. C., Flannery-Schroeder, E., Panichelli-Mindel, S. M., Southam-Gerow, M., Henin, A., & Warman, M. (1997). Therapy for youths with anxiety disorders: A second randomized clinical trial. *Journal of Consulting and Clinical Psychology, 65*, 366–380.

Kendall, P. C., Kane, M., Howard, B., & Siqueland, L. (1990). *Cognitive–behavioral therapy for anxious children: Treatment manual.* (Available from P. C. Kendall, Department of Psychology, Temple University, Philadelphia, PA 19122)

Kendall, P. C., & Southam-Gerow (1996). Long-term follow-up of a cognitive–behavioral therapy for anxiety-disordered youth. *Journal of Consulting and Clinical Psychology, 64*, 724–730.

Kerr, S. M., Jowett, S. A., & Smith, L. N. (1996). Preventing sleep problems in infants: A randomized controlled trial. *Journal of Advanced Nursing, 24*, 938–942.

King, N. J., Clowes-Hollins, V., & Ollendick, T. H. (1997). The etiology of childhood dog phobia. *Behavior Research and Therapy, 35*, 77.

King, N. J., Tonge, B. J., Heyne, D., Pritchard, M., Rollings, S., Young, D., Myerson, N., & Ollendick, T. H. (1998). Cognitive–behavioral treatment of school-refusing children: A controlled evaluation. *Journal of the American Academy of Child and Adolescent Psychiatry, 37*, 395–403.

King, S. A. (1995). Review: *DSM–IV* and pain. *Clinical Journal of Pain, 11*, 171–176.

Klorman, R., Hilpert, P. L., Michael, R., LaGana, C., & Sveen, O. B. (1980). Effects of coping and mastery modeling on experienced and inexperienced pedodontic patients' disruptiveness. *Behavior Therapy, 11*, 156–168.

Koch, D. A., Giardina, P. J., Ryan, M., MacQueen, M., & Hilgartner, M. W. (1993). Behavioral contracting to improve adherence in patients with thalassemia. *Journal of Pediatric Nursing, 8*, 106–111.

Kohen, D. G., Olness, K. N., Colwell, S. O., & Heimel, A. (1984). The use of relaxation-mental imagery (self-hypnosis) in the management of 505 pediatric behavioral encounters. *Developmental and Behavioral Pediatrics, 5*, 21–25.

Kohen, D. P. (1996). Hypnotherapeutic management of pediatric and adolescent trichotillomania. *Journal of Developmental and Behavioral Pediatrics, 17*, 328–334.

Kohen, D. P., & Botts, P. (1987). Relaxation-imagery (self-hypnosis) in Tourette syndrome: Experience with four children. *American Journal of Clinical Hypnosis, 29*, 227–237.

Kohen, D. P., Olness, K. N., Colwell, S. O., & Heimel, A. (1984). The use of relaxation-mental imagery (self-hypnosis) in the management of 505 pediatric behavioral encounters. *Journal of Developmental and Behavioral Pediatrics, 5*, 21–25.

Koot, H. M., & Verhulst, F. C. (1991). Prevalence of problem behavior in Dutch children aged 2–3. *Acta Psychiatrica Scandianvica, 83*(Suppl. 367), 1–37.

Kotagal, S., Hartse, K. M., & Walsh, J. K. (1990). Characteristics of narcolepsy in preteenaged children. *Pediatrics, 85*, 205–209.

Kotzer, A. M., Coy, J., & LeClaire, A. D. (1998). The effectiveness of a standardized educational program for children using patient-controlled analgesia. *Journal of the Society of Pediatric Nursing, 3*, 117–126.

Kovacs, M., Goldston, D., Obrosky, S., & Iyengar, S. (1992). Prevalence and predictors of pervasive noncompliance with medical treatment among youths with insulin-dependent diabetes mellitus. *Journal of the American Academy of Child and Adolescent Psychiatry, 31*, 1112–1119.

Krakow, B., Kellner, R., Neidhardt, J., Pathak, D., & Lambert, L. (1993). Imagery rehearsal treatment of chronic nightmares: With a thirty month follow-up. *Journal of Behavior Therapy and Experimental Psychiatry, 24*, 325–330.

Kurtz, S. M. (1990). Adherence to diabetes regimens: Empirical status and clinical applications. *The Diabetes Educator, 16*, 50–57.

Kuttner, L. (1988). Favorite stories: A hypnotic pain-reduction technique for children in acute pain. *American Journal of Clinical Hypnosis, 30*, 289–295.

Kuttner, L. (1997). Mind–body methods of pain management. *Child and Adolescent Psychiatric Clinics of North America, 6*, 783–796.

Labellarte, M. J., Ginsburg, G. S., Walkup, J. T., & Riddle, M. A. (1999). The treatment of anxiety disorders in children and adolescents. *Biological Psychiatry, 46*, 1567–1598.

LaClave, L. J., & Blix, S. (1989). Hypnosis in the management of symptoms in a young girl with malignant astrocytoma: A challenge to the therapist. *International Journal of Clinical and Experimental Hypnosis, 37*, 6–14.

La Greca, A. M. (1983). Interviewing and behavioral observations. In C. E. Walker & M. C. Roberts (Eds.), *Handbook of clinical child psychology* (pp. 109–131). New York: Wiley.

Lalonde, J., Turgay, A., & Hudson, J. I. (1998). Attention-deficit hyperactivity disorder subtypes and comorbid disruptive behaviour disorders in a child and adolescent mental health clinic. *Canadian Journal of Psychiatry, 43*, 623–628.

Landman, G. B., Levine, M. D., & Rappaport, L. (1983). A study of treatment resistance among children referred for encopresis. *Clinical Pediatrics, 23*, 449–452.

Larsson, B., & Carlsson, J. (1996). A school-based, nurse-administered relaxation training for children with chronic tension-type headache. *Journal of Pediatric Psychology, 21,* 603–614.

Larsson, B., Daleflod, B., Hakansson, L., & Melin, L. (1987). Therapist assisted versus self-help relaxation treatment of chronic headaches in adolescents: A school-based intervention. *Journal of Child Psychology, Psychiatry, and Allied Disciplines, 28,* 127–136.

Larsson, B., & Melin, L. (1986). Chronic headaches in adolescents: Treatment in a school setting with relaxation training as compared with information-contact and self-regulation. *Pain, 25,* 325–336.

Last, C. G., Hansen, C., & Franco, N. (1998). Cognitive–behavioral treatment of school phobia. *Journal of the American Academy of Child and Adolescent Psychiatry, 37,* 404–411.

Last, C. G., Perrin, S., Hersen, M., & Kazdin, A. E. (1992). *DSM–III–R* anxiety disorders in children: Sociodemographic and clinical characteristics. *Journal of the American Academy of Child and Adolescent Psychiatry, 31,* 1070–1076.

Lavigne, J. V., Arend, R., Rosenbaum, D., Smith, A., Weissbluth, M., Binns, H. J., & Christoffel, K. K. (1999). Sleep and behavior problems among preschoolers. *Journal of Developmental and Behavioral Pediatrics, 20,* 164–169.

Lavigne, J. V., Ross, C. K., Berry, S. L., Hayford, J. R., & Pachman, L. M. (1992). Evaluation of a psychological treatment package for treating pain in juvenile rheumatoid arthritis. *Arthritis Care and Research, 5,* 101–110.

Lazarus, A., & Abramovitz, A. (1962). The use of emotive imagery in the treatment of child's phobia. *Journal of Mental Science, 108,* 191–192.

LeBaron, S., & Zeltzer, L. (1984). Assessment of acute pain and anxiety in children and adolescents by self-reports, observer reports, and a behavior checklist. *Journal of Consulting and Clinical Psychology, 52,* 729–738.

Leckman, J. F., Riddle, M. A., Hardin, M. T., Ort, S. I., Swartz, K. L., Stevenson, J., & Cohen, D. J. (1989). The Yale Global Tic Severity Scale: Initial testing of a clinician-rated scale of tic severity. *Journal of the American Academy of Child and Adolescent Psychiatry, 28,* 566–573.

Lee, L. W., & White-Traut, R. C. (1996). The role of temperament in pediatric pain response. *Issues in Comprehensive Pediatric Nursing, 19,* 49–63.

Legrand, L. N., McGue, M., & Iacono, W. G. (1999). A twin study of state and trait anxiety in childhood and adolescence. *Journal of Child Psychology and Psychiatry, 40,* 953–958.

Leith, P. J., & Weisman, S. J. (1997a). The management of painful procedures in children. *Child and Adolescent Psychiatric Clinics of North America, 6,* 829–842.

Leith, P. J., & Weisman, S. J. (1997b). Pharmacologic interventions for pain management in children. *Child and Adolescent Psychiatric Clinics of North America, 6,* 797–815.

Lemanek, K. (1990). Adherence issues in the medical management of asthma. *Journal of Pediatric Psychology, 15,* 437–458.

Lerner, J., Franklin, J. E., Meadows, E. A., Hembree, E., & Foa, E. B. (1998). Effectiveness of a cognitive behavioral treatment program for trichotillomania: An uncontrolled evaluation. *Behavior Therapy, 29,* 157–171.

Leventhal, H. (1993). Theories of compliance, and turning necessities into preferences: Application to adolescent health action. In N. A. Krasnegar, L. Epstein, S. B. Johnson, & S. J. Yaffe (Eds.), *Developmental aspects of health compliance behavior* (pp. 91–124). New York: Plenum.

Levine, M. D. (1975). Children with encopresis: A descriptive analysis. *Pediatrics, 56,* 412–416.

Levine, M. D. (1976). Children with encopresis: A study of treatment outcome. *Pediatrics, 56,* 845–852.

Levine, M. D. (1982). Encopresis: Its potentiation, evaluation, and alleviation. *Pediatric Clinics of North America, 29,* 315–330.

Levine, M. D. (1983). Encopresis. In M. D. Levine, W. B. Carey, & A. C. Crocker (Eds.), *Developmental–behavioral pediatrics* (2nd ed., pp. 389–397). Philadelphia: Saunders.

Ley, P. (1977). Psychological studies of doctor-patient communication. In S. Rachman (Ed.), *Contributions to medical psychology* (pp. 9–42). New York: Pergamon.

Lezak, M. D. (1983). *Neuropsychological assessment* (2nd ed.). New York: Oxford University Press.

Ling, W., Cox, D. J., Sutphen, J., & Borowitz, S. (1996). Psychological factors in encopresis: Comparison of patients to nonsymptomatic siblings. *Clinical Pediatrics, 35,* 427.

Liptak, G. S. (1996). Enhancing patient compliance in pediatrics. *Pediatrics in Review, 17,* 128–134.

Liss, D. S., Waller, D. A., Kennard, B. D., Capra, P., & Stephens, J. (1998). Psychiatric illness and family support in children and adolescents with diabetic ketoacidosis: A controlled study. *Journal of the American Academy of Child and Adolescent Psychiatry, 37,* 536–544.

Loening-Baucke, V. A. (1994). Management of chronic constipation in infants and toddlers. *American Family Physician, 49,* 397–400, 403–406, 411–413.

Loening-Baucke, V. A. (1996). Encopresis and soiling. *Pediatric Clinics of North America, 43,* 279–298.

Loening-Baucke, V. A., Cruikshank, B. M., & Savage, C. (1987). Defecation dynamics and behavior profiles in encopretic children. *Pediatrics, 80,* 672–679.

Lombroso, P. J., Scahill, L., King, R. A., Lynch, K. A., Chappell, P. B., Peterson, B. S., McDougle, C. J., & Leckman, J. F. (1995). Risperidone treatment of children and adolescents with chronic tic disorders: A preliminary report. *Journal of the American Academy of Child and Adolescent Psychiatry, 34,* 1147–1152.

Long, P., Forehand, R., Wierson, M., & Morgan, A. (1994). Does parent training with young noncompliant children have long term effects? *Behavior Research and Therapy, 32,* 101–107.

Lovibond, S. H. (1964). *Conditioning and enuresis.* Oxford, England: Pergamon.

Lowe, K., & Lutzker, J. R. (1979). Increasing compliance to a medical regimen with a juvenile diabetic. *Behavior Therapy, 10,* 57–64.

Lozoff, B., Wolf, A. W., & Davis, N. S. (1985). Sleep problems seen in pediatric practice. *Pediatrics, 75,* 477–483.

Lutfey, K. E., & Wishner, W. J. (1999). Beyond "compliance" is "adherence": Improving the prospect of diabetes care. *Diabetes Care, 22,* 635–639.

Luxem, M. C., & Christophersen, E. R. (1999). Elimination disorders. In S. Netherton, D. Holmes, & C. E. Walker (Eds.), *Child and adolescent psychological disorders: A comprehensive textbook.* New York: Oxford University Press.

Luxem, M. C., Christophersen, E. R., Purvis, P. C., & Baer, D. M. (1997). Behavioral–medical treatment of pediatric toileting refusal. *Journal of Developmental and Behavioral Pediatrics, 18,* 34–41.

Macknin, M. L., Medendorp, S. V., & Maier, M. C. (1989). Infant sleep and bedtime. *American Journal of Diseases of Children, 143,* 1066–1068.

Magill, M. K., & Garrett, R. W. (1988). Behavioral and psychiatric problems. In R. B. Taylor (Ed.), *Family medicine* (3rd ed., pp. 534–562). New York: Springer-Verlag.

Mailman-Sosland, J. E., & Christophersen, E. R. (1991). Does SleepTight work? A preliminary behavioral analysis of the effectiveness of SleepTight for the management of infant colic. *Journal of Applied Behavior Analysis, 24,* 161–166.

Maiman, L. A., Becker, M. H., Liptak, G. S., Nazarian, L. F., & Rounds, K. A. (1988). Improving pediatricians' compliance-enhancing practices. *American Journal of Diseases of Children, 142,* 773–779.

Malone, A. B. (1996). The effects of live music on the distress of pediatric patients receiving intravenous starts, venipunctures, injections, and heel sticks. *Journal of Music Therapy, 33,* 19–33.

Manassis, K., & Hood, J. (1998). Individual and familial predictors of impairment in childhood anxiety disorders. *Journal of the American Academy of Child and Adolescent Psychiatry, 37,* 428–434.

Manne, S. L., Redd, W. H., Jacobsen, P. B., Gorfinkle, K., Schorr, O., & Rapkin, B. (1990). Behavioral intervention to reduce child and parent distress during venipuncture. *Journal of Consulting and Clinical Psychology, 58,* 565–572.

March, J. S., & Albano, A. M. (1998). New developments in assessing pediatric anxiety disorders. In T. H. Ollendick & R. J. Prinz (Eds.), *Advances in clinical child psychology* (Vol. 20, pp. 213–241). Plenum: New York.

March, J. S., Conners, C., Arnold, G., Epstein, J., Parker, J., Hinshaw, S., Abikoff, H., Molina, B., Wells, K., Newcorn, J., Schuck, S., Pelham, W. E., & Hoza, B. (1999). The Multidimensional Anxiety Scale for Children (MASC): Confirmatory factor analysis in a pediatric ADHD sample. *Journal of Attention Disorders, 3,* 85–89.

March, J. S., & Mulle, K. (1996). Banishing OCD: Cognitive–behavioral psychotherapy for obsessive–compulsive disorders. In E. D. Hibbs & P. S. Jensen (Eds.), *Psychosocial treatments for child and adolescent disorders: Empirically based strategies for clinical practice* (pp. 83–102). Washington, DC: American Psychological Association.

March, J. S., Parker, J. D., Sullivan, K, Stallings, P., & Conners, K. (1997). The Multidimensional Anxiety Scale for Children (MASC): Factor structure, reliability, and validity. *Journal of the American Academy of Child and Adolescent Psychiatry, 36,* 554–565.

March, J. S., Sullivan, K., & Parker, J. (1999). Test–retest reliability of the Multidimensional Anxiety Scale for Children. *Journal of Anxiety Disorders, 13,* 349–358.

Mash, E. J., & Terdal, L. G. (1988). Behavioral assessment of child and family disturbance. In E. J. Mash & L. G. Terdal (Eds.), *Behavioral assessment of childhood disorders: Selected core disorders* (2nd ed., pp. 3–65). New York: Guilford Press.

Masters, K. J. (1996). Melatonin for sleep problems. *Journal of the American Academy of Child & Adolescent Psychiatry, 35,* 704.

Matthews, J. R., McGrath, P. J., & Pigeon, H. (1993). Assessment and measurement of pain in children. In N. L. Schechter, C. B. Berde, & M. Yaster (Eds.), *Pain in infants, children, and adolescents* (pp. 97–111). Baltimore: Williams & Wilkens.

Matthey, S. (1988). Cognitive–behavioural treatment of a thunder phobic child. *Behaviour Change, 5,* 80–84.

McClung, H. J., Boyne, L. J., Linsheid, R., Heitlinger, L. A., Murray, R. D., Fyda, J., & Li, B. U. K. (1993). Is combination therapy for encopresis nutritionally safe? *Pediatrics, 91,* 591–594.

McConville, B. J., Fogelson, M. H., Norman, A. B., Klykylo, W. M., Manderscheid, P. Z., Parker, K. W., & Sanberg, P. R. (1991). Nicotine potentiation of Haloperidol in reducing tic frequency in Tourette's disorder. *American Journal of Psychiatry, 148,* 793–794.

McGrath, M. L., & Masek, B. J. (1993). Behavioral treatment of headache. In N. L. Schechter, C. B. Berde, & M. Yaster (Eds.), *Pain in infants, children, and adolescents* (pp. 555–560). Baltimore: Williams & Wilkins.

McGrath, M. L., Mellon, M. W., & Murphy, L. (2000). Empirically supported treatments in pediatric psychology: Constipation and encopresis. *Journal of Pediatric Psychology, 25,* 225–254.

McGrath, P. A. (1987). An assessment of children's pain: A review of behavioral, physiological and direct scaling techniques. *Pain, 31,* 147–176.

McGrath, P. A. (1990). *Pain in children: Nature, assessment, and treatment.* New York: Guilford Press.

McGrath, P. A. (1993). Psychological aspects of pain perception. In N. Schechter, C. Berde, & M. Yaster (Eds.), *Pain in infants, children, and adolescents* (pp. 39–63). Baltimore: Williams & Wilkins.

McGrath, P. A., deVeber, L. L., & Hearn, M. T. (1985). Multidimensional pain assessment in children. In H. L. Fields, R. Dubner, & F. Cervero (Eds.), *Advances in pain research and therapy* (Vol. 9, pp. 387–393). New York: Raven.

McGrath, P. J. (1996). Attitudes and beliefs about medication and pain management in children. *Journal of Palliative Care, 12,* 46–50.

McGrath, P. J., Humphreys, P., Keene, D., Goodman, J. T., Lascelles, M. A., Cunningham, S. J., & Firestone, P. (1992). The efficacy and efficiency of a self administered treatment for adolescent migraine. *Pain, 49,* 321–324.

McKendry, J. B., & Stewart, D. A. (1974). Enuresis. *Pediatric Clinics of North America, 21,* 1019–1020.

McKendry, J. B., Stewart, D. A., Khanna, F., & Netley, C. (1975). Primary enuresis: Relative success of three methods of treatment. *Canadian Medical Association Journal, 113,* 953–955.

McMenamy, C., & Katz, R. (1989). Brief parent-assisted treatment for children's nighttime fears. *Journal of Developmental and Behavioral Pediatrics, 10,* 145–148.

McQuaid, E. L., & Nassau, J. H. (1999). Empirically supported treatments of disease-related symptoms in pediatric psychology: Asthma, diabetes, and cancer. *Journal of Pediatric Psychology, 24,* 305–328.

Melamed, B. G., Dearborn, M., & Hermecz, D. A. (1983). Necessary considerations for surgery preparation: Age and previous experience. *Psychosomatic Medicine, 45,* 511–521.

Melamed, B. G., & Siegel, L. J. (1980). *Behavioral medicine: Practical applications in health care.* New York: Springer.

Mellon, M. W., & McGrath, M. L. (2000). Empirically supported treatments in pediatric psychology: Nocturnal enuresis. *Journal of Pediatric Psychology, 25,* 193–214.

Mendlowitz, S. L., Manassis, K, Bradley, S., Scapillato, D., Miezitis, S., & Shaw, B. F. (1999). Cognitive–behavioral group treatments in childhood anxiety disorders: The role of parental involvement. *Journal of the American Academy of Child and Adolescent Psychiatry, 38,* 1223–1229.

Merckelbach, H., & Muris, P. (1997). The etiology of childhood spider phobia. *Behaviour Research and Therapy, 35,* 1031–1034.

Meunier, P., Mollard, P., & Marechal, J. M. (1976). Physiopathology of megarectum: The association of megarectum with encopresis. *Gut, 17,* 224–227.

Miltenberger, R. G., Fuqua, R. W., & McKinley, T. (1985). Habit reversal with muscle tics: Replication and component analysis. *Behavior Therapy, 16,* 39–50.

Minde, K., Faucon, A., & Falkner, S. (1994). Sleep problems in toddlers: Effects of treatment on their daytime behavior. *Journal of the American Academy of Child and Adolescent Psychiatry, 33,* 1114–1121.

Mindell, J. A. (1993). Sleep disorders in children. *Health Psychology, 12,* 151–162.

Mindell, J. A. (1999). Empirically supported treatments in pediatric psychology: Bedtime refusal and night wakings in young children. *Journal of Pediatric Psychology, 24,* 465–481.

Minuchin, S. (1974). *Families and family therapy.* Cambridge, MA: Harvard University Press.

Miser, A. W. (1993). Management of pain associated with childhood cancer. In N. L. Schechter, C. B. Berde, & Yaster, M. (Eds.), *Pain in infants, children, and adolescents* (pp. 411–424). Baltimore: Williams & Wilkins.

Miser, A. W., Dothage, J. A., Wesley, R. A., & Miser, J. S. (1987). The prevalence of pain in a pediatric and young adult cancer population. *Pain, 29,* 73–83.

Moffatt, M. E. (1997). Nocturnal enuresis: A review of the efficacy of treatments and practical advice for clinicians. *Journal of Developmental and Behavioral Pediatrics, 18,* 49–56.

Moffatt, M. E., Harlos, S., Kirshen, A. J., & Burd, L. (1993). Desmopressin acetate and nocturnal enuresis: How much do we know? *Pediatrics, 92,* 420–425.

Moore, T., & Ucko, L. E. (1957). Night waking in early infancy: Part I. *Archives of Diseases in Childhood, 32,* 333–342.

Morgan, A. H., & Hilgard, J. R. (1979). The Stanford hypnotic clinical scale for children. *American Journal of Clinical Hypnosis, 21,* 148–169.

Morrison, D. N., McGee, R., & Stanton, W. R. (1992). Sleep problems in adolescence. *Journal of the American Academy of Child & Adolescent Psychiatry, 31,* 94–99.

Morton, N. S. (1998). Prevention and control of pain in children. *Pain Reviews, 5,* 1–15.

Mouton, S. G., & Stanley, M. A. (1996). Habit reversal training for trichotillomania: A group approach. *Cognitive and Behavioral Practice, 3,* 159–182.

Mowrer, O. H., & Mowrer, W. M. (1938). Enuresis: A method for its study and treatment. *American Journal of Orthopsychiatry, 8,* 436–459.

MTA Cooperative Group. (1999). A 14-month randomized clinical trial of treatment strategies for attention-deficit/hyperactivity disorder. *Archives of General Psychiatry, 56,* 1073–1086.

Muris, P., Merckelbach, H., Gadet, B., Moulaert, V., & Tierney, S. (1999). Sensitivity for treatment effects of the screen for child anxiety related emotional disorders. *Journal of Psychopathology and Behavioral Assessment, 21,* 323–335.

Muris, P., Merckelbach, H., Holdrinet, I., & Sijsenaar, M. (1998). Treating phobic children: Effects of EMDR versus exposure. *Journal of Consulting and Clinical Psychology, 66,* 193–198.

Muris, P., Merckelbach, H., van Haaften, H., & Mayer, B. (1997). Eye movement desensitization and reprocessing versus exposure in vivo: A single-session crossover study of spider phobic children. *British Journal of Psychiatry, 171,* 82–86.

Muris, P., Schmidt, H., & Merckelbach, H. (1999). The structure of specific phobia symptoms among children and adolescents. *Behaviour Research and Therapy, 37,* 863–868.

Mushlin, A. I., & Appel, F. A. (1977). Diagnosing potential noncompliance: Physicians' ability in a behavioral dimension of medical care. *Archives of Internal Medicine, 137,* 318–321.

National Asthma Education and Prevention Program. (1997). *Expert Panel Report 2: Guidelines for the diagnosis and management of asthma* (NIH Publication No. 97-4051, p. 73). Washington, DC: National Institutes of Health.

National Institutes of Health Task Force on the Diagnosis and Treatment of Attention Deficit Hyperactivity Disorder. (1998, November). *NIH Consensus Statement, 16*(2).

Newacheck, P. W., & Taylor, W. R. (1992). Childhood chronic illness: Prevalence, severity, and impact. *American Journal of Public Health, 82,* 364–371.

Nilzon, K. R., & Palmerus, K. (1998). Anxiety and withdrawal of depressed 9–11 year olds three years later: A longitudinal study. *School Psychology International, 19,* 341–349.

O'Brien, S., Ross, L. V., & Christophersen, E. R. (1986). Primary encopresis: Evaluation and treatment. *Journal of Applied Behavior Analysis, 19,* 137–145.

Offord, D. R., & Bennett, K. J. (1994). Conduct disorder: Long-term outcomes and intervention effectiveness. *Journal of the American Academy of Child and Adolescent Psychiatry, 33,* 1069–1078.

Ollendick, T. H. (1983). Reliability and validity of the revised Fear Survey Schedule for Children (FSSC–R). *Behaviour Research and Therapy, 21,* 685–692.

Ollendick, T. H. (2000). *Empirically-validated treatments.* Unpublished manuscript, Virginia Polytechnic Institute and State University.

Ollendick, T. H., & King, N. J. (1998). Empirically supported treatments for children with phobic and anxiety disorders: Current status. *Journal of Clinical Child Psychology, 27,* 156–167.

Olness, K. (1975). The use of self-hypnosis in the treatment of childhood enuresis. *Clinical Pediatrics, 14,* 273–279.

Olness, K. (1981). Imagery (self-hypnosis) as adjunct therapy in childhood cancer: Clinical experience with 25 patients. *American Journal of Pediatric Hematology/Oncology, 3,* 313–321.

Osborne, R. B., Hatcher, J. W., & Richtsmeier, A. J. (1989). The role of social modeling in unexplained pediatric pain. *Journal of Pediatric Psychology, 14,* 43–61.

Öst, L. G. (1996). One-session group treatment of spider phobia. *Behaviour Research and Therapy, 34,* 707–715.

Öst, L. G., Brandberg, M., & Alm, T. (1997). One versus five sessions of exposure in the treatment of flying phobia. *Behaviour Research and Therapy, 35,* 987–996.

Öst, L. G., Hellstroem, K., & Kaver, A. (1992). *Behavior Therapy, 23,* 263–282.

Ostrander, R., Weinfurt, K. P., Yarnold, P. R., & August, G. J. (1998). Diagnosing attention deficit disorders with the Behavioral Assessment System for Children and the Child Behavior Checklist: Test and construct validity analyses using optimal discriminant classification trees. *Journal of Consulting and Clinical Psychology, 66,* 660–672.

Owens-Stively, J. (1995). *Childhood constipation and soiling: A practical guide for parents and children* (2nd ed.). Minneapolis, MN: Children's Health Care.

Oxford, D. R., & Bennett, K. J. (1994). Conduct disorder: Long-term outcomes and intervention effectiveness. *Journal of the American Academy of Child and Adolescent Psychiatry, 33,* 1069–1078.

Pace, T. M., Chaney, J. M., Mullins, L. L., & Olson, R. A. (1995). Psychological consultation with primary care physicians: Obstacles and opportunities in the medical setting. *Professional Psychology: Research and Practice, 26,* 123–131.

Partin, J. C., Hamill, S. K., Fischel, J. E., & Partin, J. S. (1992). Painful defecation and fecal soiling in children. *Pediatrics, 89,* 1007–1009.

Patterson, G. R. (1971). *Families: Application of social learning to family life.* Champaign, IL: Research Press.

Patterson, G. R. (1974). Interventions for boys with conduct problems: Multiple settings, treatments, and criteria. *Journal of Consulting and Clinical Psychology, 42,* 471–481.

Patterson, G. R. (1982). *Coercive family process.* Eugene, OR: Castalia.

Patterson, G. R., & Chamberlain, P. (1994). A functional analysis of resistance during parent training therapy. *Clinical Psychology: Science and Practice, 1,* 53–70.

Patterson, G. R., & Gullion, M. D. (1968). *Living with children: New methods for parents and teachers.* Champaign, IL: Research Press.

Patterson, G. R., Reid, J. B., Jones, R. R., & Conger, R. W. (1975). *A social learning approach to family intervention* (Vol. I). Eugene, OR: Castalia.

Patterson, J. M., Budd, J., Goetz, D., & Warwick, W. J. (1993). Family correlates of 10-year pulmonary health in cystic fibrosis. *Pediatrics, 91,* 383–389.

Pear, R. (2000, March 20). White House seeks to curb pills used to calm the young. *New York Times* [On-line].

Perlmutter, A. D. (1976). Enuresis. In T. P. Kelalis & L. R. King (Eds.), *Clinical pediatric urology* (pp. 166–181). Philadelphia: Saunders.

Perrin, E. C. (1999). Commentary: Collaboration in pediatric primary care: A pediatrician's view. *Journal of Pediatric Psychology, 24,* 453–458.

Perrin, S., & Last, C. G. (1992). Do childhood anxiety measures measure anxiety? *Journal of Abnormal Child Psychology, 20,* 567–578.

Peter, B. (1997). Hypnosis in the treatment of cancer pain. *Australian Journal of Clinical and Experimental Hypnosis, 25,* 40–52.

Peterson, A. L., Camprise, R. L., & Azrin, N. H. (1994). Behavioral and pharmacological treatments for tic and habit disorders: A review. *Journal of Developmental and Behavioral Pediatrics, 15,* 430–441.

Pfefferbaum, B., Adams, J., & Aceves, J. (1990). The influence of culture on pain in Anglo and Hispanic children with cancer. *Journal of the American Academy of Child and Adolescent Psychiatry, 29,* 642–647.

Physicians' desk reference. (49th ed.). (1995). Montvale, NJ: Medical Economics Data Production Company.

Physicians' desk reference. (53rd ed.). (1999). Oradell, NJ: Medical Economics Company.

Pine, D. S., Cohen, P., Gurley, D., Brook, J., & Ma, Y. (1998). The risk for early-adulthood anxiety and depressive disorders in adolescents with anxiety and depressive disorders. *Archives of General Psychiatry, 55,* 56–63.

Pinilla, T., & Birch, L. L. (1993). Help me make it through the night: Behavioral entrainment of breast-fed infants' sleep patterns. *Pediatrics, 91*, 436–444.

Pollard, C. A., Ibe, O. I., Krojanker, D. N., Kitchen, A. D., Bronson, S. S., & Flynn, T. M. (1991). Clomipramine treatment of trichotillomania: A follow-up report on four cases. *Journal of Clinical Psychiatry, 52*, 128–130.

Pollock, J. I. (1992). Predictors and long-term associations of reported sleep difficulties in infancy. *Journal of Reproductive and Infant Psychology, 10*, 151–168.

Pollock, J. I. (1994). Night waking at five years of age: Predictor and prognosis. *Journal of Child Psychology and Child Psychiatry and Allied Disciplines, 35*, 699–708.

Porteus, S. D. (1965). *Porteus Maze Test: Fifty years application*. New York: Psychological Corporation.

Powers, S. W. (1999). Empirically supported treatments in pediatric psychology: Procedure-related pain. *Journal of Pediatric Psychology, 24*, 131–145.

Powers, S. W., Blount, R. L., Bachanas, P. J., Cotter, M. W., & Swan, S. C. (1993). Helping preschool leukemia patients and their parents cope during injections. *Journal of Pediatric Psychology, 18*, 681–695.

Prior, M., Smart, D., Sanson, A., & Oberklaid (2000). Does shy-inhibited temperament in childhood lead to anxiety problems in adolescence? *Journal of the American Academy of Child and Adolescent Psychiatry, 39*, 461–468.

Quay, H. C. (1986). Conduct disorders. In H. C. Quay & J. S. Werry (Eds.), *Psychopathological disorders of childhood* (3rd ed., pp. 35–72). New York: Wiley.

Rapoff, M. A. (1999). *Adherence to pediatric medical regimens*. New York: Kluwer Academic/Plenum.

Rapoff, M. A., & Christophersen, E. R. (1982). Improving compliance in pediatric practice. *Pediatric Clinics of North America, 29*, 339–357.

Rapoff, M. A., Christophersen, E. R., & Rapoff, K. E. (1982). The management of common childhood bedtime problems by pediatric nurse practitioners. *Journal of Pediatric Psychology, 7*, 179–196.

Rapoff, M. A., Lindsley, C. B., & Christophersen, E. R. (1984). Improving compliance with medical regimens: Case study with juvenile rheumatoid arthritis. *Archives of Physical Medicine and Rehabilitation, 65*, 267–269.

Rapoff, M. A., Purviance, M. R., & Lindsley, C. B. (1988). Improving medication compliance for juvenile rheumatoid arthritis and its effect on clinical outcome: A single-subject analysis. *Arthritis Care and Research, 1*, 12–16.

Rapoport, A. M., & Sheftell, F. D. (1996). *Headache disorders: A management guide for practitioners*. Philadelphia: Saunders.

Rapp, J. T., Miltenberger, R. G., Long, E. S., Elliott, A. J., & Lumley, V. A. (1998). Simplified habit reversal treatment for chronic hair pulling in three adolescents: A clinical replication with direct observation. *Journal of Applied Behavior Analysis, 31*, 299–302.

Rappaport, L. A., & Leichtner, A. M. (1993). Recurrent abdominal pain. In N. L. Schechter, C. B. Berde, & M. Yaster (Eds.), *Pain in infants, children, and adolescents* (pp. 561–570). Baltimore: Williams & Wilkins.

Rappley, M. D., Mullan, P. B., Alvarez, F. J., Eneli, I. U., Wang, J., & Gardiner, J. C. (1999). Diagnosis of attention-deficit/hyperactivity disorder and use of psychotropic medication in very young children. *Archives of Pediatric and Adolescent Medicine, 153*, 1039–1045.

Ravilly, S., Robinson, W., Suresh, S., Wohl, M. E., & Berde, C. B. (1996). Chronic pain in cystic fibrosis. *Pediatrics, 98*, 741–747.

Reid, M. J., Walter, A. L., & O'Leary, S. G. (1999). Treatment of young children's bedtime refusal and nighttime wakings: A comparison of "standard" and graduated ignoring procedures. *Journal of Abnormal Child Psychology, 27*, 5–16.

Reitan, R. M., & Wolfson, D. (1985). *The Halstead–Reitan Neuropsychological Test Battery.* Tucson, AZ: Neuropsychological Press.

Reynolds, C. R., & Kamphaus, R. W. (1998). *BASC: Behavior Assessment System for Children: Manual including preschool norms for ages 2–6 though 3–11.* Circle Pines, MN: American Guidance Service.

Reynolds, C. R., & Richmond, B. O. (1985). *Revised Children's Manifest Anxiety Scale (RCMAS) manual.* Los Angeles: Western Psychological Services.

Richman, N. (1981). Sleep problems in young children. *Archives of Diseases of Children, 56*, 491–493.

Richman, N. (1985). A double-blind drug trial of treatment in young children with waking problems. *Journal of Child Psychology and Psychiatry, 26*, 591–598.

Richman, N., Stevenson, J., & Graham, P. J. (1982a). *Pre-school to school: A behavior study.* New York: Academic Press.

Richman, N., Stevenson, J. E., & Graham, P. J. (1982b). Prevalence of behaviour problems in 3-year-old children: An epidemiological study in a London borough. *Journal of Child Psychology and Psychiatry, 16*, 277–287.

Richmond, J. B., Eddy, E. J., & Garrard, S. D. (1954). The syndrome of fecal soiling and megacolon. *American Journal of Orthopsychiatry, 24*, 391–401.

Ricker, J. H., Delamater, A. M., & Hsu, J. (1998). Correlates of regimen adherence in cystic fibrosis. *Journal of Clinical Psychology in Medical Settings, 5*, 159–172.

Rickert, V. I., & Johnson, M (1988). Reducing nocturnal wakening and crying episodes in infants and young children: A comparison between scheduled awakenings and systematic ignoring. *Pediatrics, 81*, 203–211.

Roberts, R. N., & Gordon, S. B. (1979). Reducing childhood nightmares subsequent to a burn trauma. *Child Behavior Therapy, 1*, 373–381.

Robins, L. N. (1966). *Deviant children grown up.* Baltimore: Williams & Williams.

Robinson, E. A., Eyberg, S. M., & Ross, A. W. (1980). The standardization of an inventory of child conduct problem behaviors. *Journal of Clinical Child Psychology, 9*, 23–29.

Robinson, L. M., Sclar, D. A., Skaer, T. L., & Galin, R. S. (1999). National trends in the prevalence of attention-deficit/hyperactivity disorder and the prescribing of methylphenidate among school-age children: 1990–1995. *Clinical Pediatrics, 38*, 209–217.

Rockney, R. M., McQuade, W. H., Days, A. L., Linn, H. E., & Alario, A. J. (1996). Encopresis treatment outcome: Long-term follow-up of 45 cases. *Journal of Developmental and Behavioral Pediatrics, 17,* 380–385.

Rolider, A., & Van Houten, R. (1984). Training parents to use extinction to eliminate nighttime crying by gradually increasing the criteria for ignoring crying. *Education and Treatment of Children, 7,* 119–124.

Romsing, J., Moller-Sonnergaard, J., Hertel, S., & Rasmussen, M. (1996). Postoperative pain in children: Comparison between ratings of children and nurses. *Journal of Pain and Symptom Management, 11,* 42–46.

Rosenbaum, J. F., Biederman, J., Bolduc, E. A., Hirshfeld, D. R., Faraone, S. V., & Kagan, J. (1992). Comorbidity of parental anxiety disorders as risk for childhood-onset anxiety in inhibited children. *American Journal of Psychiatry, 149,* 475–481.

Roter, D. L., Hall, J. A., Merisca, R., Nordstrom, B., Cretin, D., & Svarstad, B. (1998). Effectiveness of interventions to improve patient compliance. *Medical Care, 36,* 1138–1161.

Rudolph, K. D., Denning, M. D., & Weisz, J. R. (1995). Determinants and consequences of children's coping in the medical setting: Conceptualization, review, and critique. *Psychological Bulletin, 118,* 328–357.

Russo, R. M., Gururaj, V. J., & Allen, J. E. (1976). The effectiveness of diphenhydramine HCI in pediatric sleep disorders. *Journal of Clinical Pharmacology, 16,* 284–288.

Sallee, F. R., Nesbitt, L., Jackson, C., Sine, L., & Sethuraman, G. (1997). Relative efficacy of Haloperidol and Pimozide in children and adolescents with Tourette's disorder. *American Journal of Psychiatry, 154,* 1057–1062.

Sanders, M. R., & Jones, L. (1990). Behavioural treatment of injection, dental and medical phobias in adolescents. *Behavioural Psychotherapy, 18,* 311–316.

Sanders, M. R., Rebgetz, M., Morrison, M., Bor, W., Gordon, A., Dadda, M., & Shepard, R. (1989). Cognitive–behavioral treatment of recurrent nonspecific abdominal pain in children: An analysis of generalization, maintenance, and side effects. *Journal of Consulting and Clinical Psychology, 57,* 294–300.

Sanders, M. R., Shepherd, R. W., Cleghorn, G., & Woolford, H. (1994). The treatment of recurrent abdominal pain in children: A controlled comparison of cognitive–behavioral family intervention and standard pediatric care. *Journal of Consulting and Clinical Psychology, 62,* 306–314.

Satin, W., LaGraca, A., Zigo, M. A., & Skyler, J. S. (1989). Diabetes in adolescence: Effects of multifamily group intervention and parent simulation of diabetes. *Journal of Pediatric Psychology, 14,* 259–275.

Satory, G., Muller, B., Metsch, J., & Pothmann, R. (1998). A comparison of psychological and pharmacological treatment of pediatric migraine. *Behaviour Research and Therapy, 36,* 1155–1170.

Schachar, R., & Wachsmuth, R. (1990). Oppositional disorder in children: A validation study comparing conduct disorder, oppositional disorder and normal control children. *Journal of Psychology and Psychiatry, 31,* 1089–1102.

Schade, J. G., Joyce, B. A., Gerkensmeyer, J., & Keck, J. F. (1996). Comparison of three preverbal scales for postoperative pain assessment in a diverse pediatric sample. *Journal of Pain and Symptom Management, 12,* 348–359.

Schafer, L. C., Glasgow, R. E., & McCaul, K. D. (1982). Increasing the adherence of diabetic adolescents. *Journal of Behavioral Medicine, 5,* 353–362.

Schlundt, D. G., Rea, M., Hodge, M., Flannery, M. E., Kline, S., Meek, J., Kinzer, C., & Pichert, J. W. (1996). Assessing and overcoming situational obstacles to dietary adherence in adolescents with IDDM. *Journal of Adolescent Health, 19,* 282–288.

Schoenberg, N. E., Mley, C. H., & Coward, R. T. (1998). Diabetes knowledge and sources of information among African American and white older women. *The Diabetes Educator, 24,* 319–324.

Schroeder, C. S. (1999). Commentary: A view from the past and a look to the future. *Journal of Pediatric Psychology, 24,* 447–452.

Schwartz, C. E., Snidman, N., & Kagan, J. (1999). Adolescent social anxiety as an outcome of inhibited temperament in childhood. *Journal of the American Academy of Child and Adolescent Psychiatry, 38,* 1008–1015.

Seymour, R. A., Simpson, J. M., & Charlton, J. E. (1985). An evaluation of length and end-phrase of visual analogue scales in dental pain. *Pain, 21,* 177–185.

Shaffer, D. (1989). Child psychiatry. In H. I. Kaplan & B. J. Sadock (Eds.), *Comprehensive textbook of psychiatry* (5th ed., pp. 1689–1694). Baltimore: Williams & Williams.

Shaffer, D., Fisher, P., Lucas, C. P., Dulcan, M. K., & Schwab-Stone, M. E. (2000). NIMH Diagnostic Interview Schedule for Children Version IV (NIMH DISC–IV): Description, differences from previous versions, and reliability of some common diagnoses. *Journal of the American Academy of Child and Adolescent Psychiatry, 39,* 28–38.

Shannon, M., & Berde, C. B. (1989). Pharmacologic management of pain in children and adolescents. *Pediatrics Clinics of North America, 36,* 855–871.

Shapiro, A. K., & Shapiro, E. S. (1989). Tic disorders. In H. I. Kaplan & B. J. Sadock (Eds.), *Comprehensive textbook of psychiatry* (5th ed., pp. 1865–1878). Baltimore: William & Wilkins.

Shapiro, A. K., Shapiro, E. S., Young, J. G., & Feinberg, T. E. (1988). Measurement in tic disorders. In A. K. Shapiro, E. S. Shapiro, J. G. Young, & T. E. Feinberg (Eds.), *Gilles de la Tourette syndrome* (pp. 451–480). New York: Raven.

Shapiro, B. S. (1993). Management of painful episodes in sickle cell disease. In N. L. Schechter, C. B. Berde, & Yaster, M. (Eds.), *Pain in infants, children, and adolescents* (pp. 385–410). Baltimore: Williams & Wilkin.

Shapiro, F. (1995). *Eye movement desensitization and reprocessing: Basic principles, protocols, and procedures.* New York: Guilford Press.

Shelov, S. P., Gundy, G. J., Weiss, J. C., McIntire, M. S., Olness, K., Staub, H. P., Jones, D. J., Haque, M., Ellerstein, N. S., Heagarty, M. C., & Starfield, B. (1981). Enuresis: A contrast of attitudes of parents and physicians. *Pediatrics, 67,* 707–710.

Silber, K. P., & Haynes, C. E. (1992). Treating nailbiting: A comparative analysis of mild aversion and competing response therapies. *Behavior Research and Therapy, 30,* 15–22.

Silva, R. R., Munoz, D. M., Daniel, W., Barickman, J., & Friedhoff, A. J. (1996). Causes of Haloperidol discontinuation in patients with Tourette's disorder: Management and alternatives. *Journal of Clinical Psychiatry, 57,* 129–135.

Silver, A. A., Shytle, R. D., Philipp, M. K., & Sanberg, P. R. (1996). Case study: Long-term potentiation of neuroleptics with transdermal nicotine in Tourette's syndrome. *Journal of the American Academy of Child and Adolescent Psychiatry, 35,* 1631–1636.

Silverman, W. K., Kurtines, W. M., Ginsburg, G. S., Weems, C. F., Lumpkin, P. W., & Carmichael, D. H. (1999). Treating anxiety disorders in children with group cognitive–behavioral therapy: A randomized clinical trial. *Journal of Consulting and Clinical Psychology, 67,* 995–1003.

Silverman, W. K., Kurtines, W. M., Ginsburg, G. S., Weems, C. F., Rabian, B., & Serafini, L. T. (1999). Contingency management, self-control, and education support in the treatment of childhood phobic disorders: A randomized clinical trial. *Journal of Consulting and Clinical Psychology, 67,* 675–687.

Silverman, W. K., & Nelles, W. B. (1988). The anxiety disorders interview schedule for children. *Journal of the American Academy of Child and Adolescent Psychiatry, 27,* 772–778.

Simonds, J. D. (1977). Enuresis: A brief survey of current thinking with respect to pathogenesis and management. *Clinical Pediatrics, 16,* 79–82.

Simonoff, E. A., & Stores, G. (1987). Controlled trial of trimeprazine tartrate for night waking. *Archives of Diseases of Children, 62,* 253–257.

Sindou, M., Fischer, C., Derraz, S., Keravel, Y., & Palfi, S. (1996). Microsurgical vascular decompression in the treatment of facial hemispasm: A retrospective study of a series of 65 cases and review of the literature [Abstract]. *Neurochirurgie, 42,* 17–28.

Singer, H. S., Brown, J., Quaskey, S., Rosenberg, L. A., Mellits, E. D., & Denckla, M. B. (1995). The treatment of attention-deficit hyperactivity disorder in Tourette's syndrome: A double-blind placebo-controlled study with clonidine and desipramine. *Pediatrics, 95,* 74–81.

Siqueland, L., & Diamond, G. S. (1998). Engaging parents in cognitive behavioral treatment for children with anxiety disorders. *Cognitive and Behavioral Practice, 5,* 81–102.

Smith, J. T., Barabasz, A., & Barabasz, M. (1996). Comparison of hypnosis and distraction in severely ill children undergoing painful medical procedures. *Journal of Counseling Psychology, 43,* 187–195.

Smith, M. (1957). Effectiveness of symptomatic treatment of nailbiting in college students. *Psychological Newsletter, 8,* 219–231.

Smith, N. A., Seale, J. P., Ley, P., Mellis, C. M., & Shaw, J. (1994). Better medication compliance is associated with improved control of childhood asthma. *Archive of Chest Disease, 49,* 470–474.

Smith, N. A., Seale, J. P., Ley, P., Shaw, J., & Bracs, P. U. (1986). Effects of intervention on medication compliance in children with asthma. *Medical Journal of Australia, 144,* 119–122.

Snyder, J., & Patterson, G. R. (1986). The effects of consequences on patterns of social interaction: A quasi-experimental approach to reinforcement in natural interaction. *Child Development, 57,* 1257–1268.

Solnick, J. V., Rincover, A., & Peterson, C. P. (1977). Some determinants of the reinforcing and punishing effects of time-out. *Journal of Applied Behavior Analysis, 10,* 425–424.

Sonnenberg, A., & Koch, T. R. (1989). Physician visits in the United States for constipation: 1958 to 1986. *Digestive Diseases and Sciences, 34,* 606–611.

Spence, S. H. (1997). Structure of anxiety symptoms among children: A confirmatory factor-analytic study. *Journal of Abnormal Psychology, 106,* 280–297.

Spencer, J. A. D., Moran, D. J., Lee, A. & Talbert, D. (1990). White noise and sleep induction. *Archives of Diseases of Children, 65,* 135–137.

Sperling, M. (1965). Dynamic considerations and treatment of enuresis. *Journal of American Academy of Child Psychiatry, 4,* 19–31.

Spielberger, C. (1973). *Manual for the State–Trait Anxiety Inventory for Children.* Palo Alto, CA: Consulting Psychologists Press.

Stanley, K. (1999). Low-literacy materials for diabetes nutrition education. *Practical Diabetology, 18,* 36–44.

Starfield, B. (1982). Behavioral pediatrics and primary care. *Pediatric Clinics of North America, 29,* 377–390.

Stark, L. J., Allen, K. D., Hurst, M., Nash, D. A., Rigney, B., & Stokes, T. F. (1989). Distraction: Its utilization and efficacy with children undergoing dental treatment. *Journal of Applied Behavior Analysis, 22,* 297–307.

Stark, L. J., Opipari, L. C., Donaldson, D. L., Danovsky, M. B., Rasile, D. A., & Del Santo, A. F. (1997). Evaluation of a standard protocol for retentive encopresis: A replication. *Journal of Pediatric Psychology, 22,* 619–633.

Stark, L. J., Owens-Stively, J., Spirito, A., Lewis, A., & Guevremont, D. (1990). Group behavioral treatment of retentive encopresis. *Journal of Pediatric Psychology, 15,* 659–671.

Stevens, B. (1990). Development and testing of a pediatric pain management sheet. *Pediatric Nursing, 16,* 543–548.

Stine, J. J. (1994). Psychosocial and psychodynamic issues affecting noncompliance with psychostimulant treatment. *Journal of Child and Adolescent Psychopharmacology, 4,* 75–86.

Strafford, M., Cahill, C., Schwartz, T., Yee, J., Sethna, N., & Berde, C. (1991). Recognition and treatment of pain in pediatric patients with AIDS. *Journal of Pain and Symptom Management, 6,* 146.

Streichenwein, S. M., & Thronby, J. I. (1995). A long-term, double-blind, placebo-controlled trial of the efficacy of fluoxetine for trichotillomania. *American Journal of Psychiatry, 152,* 1192–1196.

Stroop, J. R. (1935). Studies of interference in serial verbal reactions. *Journal of Experimental Psychology, 18,* 643–662.

Sutphen, J. L., Borowitz, S. M., Hutchison, R. L., & Cox, D. J. (1995). Long-term follow-up of medically treated childhood constipation. *Clinical Pediatrics, 34,* 576–580.

Swansen, S., & Christophersen, E. R. (1997). *Habit reversal training for reducing children's tics.* Unpublished.

Szapocznik, J., Rio, A., Murray, E., Cohen, R., Scopetta, M., Rivas-Vazquez, A., Posada, V., & Kurtines, W. (1989). Structural family therapy versus psychodynamic child therapy for problematic Hispanic boys. *Journal of Consulting and Clinical Psychology, 57,* 571–578.

Task Force on Promotion and Dissemination of Psychological Procedures. (1995). Training in and dissemination of empirically-validated psychological treatment: Report and recommendation. *Clinical Psychologist, 48,* 3–23.

Taylor, P. D., & Turner, R. K. (1975). A clinical trial of continuous intermittent and overlearning "bell and pad" treatments for nocturnal enuresis. *Behaviour Research and Therapy, 3,* 281–293.

Thomas, A. M., Peterson, L., & Goldstein, D. (1997). Problem solving and diabetes regimen adherence by children and adolescents with IDDM in social pressure situations: A reflection of normal development. *Journal of Pediatric Psychology, 22,* 541–561.

Thomas, J. (1994). New approaches to achieving dietary change. *Current Opinion in Lipidology, 5,* 36–41.

Thompson, R. J., & Gustafson, K. E. (1996). *Adaptation to chronic childhood illness.* Washington, DC: American Psychological Association.

Thompson, S., & Rey, J. M. (1995). Functional enuresis: Is desmopressin the answer? *Journal of the American Academy of Child and Adolescent Psychiatry, 34,* 266–271.

Turner, S. M., Beidel, D. C., & Costello, A. (1987). Psychopathology in the offspring of anxiety disordered patients. *Journal of Consulting and Clinical Psychology, 55,* 229–235.

Turner, S. M., Biedel, D. C., & Epstein, L. H. (1991). Vulnerability and risk for anxiety disorders. *Journal of Anxiety Disorders, 5,* 151–166.

Tyler, D. C. (1990). Patient-controlled analgesia in adolescents. *Journal of Adolescent Health Care, 11,* 154–158.

van Londen, A., van Londen-Barentsen, M. W., van Son, M. J., & Mulder, G. A. (1993). Arousal training for children suffering from nocturnal enuresis: A 2 1/2-year follow-up. *Behaviour Research and Therapy, 31,* 613–615.

Van Sciver, M. M., D'Angelo, E., Rappaport, L., & Woolf, A. D. (1995). Pediatric compliance and the roles of distinct treatment characteristics, treatment attitudes, and family stress: A preliminary report. *Developmental and Behavioral Pediatrics, 16,* 350–358.

van Son, M. J., Mulder, G., & van Londen, A. (1990). The effectiveness of dry bed training for nocturnal enuresis in adults. *Behaviour Research and Therapy, 28,* 347–349.

Varni, J. W., & Bernstein, B. H. (1991). Evaluation and management of pain in children with rheumatic diseases. *Pediatric Rheumatology, 17,* 985–1000.

Varni, J. W., Thompson, K. L., & Hanson, V. (1987). The Varni/Thompson Pediatric Pain Questionnaire: I. Chronic musculoskeletal pain in juvenile rheumatoid arthritis. *Pain, 28,* 27–38.

Varni, J. W., & Walco, G. A. (1988). Chronic and recurrent pain associated with pediatric chronic diseases. *Issues in Comprehensive Pediatric Nursing, 11,* 145–158.

Vaughn, M. L., Riccio, C. A., Hynd, G. W., & Hall, J. (1997). Diagnosing ADHD (predominantly Inattentive and Combined type subtypes): Discriminant validity of the Behavior Assessment System for Children and the Achenbach parent and teacher rating scales. *Journal of Clinical Child Psychology, 26,* 349–357.

Velosa, J. F., & Riddle, M. A. (2000). Pharmacologic treatment of anxiety disorders in children and adolescents. *Child and Adolescent Clinics of North America, 9,* 119–133.

Villarruel, A. M., & Denyes, M. J. (1991). Pain assessment in children: Theoretical and empirical validity. *Advances in Nursing Science, 14,* 32–41.

Vitiello, B., & Jensen, P. (1995). Disruptive behavior disorders. In H. I. Kaplan & B. J. Sadock (Eds.), *Comprehensive textbook of psychiatry* (6th ed., pp. 2311–2319). Baltimore: Williams & Wilkins.

Vogel, W., Young, M., & Primack, W. (1996). A survey of physician use of treatment methods for functional enuresis. *Journal of Developmental and Behavioral Pediatrics, 17,* 90–93.

Walco, G. A., & Oberlander, T. F. (1993). Musculoskeletal pain syndromes in children. In N. L. Schechter, C. B. Berde, & M. Yaster (Eds.), *Pain in infants, children, and adolescents* (pp. 459–471). Baltimore: Williams & Wilkin.

Walco, G. A., Sterling, C. N., Conte, P. M., & Engel, R. G. (1999). Empirically supported treatments in pediatric psychology: Disease-related pain. *Journal of Pediatric Psychology, 24,* 155–167.

Walco, G. A., Varni, J., & Ilowite, N. T. (1992). Cognitive–behavioral pain management in children with juvenile rheumatoid arthritis. *Pediatrics, 89,* 1075–1079.

Walker, L. S., Garber, J., & Greene, J. W. (1993). Psychosocial correlates of recurrent childhood pain: A comparison of pediatric patients with recurrent abdominal pain, organic illness, and psychiatric disorders. *Journal of Abnormal Psychology, 102,* 248–258.

Walker, L. S., Garber, J., Van Slyke, D. A., & Greene, J. W. (1995). Long-term health outcomes in patients with recurrent abdominal pain. *Journal of Pediatric Psychology, 20,* 233–245.

Walkup, J. T., Rosenberg, L. A., Brown, J., & Singer, H. S. (1992). The validity of instruments measuring tic severity in Tourette's syndrome. *Journal of the American Academy of Child and Adolescent Psychiatry, 31,* 472–477.

Warzak, W. J. (1993). Psychosocial implications of nocturnal enuresis. *Clinical Pediatrics* (Special Suppl.), 38–40.

Wasserman, R. C., Kelleher, K. J., Bocian, A., Baker, A., Childs, G. E., Indacochea, F., Stulp, C., & Gardner, W. P. (1999). Identification of attentional and hyperactivity problems in primary care: A report from Pediatric Research Office Settings and the Ambulatory Sentinel Practice Network. *Pediatrics, 103,* 1–7.

Watson, T. S., & Allen, K. D. (1993). Elimination of thumb-sucking as a treatment for severe trichotillomania. *Journal of the American Academy of Child and Adolescent Psychiatry, 32,* 830–834.

Webster-Stratton, C. H. (n.d.). *The parents and children series: A comprehensive course divided into four programs.* Seattle, WA: Author.

Webster-Stratton, C. H. (1990). Long-term follow-up of families with young conduct problem children: From preschool to grade school. *Journal of Clinical Child Psychology, 19,* 144–149.

Webster-Stratton, C. H. (1996). Early intervention with videotaped modeling: Programs for families of children with oppositional defiant disorder or conduct disorder. In E. D. Hibbs & P. S. Jensen (Eds.), *Psychosocial treatments for child and adolescent disorders: Empirically based strategies for clinical practice* (pp. 435–474). Washington, DC: American Psychological Association.

Webster-Stratton, C. H. (1998). Preventing conduct problems in Head Start children: Strengthening parenting competencies. *Journal of Consulting and Clinical Psychology, 66,* 715–730.

Webster-Stratton, C. H., & Hammond, M. (1997). Treating children with early-onset conduct problems: A comparison of child and parent training interventions. *Journal of Consulting and Clinical Psychology, 65,* 93–109.

Weems, C. F., Silverman, W. K., Saavedra, L. M., Pina, A. A., & Lumpkin, P. W. (1999). The discrimination of children's phobias using the Revised Fear Survey Schedule for Children. *Journal of Child Psychology and Psychiatry, 40,* 941–952.

Weinstein, S. R., Noam, G. G., Grimes, K., Stone, J., & Schwab-Stone, M. (1990). Convergence of *DSM–III* diagnoses and self-reported symptoms in child and adolescent patients. *Journal of the American Academy of Child and Adolescent Psychiatry, 29,* 627–634.

Weissbluth, M. (1984). Is drug treatment of night terrors warranted? *American Journal of Diseases in Children, 138,* 1086.

Weller, E. B., Weller, R. A., Fristad, M. A., Rooney, M. T., & Schecter, J. (2000). Children's Interview for Psychiatric Syndromes (ChIPS). *Journal of the American Academy of Child and Adolescent Psychiatry, 39,* 76–84.

Werry, J. S., & Cohrssen, J. (1965). Enuresis: An etiologic and therapeutic study. *Journal of Pediatrics, 67,* 423–431.

Westenberg, P. M., Siebelink, B. M., Warmenhoven, N. J., & Treffers, P. D. (1999). Separation anxiety and overanxious disorders: Relations to age and level of psychosocial maturity. *Journal of the American Academy of Child and Adolescent Psychiatry, 38,* 1000–1007.

Whaley, S. E., Pinto, A., & Sigman, M. (1999). Characterizing interactions between anxious mothers and their children. *Journal of Consulting and Clinical Psychology, 67,* 826–836.

Williams, C. (1996). Patient-controlled analgesia: A review of the literature. *Journal of Clinical Nursing, 5*, 139–147.

Williams, C. L., Bollella, M., & Wynder, E. L. (1995). A new recommendation for dietary fiber in childhood. *Pediatrics, 96*, 985–988.

Wishnie, E., & Weisman, S. J. (1997). Children with AIDS: Pain syndromes and unique issues of assessment and management. *Child and Adolescent Psychiatric Clinics of North America, 6*, 863–878.

Wolf, A. W., & Lozoff, B. (1989). Object attachment, thumbsucking, and the passage to sleep. *Journal of the American Academy of Child and Adolescent Psychiatry, 28*, 287–292. .

Wolf, M. M., Kirigan, K. A., Fixsen, D. G., Blasé, K. A., & Braukmann, C. J. (1995). The teaching-family model: A case study in data-based program development and refinement (and dragon wrestling). *Journal of Organizational Behavior Management, 15*, 11–68.

Woodgate, R., & Kristjanson, L. J. (1996). A young child's pain: How parents and nurses "take care." *International Journal of Nursing Studies, 33*, 271–284.

Woods, D. W., & Miltenberger, R. G. (1996). A review of habit reversal with childhood habit disorders. *Education and Treatment of Children, 19*, 197–214.

Woods, D. W., Miltenberger, R. G., & Lumley, V. A. (1996). Sequential application of major habit-reversal components to treat motor tics in children. *Journal of Applied Behavior Analysis, 29*, 483–493.

World Health Organization. (1993). *The ICD-10 classification of mental and behavioural disorders: Diagnostic criteria for research.* Geneva: Author.

Wright, L. (1975). Outcome of a standardized program for treating psychogenic encopresis. *Professional Psychology, 6*, 453–456.

Wysocki, T. (1997). *The ten keys to helping your child grow up with diabetes.* Alexandria, VA: American Diabetes Association.

Wysocki, T., Green, L., & Huxtable, K. (1989). Blood glucose monitoring by diabetic adolescents: Compliance and metabolic control. *Health Psychology, 8*, 267–284.

Yunas, M. B. (1992). Fibromyalgia. In F. Sicuteri, L. Terenius, L. Vecchiet, C. A. Maggi, M. Nicolodi, & M. Alessandri (Eds.), *Advances in pain research and therapy* (Vol. 20, pp. 133–140). New York: Raven.

Zito, J. M., Safer, D. J., dosReis, S., Gardner, J. F., Boles, M., & Lynch, F. (2000). Trends in the prescribing of psychotropic medications to preschoolers. *Journal of the American Medical Association, 283*, 1025–1030.

Zuckerman, B. (1995). Sleep problems. In S. Parker & B. Zuckerman (Eds.), *Behavioral and developmental pediatrics* (pp. 289–293). Boston: Little, Brown.

Zuckerman, B., Stevenson, J., & Bailey, V. (1987). Stomachaches and headaches in a community sample of preschool children. *Pediatrics, 79*, 677–682.

AUTHOR INDEX

A

Abbott, F. V., 160
Abikoff, H., 100
Abramovitz, A., 185
Abramson, H., 150
Aceves, J., 175
Achenbach, T. M., 23, 24, 25, 65, 106, 107, 127, 132, 147, 205
Ackerson, L., 206
Acute Pain Management Guideline Panel, 180, 183
Adair, R., 105, 109
Adams, J., 175
Adams, L. A., 116
Agency for Health Care Policy and Research, 170
Ahmann, P. A., 41, 42, 43
Alario, A. J., 133
Albano, A. M., 58, 60, 61, 64
Aljazireh, L., 105
Allen, J. E., 110, 111
Allen, J. S., Jr., 4
Allen, K. D., 91, 105, 194, 199
Allen, K. W., 94
Alm, T., 75
Amdorfer, R. E., 105
American Academy of Child and Adolescent Psychiatry, 23, 58, 59, 67
American Academy of Pediatrics, 23
American Psychiatric Association, 9, 12, 13, 14, 16, 17, 18, 49, 50, 53, 54, 60, 79, 80, 81, 101, 102, 103, 104, 123, 124, 132, 145, 146, 160, 162
Amir, S., 218
Anastopoulos, A. D., 15, 26, 33, 40, 44
Anders, R. F., 99, 101, 104, 106
Andrea, H., 57
Andrews, K., 177
Angold, A., 53, 55, 56, 61
Aponte, H. J., 34
Appel, F. A., 202
Aradine, C. R., 174, 175
Armstrong, F. D., 165
Arnold, C. M., 33
Ashley, L., 21
Attanasio, V., 194

August, G. J., 26

August, G. J., 26
Auslander, W. F., 206
AvRushkin, T. W., 218
Ayers, W. A., 4
Azrin, N. H., 6, 82, 83, 84, 87, 91, 92, 94, 95, 96, 97, 152, 154, 155, 156, 157

B

Bachanas, P. J., 190
Baer, D. M., 124
Baer, R. A., 208, 210
Bailey, V., 162
Baker, S. S., 135, 143
Ballmer, R. S., 135
Banerjee, S., 155
Barabasz, A., 189, 190
Barabasz, M., 189, 190
Baren, M., 27
Barickman, J., W. 86
Barkley, R. A., 15, 24, 27, 33, 34, 35, 40, 41, 42, 43, 44, 67
Barnard, J. D., 33
Barnard, S. R., 33
Barone, V. J., 89, 90
Barr, R. G., 130, 131, 133
Barrett, P. M., 65, 69, 72, 73
Barry, J., 192
Barzilai, A., 96
Bass, D., 4, 33, 36
Bass, J. W., 208
Bauchner, H., 105, 109, 163
Bauer, C. H., 128
Baum, C. G., 11
Baum, D., 221
Bax, M., 21
Becker, M. H., 206, 208
Beidel, D. C., 57
Bell-Dolan, D. J., 57, 61
Bellman, M., 125
Bender, B., 206, 217, 218
Bennett, K. J., 21, 39
Benson, H., 191
Benton, A. L., 27
Benton, C. M., 33
Berde, C. B., 182, 183
Bergin, A., 94
Berman, J. S., 150

Bernstein, B. A., 164
Bernstein, B. H., 182
Bernstein, G. A., 58
Berry, S. L., 197
Beyer, J. E., 174, 175
Bezman, R. J., 16
Biederman, J., 19, 24, 57
Binderglas, P. M., 145
Birch, L. L., 110, 111
Birmaher, B., 62, 63, 64, 66
Blader, J. C., 100, 105
Blampied, N. M., 115
Blanchard, E. R., 193
Blasé, K. A., 33
Blix, S., 196
Blount, R. L., 168, 175, 179, 184, 190, 208,
    210
Blum, N. J., 106
Bobrow, E. S., 218
Boggs, S. R., 46
Bollella, M., 137
Bond, L. A., 21
Borowitz, S., 127, 137, 140
Borowitz, S. M., 124
Botts, P., 94
Bracs, P. U., 206
Bradley-Johnson, S., 120
Brandberg, M., 75
Braswell, L., 45, 46
Braukmann, C. J., 33
Brody, J. E., 125, 142
Brook, J., 55
Broughton, R. J., 101
Brown, J., 85, 94
Brown, R. T., 177
Brownbridge, G., 217
Bruun, R. D., 87
Budd, J., 218
Budman, C. L., 87
Burd, L., 150
Bush, P. J., 206, 208, 219
Bushell, D., Jr., 33
Butler, R. J., 151

C
Caldwell, A. B., 101, 102
Caldwell, S., 167
Campbell, S. B., 18, 20, 21, 28
Camprise, R. L., 87
Canadian Task Force on Periodic Health
    Examination, 4
Cantwell, D. P., 12, 13, 16, 28

Capra, B. D., 217
Carey, W. B., 106
Carlsson, J., 191, 192
Carmichael, D. H., 65, 72
Carr, T., 165
Carson, K., 94
Carton, J., 205
Casey, R., 211
Cassidy, R. C., 177, 183
Castelanos, D., 53, 55
Cataldo, M. F., 10, 194
Cavior, N., 120
Cendron, M., 154, 155
Chadwick, B. A., 219
Chamberlain, P., 46
Chambless, D. L., 4, 183
Chandra, R., 127
Chaney, J. M., 9
Chappell, P. B., 85
Charlton, J. E., 176
Chiponis, D., 127
Christophersen, E. R., 6, 10, 30, 31, 32, 33,
    84, 89, 90, 93, 105, 113, 117, 118,
    120, 122, 124, 126, 127, 128, 131,
    132, 133, 136, 141, 142, 149, 156,
    157, 204, 205, 206, 208, 212, 214,
    215
Ciminero, A. R., 151
Cipes, M. H., 212
Clark, J. H., 134
Clark, L. A., 6
Clay, R. A., 42
Cleghorn, G., 192, 193
Clowes-Hollins, V., 57
Cobham, V. E., 77
Cohen, D. J., 83, 85, 86
Cohen, H. A., 96
Cohen, L. L., 175, 185, 190
Cohen, M. W., 146, 147, 150
Cohen, P., 55
Cohrssen, J., 147, 151
Colcher, I. S., 208
Coleman, J., 21
Collins, M., 193
Colwell, S. O., 154, 191
Conger, R. W., 30
Conners, C. K., 24, 25, 27
Conners, K., 62, 63, 64
Conner-Warren, R. L., 165, 175
Connor, D. F., 35
Conrad, P., 74
Conte, P. M., 196

Costello, A., 57
Costello, A. J., 55, 56, 60
Costello, E. J., 53, 55, 56, 61
Cotter, M. W., 184, 190
Coward, R. T., 206
Cox, D. J., 124, 127, 137, 140
Coy, J., 181
Coyle, J. T., 35, 40
Craig, K. D., 180
Creer, T. L., 221
Crowther, J. K., 21
Cruikshank, D. M., 127
Cummings, E. A., 160, 163
Curry, S. L., 166
Curtis, A. C., 135

D
da Costa, I. G., 213
Dadds, M., 74, 193
Dadds, M. R., 69, 72, 73, 77
Dahlquist, L. M., 187, 188, 208, 210
Daleflod, B., 192
D'Angelo, E., 214
Daniel, W. 86
D'Astous, J., 168
Davidson, M., 125, 128, 133
Davis, D. M., 112
Davis, N. S., 104
Davis, R. T., 35
Daviss, W. B., 214, 217
Days, A. L., 133
Dearborn, M., 188
Deichmann, M. M., 190
De Jong, P. J., 57
Delamater, A. M., 201, 219
Denning, M. D., 166
Denyes, M. J., 175
Derraz, S., 82
Detlor, J., 85
Deutsch, A., 120
DeVane, C. L., 35
deVeber, L. L., 175, 177, 179, 180
Diamond, G. S., 77
Dinges, D. F., 196
Doepke, K., 193
Doleys, D. M., 151
Dothage, J. A., 163
Drabman, R. S., 4, 45, 114
Dragisic, K., 162
Dreitzer, D., 206
Dulcan, M. K., 24, 60
Dunbar-Jacob, J., 202, 205

Dunn-Geier, B. J., 168
Dunning, E. J., 202
DuPaul, G. J., 26, 40
DuRant, R. H., 219
Dwyer, K., 202

E
Eckman, J., 193
Eddy, E. J., 125
Edelbrock, C., 106, 107, 205
Edelbrock, C. S., 41, 43, 60
Edens, J. L., 166
Edwards, A., 112
Edwards, D., 46
Edwards, K. J., 113, 117
Eifert, G. H., 6
Eisen, A. R., 60
Elliott, A. J., 92
Elliott, C. H., 165, 167, 174, 185, 186, 198
Elliott, D., 4
Eney, R. D., 211
Engel, R. G., 196
Epstein, L. H., 217
Erenberg, G., 82, 86
Evidence-Based Working Group, 4
Ewing, L. J., 28
Eyberg, S. M., 22, 46, 127

F
Falkner, S., 106
Falvo, D. R., 206, 208, 212, 214
Faraone, S. V., 24
Farrington, D. P., 21
Faucon, A., 106
Faust, J., 167, 187, 188
Favaloro, R., 165
Feber, R., 104, 105
Feinberg, T. E., 85
Fentress, D. W., 191
Ferber, R., 99, 109, 116
Fielding, D. M., 217
Finley, A., 160
Finley, G. A., 160
Finney, J. W., 6, 84, 91, 92, 127, 190, 191, 194, 204, 208, 213
Fischel, J. E., 125
Fischer, C., 82
Fisher, C., 112
Fisher, P., 24
Fitzgerald, J. F., 134
Fitzgerald, M., 177
Fitzgerald, P., 160

Fitzgibbons, I., 174
Fixsen, D. G., 33
Fleischman, M. H., 29
Fletcher, K. E., 33
Foa, E. B., 96
Foley, C., 100
Foote, R., 46
Forbes, G. B., 27
Forehand, R. L., 29, 30, 44
Forsythe, W. T., 151
Forward, S. P., 160
Foster, R., 174
Fox, J. E., 61
Foxx, R. M., 6, 152, 154, 155, 156
France, K. G., 115
Franco, N., 74
Frank, N. C., 121
Franklin, J. E., 96
Frantz, S. E., 94, 95, 96
Frantz-Renshaw, S. E., 82
Free, K., 184
Friedhoff, A. J., 86
Friman, P. C., 89, 90, 91, 127, 147, 208
Fristad, M. A., 24
Fuqua, R. W., 6, 92, 194

G
Gabel, S., 127
Gadet, B., 64
Gadin, R. S., 40
Galatzer, A., 218
Garber, J., 168, 190
Garrard, S. D., 125
Garrett, R. W., 10
Genel, M., 16
Genuis, M. L.197
Gerkensmeyer, J., 168
Giardina, P. J., 213
Giebehain, J. E., 117
Gil, K. M., 166
Gil, R., 218
Ginsburg, G. S., 50, 65, 72, 74, 75
Glasgow, R. E., 216
Glick, B. S., 112
Glowasky, A., 211
Goetz, D., 218
Gold, D. M., 128
Goldman, L. S., 16, 40
Goldstein, D., 219
Goldstein, E. O., 211
Goldstein, G. L., 213
Goldston, D., 214

Goodman, W. K., 85
Gordon, A., 193
Gordon, M., 27
Gordon, S. B., 120
Goyette, C. H., 107
Graham, P. J., 18, 145
Gray-Donald, I., 160
Green, J. P., 196
Green, L., 216
Green, W. H., 86
Greenan-Fowler, E., 216
Greene, J. W., 168, 190
Greenhill, L. L., 64
Grimes, K., 24
Grodzinsky, G. M., 27
Gross, A. M., 217, 218
Grunau, R. V., 180
Gudas, L. L., 219
Guevremont, A. D., 33
Guevremont, D., 136
Guevremont, D. C., 26
Gullion, M. D., 29
Gurley, D., 55
Gururaj, V. J., 110, 111
Gustafson, K. E., 201

H
Haaften, H., 75
Hadjistavropoulos, H. D., 180
Hakansson, L., 192
Hall, C. C. I., 7, 8
Hall, C. L., 6, 84
Hall, J., 26
Halpern, L. F., 106
Hamill, S. K., 125
Hammond, M., 38
Hamsher, K., 27
Handwerk, M. L., 147
Hansen, C., 74
Hanson, V., 168
Harcherik, D. F., 85
Harlos, S., 150
Hart, H., 21
Hartse, K. M., 105
Hatcher, J. W., 168
Hauser, S. T., 218
Hayford, J. R., 197
Haynes, C. E., 92
Haynes, R. B., 214
Hays, R. D., 204
Hazzard, A., 206
Heard, P. M., 74

288   *AUTHOR INDEX*

Hearn, M. T., 175, 177, 179, 180
Heaton, R. K., 27
Hegedus, A. M., 127
Heimel, A., 154, 191
Hellstrom, K., 75
Hembree, A., 96
Hermann, C., 193
Hermecz, D. A., 188
Hersen, M., 55
Hertel, S., 163
Hester, N., 174
Heyman, M. B., 126
Hibbs, E. D., 5, 9, 18
Hilgard, J., 165, 196
Hilgard, J. R., 190
Hilgartner, M. W., 213
Hill, D. W., 33
Hilpert, P. L., 167
Hirshfeld, D. R., 57, 162
Hjalmas, K., 146
Hoder, E. L., 83, 86
Hodgins, M. J., 165
Holden, E. W., 190, 191, 193
Holdrinet, I., 75
Holland, D. E., 72, 73
Hood, J., 56, 57, 58
Hornyak, L. M., 196
Horton, L., 180
Houston, B. K., 61
Houts, A. C., 137, 150, 151
Hove, G., 89, 91
Howard, B., 68, 69
Hsu, J., 219
Hua, J., 106
Hudson, J. I., 19
Hudson, S. M., 115
Hudziak, J. J., 149
Hufford, M. R., 6
Hunter, T., 53, 55
Hurley, R. M., 147
Hutchinson, R. L., 124
Hutchinson, S. J., 206
Huxtable, K., 216
Hynd, G. W., 26

I
Iacono, W. G., 55, 56
Iancu, I., 88
Iannotti, R. J., 206, 208, 219
Ilowite, N. T., 176
Ingebo, K. P., 126
Iwamasa, G. Y., 6

Iyanger, S., 214

J
Jackson, C., 87
Jacobsen, P. B., 165, 214
Jacobson, A. M., 217
Janicke, D. M., 190, 191
Jarecke, R., 35
Jarvie, G., 45, 114
Jaspers, J. P. C., 88
Jaworski, T. M., 163
Jay, M. S., 219
Jay, S. M., 165, 167, 174, 180, 185, 187, 189, 198
Jeans, M. E., 160
Jenkins, S., 21
Jensen, P., 12, 13, 17, 18, 19, 35
Jensen, P. S., 9, 18, 40, 65
Johnson, C. M., 120
Johnson, M., 116, 194
Johnson, S. B., 204, 219
Johnston, C. C., 160, 180
Jones, L., 74
Jones, P. K., 206
Jones, R. R., 30
Jones, S. L., 206
Jowett, S. A., 110
Joyce, B. A., 168, 179
Joyette, C. H., 24, 25

K
Kagan, J., 27, 56
Kahn, A., 113
Kahn, E., 112
Kalas, R., 60
Kales, J. D., 101, 102
Kamphaus, R. W., 24, 25, 26, 65, 66, 132, 205
Kane, M., 68, 69
Kaplan, R. M., 219
Karp, M., 218
Kaslow, N., 193
Kataria, S., 100
Katz, E., 165
Katz, E. R., 165, 167
Katz, H. P., 194
Katz, J., 206
Katz, R., 117, 118
Kaufman, A. S., 27
Kaufman, N. L., 27
Kaver, A., 75
Kazak, A. E., 179, 185, 186, 189

Kazdin, A. E., 4, 19, 24, 29, 33, 36, 37, 38, 48, 55
Kearney, C. A., 60, 66, 67
Keck, J. F., 168
Keefe, F. J., 183
Kellerman, J., 120, 165
Kemph, J. P., 35
Kemphaus, R. W., 147
Kendall, P. C., 7, 45, 46, 53, 55, 65, 68, 69, 70-71, 73, 74, 76, 77
Kennard, B. D., 217
Keravel, Y., 82
Kerr, S. M., 110
Kessler, B. H., 128
Khanna, F., 151
Kim, M., 193
Kindler, S., 88
King, N. J., 22, 57, 68, 73, 74, 76
King, S. A., 160
Kirgian, K. A., 33
Kirshen, A., 150
Klaric, S. H., 60
Klorman, R., 167
Koch, D. A., 213
Koch, T. R., 125
Kohen, D. G., 191
Kohen, D. P., 81, 94, 96, 154
Koocher, G. P., 219
Koot, H. M., 18
Koplewicz, H. S., 100
Kotagal, S., 105
Kotzer, A. M., 181
Kovacs, M., 214
Kovatchev, B., 137, 140
Krakow, B., 120
Krawiecki, N., 206
Kristensen, K., 174
Kristjanson, L. J., 163, 179
Kugler, M. M., 128
Kurtines, W. M., 65, 72, 74, 75
Kurtz, S. M., 214, 219
Kuttner, L., 180, 189, 192, 194

L
Labellarte, M. J., 50, 68
LaClave, L. J., 196
LaGana, C., 167
La Greca, A. M., 23
LaGreca, W., 218
Lahat, E., 96
Lalonde, J., 19
Lander, J., 165

Landman, G. B., 140
Laron, Z., 218
Larsson, B., 191, 192
Last, C. G., 55, 56, 57, 58, 74
Latter, J., 168
Lau, A. W., 6
Laurens, K. R., 72
Lavigne, J. V., 106, 197
Lazarus, A., 185
LeBaron, S., 165, 174, 196
Leckman, J. F., 85
LeClaire, A. D., 181
Lee, A., 119
Lee, L. W., 166
Legrand, L. N., 55, 56
Leibowitz, J. M., 89
Leibowitz, M., 127
Leichtner, A. M., 162
Leith, P. J., 180, 181
Lejuez, C. W., 6
Lemanek, K., 202, 213
Lemanek, K. L., 165, 194
Lerner, J., 96
Levenson, S., 105, 109
Leventhal, H., 206
Levin, G. M., 35
Levine, J., 123, 128
Levine, M. D., 125, 130, 131, 133, 134, 135
Levy, J. D., 190
Lewis, A., 136
Ley, P., 206, 213
Lezak, M. D., 27
Liebert, R. M., 151
Linder, C., 219
Lindsley, C. B., 215, 216
Ling, W., 127, 137
Linn, H. E., 133
Linton, L., 180
Liptak, G. S., 201, 208, 220
Liss, D. S., 217, 218
Litt, I. F., 219
Loening-Baucke, V. A., 123, 127
Lombroso, P. J., 87
Long, E. S., 92
Long, P., 29
Lovibond, S. H., 150
Lowe, K., 215, 216, 217
Lozoff, B., 100, 104
Lucas, C. P., 24
Ludwig, S., 211
Lumley, V. A., 92
Lumpkin, P. W., 61, 65, 72

Lutfey, K. E., 201
Lutzker, J. R., 215, 216, 217
Luxem, M. C., 124, 128, 131, 133

M
Ma, Y., 55
Macknin, M. L., 113
MacQueen, M., 213
Magalnick, L. J., 218
Magill, M. K., 10
Maier, M. C., 113
Mailman-Sosland, J. E., 120
Maiman, L. A., 208
Malone, A. B., 185
Manassis, K., 56, 57, 58
Manne, S. L., 179
March, J., 64
March, J. S., 58, 60, 61, 62, 63, 64, 81
Marechal, J. M., 126
Masek, B. J., 191, 194
Mash, E. J., 22
Massie, E. D., 58
Masters, K. J., 113
Mathews, J. R., 127
Matthey, S., 74
Mayer, B., 75
McCaul, K. D., 216
McClung, H. J., 135
McConaughy, S. H., 23, 24, 25
McConville, B. J., W. 86
McGee, R., 105
McGinnis, J. C., 147
McGrath, M. L., 8, 157, 194
McGrath, P. A., 159, 160, 165, 167, 168,
        169, 171, 175, 177, 179, 180, 182,
        183, 194
McGrath, P. J., 160, 168, 173, 183, 191, 192
McGue, M., 55, 56
McKendry, J. B., 146, 151
McKinley, T., 6, 92
McMahon, R. J., 30, 44
McMenamy, C., 117, 118
McMurray, M. B., 41, 43
McNeill, G., 160
McQuade, W. H., 133
McQuaid, E. L., 198
Meadows, E. A., 96
Mehegan, J. E., 191
Melamed, B. G., 167, 187, 188
Melin, L., 192
Mellis, C. M., 213
Mellon, M. W., 8, 137, 157

Mendendorp, S. V., 113
Mendlowitz, S. L., 73
Merckelbach, H., 56, 57, 64, 75
Metevia, L., 26
Metsch, J., 194
Meunier, P. P., 126
Michael, R., 167
Milgrom, H., 206
Miller, R. L., 35
Miltenberger, R. G., 6, 92
Minde, K., 106, 116
Mindell, J. A., 100, 101, 102, 113, 121
Minuchin, S., 34
Miraglia, M., 212
Miser, A. W., 163, 181, 195
Miser, J. S., 163
Mley, C. H., 206
Moffatt, M. E., 150, 151, 152
Mollard, P., 126
Moller-Sonnergaard, J., 163
Moore, T., 100
Moran, D. J., 119
Morgan, A., 29
Morgan, A. H., 190
Morrison, D. N., 105
Morrison, M., 193
Morton, N. S., 181, 182
Moss, H., 162
Moulaert, V., 64
Mouton, S. G., 94
Mowrer, O. H., 151
Mowrer, W. M., 151
Mozin, M. J., 113
MTA Cooperative Group, 41, 44, 47
Mulder, G., 154
Mulder, G. A., 154
Mulle, K., 81
Muller, B., 194
Muller, M. F., 113
Mullins, L. L., 9
Mulvihill, D., 130, 131, 133
Munoz, D. M., 86
Muris, P., 56, 64, 75
Murphy, L., 8
Mushlin, A. I., 202

N
Nagamori, K. E., 134
Nassau, J. H., 198
National Institutes for Health Task Force,
        40
National Institutes of Health, 209

Nazarien, L. F., 208
Nelles, W. B., 60, 65
Nesbitt, L., 87
Netley, C., 151
Newacheck, P., 162
Nilzon, K. R., 55, 56
Noam, G. G., 24
Nunn, R. G., 82, 83, 84, 91, 94, 95, 96, 97

O
Oberlander, T. F., 182
O'Brien, S., 136, 137, 140
Obrosky, S., 214
O'Dell, S. L., 117
Offord, D. R., 39
O'Leary, S. G., 116
Ollendick, T., 75
Ollendick, T. H., 22, 57, 61, 62, 68, 73, 74
Olness, K., 147, 196
Olness, K. N., 154, 191
Olson, R. A., 9, 185, 186
Orsillo, S. M., 6
Osborne, R. B., 168
Öst, L. G., 75
Ostrander, R., 26
Owens-Stively, J., 121, 136, 137, 139
Oxford, D. R., 21
Ozolins, M., 167, 185

P
Pace, T. M., 9, 10
Pachman, L. M., 197
Pachter, L. M., 164
Padawer, M., 151
Palan, B. M., 155
Palfi, S., 82
Palmerus, K., 55, 56
Panopoulos, G., 175
Parker, J. D., 62
Partin, J. C., 125
Patterson, G. R., 22, 24, 30, 36, 38, 45, 46, 218
Patterson, J. M., 29
Perlmutter, A. D., 147
Perrin, E. C., 10, 61
Perrin, S., 55
Peter, B., 196
Peterson, A. L., 82, 87, 92
Peterson, C. P., 30
Peterson, L., 219
Pettei, M. J., 128

Pfefferbaun, B., 175
Philipp, B., 105, 109
Philipp, M. K., W. 86
Pigeon, H., 173
Pina, A. A., 61
Pine, D., 64
Pine, D. S., 55
Pinilla, T., 110, 111
Pinto, A., 58
Pizzo, P. A., 162
Pollard, C. A., 87
Pollock, J. I., 100
Porteus, S. D., 27
Pothmann, R., 194
Powell, C., 216
Powers, S. W., 168, 183, 184, 190
Price, L. H., 85
Primack, W., 153
Prior, M., 56
Pruitt, S. D., 185
Purtin, J. S., 125
Purviance, C. B., 216
Purvis, P. C., 124, 149

Q
Quay, H. C., 18, 20
Quiltich, H. R., 33

R
Rabian, B., 74, 75
Rand, C., 206
Rapee, R. M., 69
Rapoff, K. E., 105
Rapoff, M. A., 6, 84, 105, 114, 204, 205, 206, 208, 210, 212, 213, 214, 215, 216
Rapoport, A. M., 190, 191
Rapoport, J. L., 85
Rapp, M. A., 92
Rappaport, G. B., 134, 135
Rappaport, L., 214
Rappaport, L. A., 162
Rappley, M. D., 40
Rappoff, M. A., 202
Rasmussen, M., 163
Rasmussen, S. A., 85
Ravilly, S., 182
Rebgetz, M., 193
Rebuffat, E., 113
Reid, G. J., 160
Reid, J. B., 30
Reid, M. J., 116

Reitan, R. M., 27
Rey, J. M., 151
Reynolds, C. R., 24, 25, 26, 61, 62, 65, 66,
    132, 147, 205
Reynolds, S., 7
Riccio, C. A., 26
Richardson, P., 218
Richman, N., 18, 21, 101, 112, 145
Richmond, B. O., 61, 62
Richmond, J. B., 125
Richters, J. E., 65
Richtsmeier, A. J., 168
Ricker, J. H., 219
Rickert, V. I., 116
Riddle, M. A., 50, 64, 66, 67, 85
Rincover, A., 30
Ritchie, J. A., 160
Robbins, K., 41, 43
Roberts, R. N., 120
Robins, L. N., 11
Robinson, E. A., 127
Robinson, L. M., 40
Robinson, W., 182
Rockney, R. M., 133
Rodgers, A., 4
Rolf, J. E., 21
Rolider, A., 115
Romsing, J., 163, 174
Rooney, M. T., 24
Rosen, B., 211
Rosenbaum, J. E., 57
Rosenberg, L. A., 85
Ross, A. W., 127
Ross, C. K., 197
Ross, L. V., 136
Roter, D. L., 216, 221
Rounds, K. A., 208
Rourke, B. P., 168
Rudolph, K. D., 166
Russ, S. W., 166
Russell, G. J., 134
Russo, D. C., 10
Russo, R. M., 110, 111
Ryan, M., 213

S
Saavedra, L. M., 61
Sackett, D. L., 214
Sallee, F. R., 87
Salzberg, A. D., 65
Sanberg, P. R., W. 86
Sanders, M. R., 74, 192, 193

Sanson, A., 56
Santiago, J. V., 206
Sartory, G., 194
Sasson, Y., 88
Satin, W., 218
Savage, C., 127
Schachar, R., 13
Schade, J. G., 168, 179
Schafer, L. C., 216
Schecter, J., 24
Schimmel, L. E., 219
Schlundt, D. G., 219, 220
Schmidt, H., 56
Schoenberg, N. E., 206
Schroeder, C. S., 10
Schulte, M. J., 6
Schwab-Stone, M., 24
Schwab-Stone, M. E., 24
Schwartz, C. E., 56, 57
Schweitzer, J. B., 205
Sclar, D. A., 40
Seale, J. P., 206, 213
Serafini, L. T., 74, 75
Sethuraman, G., 87
Seymour, R. A., 176
Shaffer, D., 11, 24, 60
Shannon, M., 183
Shapiro, A. K., 82
Shapiro, B. S., 182
Shapiro, E. S., 82, 85
Shapiro, F., 75
Shaw, J., 206, 213
Sheftell, F. D., 190, 191
Shelov, S. P., 146
Shelton, T. L., 15, 26, 44
Shephard, R., 193
Shepherd, R. W., 192
Shoffitt, T., 219
Shriver, M. D., 194, 199
Shulman, D., 112
Shytle, R. D., W. 86
Siebelink, B. M., 55
Siegel, L. J., 187, 188
Siegel, S., 165, 174
Siegel, T., 36
Siegel, T. C., 33
Sigman, M., 58
Sijsenaar, M., 75
Silber, K. P., 92
Siller, J., 218
Silva, R. R., 86
Silver, A. A., W. 86

Silverman, W. K., 60, 61, 65, 66, 67, 72, 74, 75
Simonds, J. D., 146
Simonian, S. J., 4
Simonoff, E. A., 112
Simpson, J. M., 176
Sindou, M., 82
Sine, L., 87
Singer, H. S., 85, 87, 94
Siqueland, L., 68, 69, 77
Skaer, T. L., 40
Skyler, J. S., 218
Slanetz, P. J., 16
Smart, D., 56
Smith, J. A., 219
Smith, J. T., 189, 190
Smith, L. N., 110
Smith, M., 94
Smith, N. A., 206, 213
Smith, W., 162
Sneed, T. J., 152, 154
Snidman, N., 56
Snyder, J., 24
Soldatos, C. R., 101, 102
Solnick, J. V., 30
Sonnenberg, A., 125
Sottiaux, M., 113
Spence, S. H., 56, 72, 77
Spencer, J. A. D., 119
Sperling, M., 150
Spielberger, C., 61, 63
Spirito, A., 121, 136
Srivastav, A., 155
Stack, J. M., 120
Stallings, P., 62
Stanley, K., 208, 209, 211
Stanley, M. A., 94
Stanton, W. R., 105
Starfield, B., 3
Stark, L., 121
Stark, L. J., 136, 140, 185
Stephens, P., 217
Sterling, C. N., 196
Stevens, B., 178
Stevens, B. J., 180
Stevenson, J., 162
Stevenson, J. E., 18, 145
Stewart, D. A., 146, 151
Stine, J. J., 206, 219
Stone, J., 24
Stores, G., 112
Strauss, C. C., 57

Streichenwein, S. M., 87
Stroop, J. R., 27
Sturges, J. W., 168
Sullivan, K., 62
Suresh, S., 182
Sutphen, J., 127, 137, 140
Sutphen, J. L., 124, 134
Sveen, O. B., 167
Swan, S., 184
Swan, S. C., 190
Swanson, J. M., 27
Swanson, M. S., 100
Swanson, S., 93
Swearer, S. M., 147
Szapocznik, J., 34

T
Talbert, D., 119
Tarnowski, K. J., 4
Task Force on Promotion and
    Dissemination of Psychological
    Procedures, 183
Taylor, P. D., 151
Taylor, W. R., 162
Taylow, D. W., 214
Terdal, L. G., 22
Thomas, A. M., 219
Thomas, C., 36
Thomas, J., 206, 214
Thompson, K. L., 168, 171
Thompson, R. J., 201
Thompson, S., 151
Thompson, S. J., 206
Thornby, J. I., 87
Thuras, P. D., 58
Tierney, S., 64
Tollison, J. W., 151
Touzel, B., 165
Treffers, P. D., 55
Trevathan, G. E., 100
Turecki, S., 112
Turgay, A., 19
Turner, R. K., 151
Turner, S. M., 57
Tyler, D. C., 181

U
Ucko, L. E., 100
Ulrich, R. F., 24, 25

V
Van Deusen, J. M., 34

Van Houten, R., 115
van Londen, A., 154
van Londen-Barentsen, M. W., 154
van Sciver, M. M.
Van Slyke, D. A., 190
van Son, M. J., 154
Varni, J., 176, 216
Varni, J. W., 10, 160, 168, 171, 182, 198
Vaughn, M. L., 26
Velosa, J. F., 66, 67
Verhulst, F. C., 18
Villarruel, A. M., 175
Vitiello, B., 12, 13, 17, 18, 19, 35
Vogel, W., 153
von Baeyer, C. L., 192

W
Wachsmuth, R., 13
Walco, G. A., 160, 176, 177, 182, 183,
    196
Wald, A., 127
Walker, L. S., 168, 190
Walkup, J. T., 50, 85
Waller, D. A., 217
Walsh, J. K., 105
Walter, A. L., 116
Warmenhoven, N. J., 55
Warren, S. L., 58
Warwick, D. J., 218
Warzak, W. J., 147, 157
Wassell, G., 38, 337
Wasserman, R. C., 16, 19
Watanabe, H. K., 65
Watson, D., 6
Watson, T. S., 91
Webster-Stratton, C. H., 21, 22, 38, 48
Weems, C. F., 61, 65, 66, 72, 74, 75
Weinfurt, K. P., 26
Weinstein, S. R., 24
Weinstein, T. A., 128
Weisman, S. J., 180, 181, 182
Weissbluth, M., 112
Weist, M. D., 204
Weisz, J. R., 4, 48, 166
Weizman, A., 88
Weller, E. B., 24
Weller, R. A., 24
Wells, K. C., 151

Werry, J. S., 147, 151
Wesley, R. A., 163
Westenberg, P. M., 55
Whaley, S. E., 58
Whelan, J. P., 137
White, N. H., 219
White-Traut, R. C., 166
Whitfield, M. F., 180
Wierson, M., 29
Wilkinson, P., 115
Wilkinson, R. H., 130, 131, 133
Williams, C. L., 137, 181
Williams, D. L., 151
Wilson, J. J., 166
Wishner, W. J., 201
Wishnie, E., 182
Wohl, M. E., 182
Wolf, A. W., 100, 104
Wolf, M. M., 33
Wolfson, D., 27
Wolkind, S., 21
Woodgate, R., 163, 179
Woods, D. W., 92
Woody, P., 174
Woolf, A. D., 214
Woolford, H., 192, 193
World Health Organization, 60
Wranch, H. R., 94
Wright, L., 136
Wuori, D., 208, 210
Wynder, E. L., 137
Wypij, D., 219
Wysocki, T., 206, 216

Y
Yang, F., 180
Yarnold, P. R., 26
Young, J. G., 85
Young, M., 153
Yunas, M. B., 163

Z
Zeltzer, L., 165, 174
Zigo, M. A., 218
Zito, J. M., 35, 40, 47
Zohar, J., 88
Zuckerman, B., 105, 107, 109, 162
Zvolensky, D., 6

SUBJECT INDEX

A

Abdominal pain, prevalence of, 162
Achenbach Child Behavior Checklist, in
enuresis, 147
Acquired immunodeficiency syndrome
(AIDS)
pain in, 163
ADHD. See Activity deficit hyperactivity
disorder (ADHD)
Adherence
assessment of
direct measures in, 203–204
general behavioral adherence in,
204–205
indirect measures in, 204
communication of illness and regimen
information for, 205–210
to complex treatment regimen,
214–217
child–related barriers to, 217
comprehensive strategies for
complex treatment regimens,
216–217
contingency contracting in, 216
motivation and cooperation for,
214
reinforcement and reminder
strategies in, 214–215
tailoring to individual need and,
214
token economies in, 215–216
comprehensive strategies for
medication regimens, 213
definitions of, 201
factors influencing, 202–203
family and, 217–218
importance of, 201–202
interventions for, 204–220
to medication regimen, 210–213
comprehensive strategies for, 213
contracting, 212–213
cues for, 212
increased follow-up, 210–211
reinforcement, 212
token economies in, 212–213
parental, 45

patient education for
asthma inhaler instruction sheet,
209
cognitive concepts and, 207, 208
developmentally appropriate
information in, 206, 208
literacy levels and, 208, 209, 211
pill–swallowing handout, 210
strategies for effective, 206
written materials in, 208, 209, 210
peer interventions in, 219–220
prevalence of, 202
research in, 205
social barriers to, 218–219
Adult reports
in anxiety disorders, 64–65
of child's pain, 177–179
Aggressive behavior
prognostic value of, 13–14
risperidone for, 35
AIDS. See Acquired immunodeficiency
syndrome
Alprazolam (Xanax), for anxiety disorders,
67
American Academy of Child and
Adolescent Psychiatry, practice
guidelines for anxiety disorders,
58–59, 67
Analgesic ladder
for AIDS pain, 180
for cancer pain, 182
for recurrent/disease–state pain, 180
Analgesics, for procedure–related pain, 181
Antidepressants. See also Tricyclic
antidepressants
increased usage of, 40
Anxiety, adherence to complex treatment
regimen and, 217
Anxiety disorders
assessment of, 58–66
adult reports in, 64–65
child's self–report in, 61–64,
62t–63t
components of, 58–59
structured and semistructured
interview in, 60–61

causes and correlates of, 55–58
cognitive-behavioral therapy for,
    68–69, 70t–71t, 72
    group sessions in, 72–73
    for specific phobias, 73–75
comorbidity with other disorders, 50,
    53, 55
comorbid with conduct disorder, 19
defined, 49
differential diagnoses of, 50–55
in *DSM–III–R*
    DSM–IV and, 50
in *DSM–IV*, 49
environmental factors in, 57–58
parent and teacher rating scales, 64–65
pharmacologic interventions in, 66–68
    need for evaluation of, 67
    pharmaceutical studies of, 66–67
    practice guidelines for, 67
prevalence of, 55
risk factors for, 55
    behavioral inhibition, 56–57
    genetic, 56
Anxiety Disorders Interview Schedule for
    Children (ADIS–C), 60
Anxiety Disorders Interview Schedule for
    Parents (ADIS–P), 60
Arousal training, for enuresis, 154
Attention deficit hyperactivity disorder
    (ADHD), 39–47
    assessment of
        neuropsychological tests in, 27
    behavioral interventions in, 44–45
        barriers to, 45–46
    clinical features of, 15
    comorbid oppositional defiant disorder
        and conduct disorder with, 19–20
    comorbid with anxiety, 55
    defined, 14–15
    developmental changes in, 16
    DSM–IV criteria for, 15–16
    DSM–IV differential diagnosis criteria
        for, 17t
    parent training program for, 44
    pharmacologic intervention in, 40–43
        efficacy study of, 41
        medication recommendations for,
            42
        medication side effects and, 41–42
        overprescription issue in, 40
    prevalence of, 18–19
    treatments for, 39–40

Attention disorders, adherence to complex
    treatment regimen and, 217
Aversive responding, in conduct problem
    development, 22
Aversive–taste procedure, for thumb
    sucking, 90–91
Awareness training, in habit reversal
    training, 93

B
Barkley, R. A., 27
Barkley Side Effects Questionnaire (BSEQ),
    41, 42, 43
Bedtime resistance, 100, 105
Bedtime routines
    comparison with graduated extinction
        for bedtime tantrums, 116–117
    for sleep problems, 110
Behavioral Assessment System for Children
    (BASC)
    in anxiety disorders
        adult assessment of, 65, 66
    in disruptive behavior disorders, 24,
        25t, 26
    in encopresis, 132
    in enuresis, 147
Behavioral problems
    interventions in
        efficacy research in, 3–4
    prevalence of, 3
Behavior rating scales
    for disruptive behavior disorders,
        24–26
        diagnostic utility of, 26
Bell–and–pad training. *See* Urine–alarm
    training
Benadryl Elixir (diphenhydramine
    hydrochloride)
    for sleep problems, 110–111
Benzodiazepines, for anxiety disorders, 66,
    67
Biofeedback
    for encopresis, 137
    for headache pain, 192–194
    for pain in chronic disease states, 197
    for pain in recurrent medical
        conditions, 192–193
    thermal, 193–194
    with and without cognitive-behavioral
        therapy
        for disease–related pain, 197
Bowel control, muscle training for, 140

Breast feedings, timing of, for sleep
    problems, 110
Breathing exercises
    for disease–related pain, 196
    for procedure–related pain and anxiety,
        184t, 184–185
Brief interventions, for simple tics, 89, 90
Busipone, for anxiety disorders, 66

C
Cambridge Study in Delinquent
    Development, 21
Cancer
    pain in, 163, 182
Child Behavior Checklist (CBCL)
    in anxiety disorders
        adult assessment of, 65
    in correlation of daytime behavior and
        sleep problems, 106
    in disruptive behavior disorders, 24,
        25t, 25–26
    in encopresis, 132
    in enuresis, 147
Children's Interview for Psychiatric
    Syndromes, 24
Children's Yale-Brown Obsessive
    Compulsive Scale (CY–BOCS)
    for tic severity rating, 85
Clinical Global Impression Scale for
    Tourette's syndrome, 85
Clonidine
    comparison with desipramine
        for Tourette's syndrome, 87
    for conduct disorder, 34–35
    increased usage of, 40
    with methylphenidate
        for conduct disorder and opposi-
            tional defiant disorder, 35
Coercive behavior, parental, 45
Coercive process model, in conduct
    problem development, 22
Cognitive-behavioral therapy (CBT)
    for anxiety
        Screen for Child Anxiety Related
            Emotional Disorders
            monitoring of, 64
    for anxiety disorders, 60–61
        Kendall model, 68–69, 70t–71t, 76
    in attention deficit/hyperactivity
        disorder, 45, 46
    comparison with diazepam (Valium)
        during painful procedures, 188–189

in conduct disorder, 36–38
group format
    components of, 72
    pain in recurrent medical conditions,
        190–192
    effectiveness of, 192
    relaxation training in, 191
parent training with, 72, 73
Cohen, D. J.
    etiology of tic and Tourette's disorder,
        83
Communication skills, parental, 46
Comorbidity
    with anxiety disorders, 50, 53, 55
    attention deficit/hyperactivity disorder
        and oppositional defiant disorder,
        28
    with disruptive behavior disorders,
        19–20
Competing response, in habit reversal
    training, 93
Compliance. *See also* Adherence
    meanings of term, 201
Conditioned reinforcers, defined, 30
Conduct disorder (CD)
    associated diagnoses, 13
    behavioral interventions in, 36–39
    comorbid depression and anxiety in,
        19
    defined, 13
    differential diagnosis criteria for, 17t
    DSM–IV criteria for, 13, 14
    pharmacological intervention in,
        34–36
    prevalence of, 18
Constipation
    chronic, 128
    digital rectal examination for, 128
    in encopresis, 125
    functional, 125
    medication–related, 128
    stooling abnormalities with, 126
Contingency contracting
    for adherence to treatment regimen
        in diabetes, Type I, 216
    for medication adherence, 212–
        213
Contingency management
    in cognitive behavioral therapy
        for school phobia, 74
    in cognitive behavioral therapy group,
        72, 75

Continuous Performance Task (CPT)
in assessment
of disruptive behavior disorders, 27
Coping skills, family, adherence and, 218
Coping strategies
for pain, 165
behavioral, 166
cognitive, 166
Covariance
habit, defined, 89
thumb sucking and hair pulling, 89–90, 91
Coyle, J. T., 35–36
Cues, for medication adherence, 212
Cultural diversity
adherence and, 218–219
importance of, 7–8
research deficiency in, 7
sleep disorders and, 87
Cystic fibrosis, pain in, 163

D
Amphetamine (Dexedrine)
in comorbid conduct disorder and attention deficit/hyperactivity disorder, 35
Day wetting
as behavioral problem, 147
evaluation of, 149
positive practice training for, 155–157
prevalence of, 147
DDAVP. See Desmopressin (DDAVP)
Depression
adherence to complex treatment regimen and, 217
comorbid
with anxiety, 55
with conduct disorder, 19
parental
patient adherence and, 217
Desmopressin (DDAVP)
cost–benefit considerations with, 150
for enuresis, 149, 150–151
Dexedrine. See Amphetamine (Dexedrine)
Diabetes, dietary adherence in, peer interventions in, 219–220
Diabetes, Type I
adherence to treatment regimen and contingency contracting for, 216
token economies for, 216

Diagnostic and Statistical Manual of Mental Disorders (4th ed, DSM–IV)
use of diagnostic symptoms, criteria, codes, 9
Diagnostic Interview Schedule for Children (DISC), 24
in anxiety assessment
versions of, 60
Diaries
pain, 173t, 177–178
sleep, 107–108, 109
Diazepam (Valium)
adjunctive to cognitive-behavioral therapy for pain, 188–189
cognitive-behavioral therapy comparison with
during painful procedures, 188–189
for sleep terrors, 112–113
Diet
constipation and, 133, 134
sleep problems and, 113
Dietary fiber
in encopresis treatment, 134, 135, 137, 138t–139t
Dietary problems
in diabetes
peer interventions in, 219–220
Discipline problems, prevalence of, 3
Disruptive behavior disorder(s)
age and, 20–21
assessment of, 22–28
behavior rating scales in, 24–26
clinical utility of, 22
clinic–based diagnostic procedures, 26–28
empirically based and DSM–IV diagnostic criteria in, 23
functions in, 22
interviewing in, 23–24
multimodal, 22–23
attention deficit/hyperactivity disorder, 14–16
causes and correlates of, 20–22
classification of, 11
comorbidity with, 19–20
conduct disorder, 13–14
differential diagnosis of, 16–17, 17t
family functioning in, 21–22
gender and, 18, 20, 21

interventions in, 28–47
longitudinal study of, 21
oppositional defiant disorder, 12–13
pharmacologic therapies in
    effectiveness of, 47
prevalence of, 11, 18–19
Distraction, for procedure–related pain and
    anxiety, 184t, 185
Doctoral trainees, 9
Dry–bed training. *See also* Urine–alarm
    training
physician training in, 152–153
procedures in, 152, 153–154
DSM–IV. *See Diagnostic and Statistical
    Manual of Mental Disorders*

E
Educational-supportive therapy
    comparison of cognitive behavioral
        therapy with, 74, 75
Empirically supported treatments
    advantages of, 4–5
    comorbidity *versus* single diagnoses
        and, 6
    movement for, 4
Encopresis
    absence of behavioral problems in, 127
    assessment of
        behavioral, 131–133, 132t
        medical, 127–131, 132t
    associated terminology, 123–124
    biological factors in, 126–127
    bowel problem intake form in,
        129–130
    causes of, 125
    constipation in, 125, 126
        digital rectal examination for, 128
        medication–related, 128
    defined, 123, 124
    differential diagnosis of, 130–131, 132t
    DSM–IV diagnostic criteria for, 132t
    group interventions in, 136
    versus Hirschsprung disease, 130, 131t
    medical-behavioral treatment of
        parent education in, 136
    medical treatment of, 133
        colon cleanout in, 133, 135
        demystification process in, 134, 135f
        dietary fiber in, 134, 135, 137,
            138t–139t
        long–term follow–up of, 133–134

mineral oil in, 133, 134–135
    safety studies of, 134–135
    as treatment of choice, 134
outcome studies of, 8
prevalence of, 125
rectal insensitivity in, 126
symptoms of, 131
treatment of
    adherence in, 140–141
    bowel symptom rating sheet in,
        141–142
    procedures for, 137
    resistance to, 137, 140
Enhanced toilet training (ETT), in
    encopresis, 137, 140
Enuresis
    arousal training for, 154
    assessment of, 147–149
    behavioral assessment of
        enuresis intake form in, 148–149
        interview and rating scales in, 147
    behavioral treatment of, 151–157
    causes of, 146–147
    defined, 145
    dry–bed training for, 152–154
    DSM–IV diagnostic criteria for, 145,
        146
    family history of, 147
    hypnotherapy for, 154–155
    intervention in, 149–157
    medical assessment of, 147
    medical *versus* psychological
        treatments of, 148–150
    outcome studies of, 8
    overlearning for, 151–152
    pharmacological treatment of, 149, 150
    positive practice for, 155–157
    prevalence of
        for day wetting, 146
        for nocturnal, 145–146
    social and interpersonal treatments for,
        157
    treatment options for, 157
    urine–alarm training for, 151, 154,
        155t, 157
Eskalith. *See* Lithium carbonate (Eskalith)
Exposure, for anxiety disorders, 69, 75, 76
Extinction
    for prevention of sleep problems,
        113–114
    for sleep onset problems, 115–116

Eyberg Child Behavior Inventory, in encopresis, 127

Eye movement desensitization and reprocessing (EMDR), for simple phobias, 75

F

Faces scale, in pain assessment, 172t, 174–175

Family, adherence to medical regimen and, 203

Family dysfunction, child anxiety and, 57

Family history
in anxiety disorders, 59
in disruptive behavior disorders, 23–24

Fear Survey Schedule for Children–Revised (FSSC–R), in anxiety assessment, 61, 62t

Fibromyalgia, pain in, 163

Fluoxetine, comparison with placebo, for trichotillomania, 87

Freeze–frame technique, for anxiety disorders, 69

G

General anesthesia, for procedure–related pain, 181

Generalized anxiety disorder
defined, 50
DSM–IV criteria for, 51–52

Grodzinsky, G. M., 27

Guided imagery, for procedure–related pain and anxiety, 186

H

Habit covariance
defined, 89
thumb sucking and hair pulling, 89–91

Habit disorders
assessment of, 84
behavioral observations in, 84
severity rating scales in, 84–85
behavioral treatments for
comparison of, 95t
defined, 79
differential from organically caused movement disorders, 82
pharmacological treatments for, 86–88, 88t

Habit reversal
components in, 91

group training in
for trichotillomania, 94
long–term follow–up of, 96
versus negative practice
for self–destructive oral habits, 95
simplification of, 91–92
for Tourette's syndrome, 92

Hair pulling. *See* Trichotillomania (hair pulling)

Haldol. *See* Haloperidol (Haldol)

Hall, C. C. I., 7

Haloperidol (Haldol)
for Tourette's syndrome, 86
versus clonidine, 87
with nicotine, 86–87
versus pimozide, 87

Headache
biofeedback for, 192
combination psychological interventions for
comparison with pharmacological treatments, 194–195
prevalence of, 160, 162
relaxation training for
school–based, 191–192
thermal biofeedback for, 193–194

Health care providers, pain assessment and, 178, 179

Health care system, adherence to medical regimen and, 203

Hirschsprung disease
definition and characteristics of, 123–124
symptoms of, 131

Hoder, E. L., etiology of tic disorder and Tourette's syndrome, 83

Hyperactivity
in attention deficit/hyperactivity disorder, 15
cultural diversity and, 8

Hypersomnia, primary
DSM–IV criteria for, 101, 102t
DSM–IV differential criteria for, 104t

Hypnotherapy
for disease–related pain, 196–197
for enuresis, 154–155, 157
for procedure–related pain, 189–190
for trichotillomania (hair pulling), 95–96

I

Ignoring, for sleep resistance, 114–115

Illness, adherence to medical regimen and, 203

Imagery
    for disease–related pain, 196
    for procedure–related pain and anxiety,
        184t, 185–186
        emotive, 185–186
        guided, 186
Imagery rehearsal, for nightmare disorder,
    120
Imipramine (Tofranil)
    for enuresis
        as adjunctive therapy, 150
        comparison with hypnosis, 155
Impulsivity, in attention
    deficit/hyperactivity disorder, 15–
    16
Inattention, in attention
    deficit/hyperactivity disorder, 15
Infant, pain assessment for, 177–178
Insomnia, primary. *See also* Sleep onset
    (primary insomnia)
    DSM–IV criteria for, 101, 102t
    DSM–IV differential criteria for, 104t
Intensive medical care, in encopresis, 137
Internalizing and externalizing factors
    Behavior Assessment System for
        Children and, 65
    in Child Behavior Checklist, 65
Interns, 9
Interviews
    for disruptive behavior disorders,
        23–24
    for pain, 169–171
    for sleep problems, 107

J
Jensen, P., 12
Juvenile rheumatoid arthritis
    adherence to treatment regimen and
        token economies for, 215–216
    pain management in, 163, 176, 182

K
Kendall cognitive-behavioral program
    for anxiety, avoidant, and overanxious
        disorders
        educational strategies in, 69
        effectiveness of, 69
        exposure strategies in, 69
        format for, 68
        freeze–frame technique in, 69
        participants in, 68

L
Learning disorders, adherence to complex
    treatment regimen and, 217
Literacy level
    parental
        and patient adherence, 218
        patient education materials and, 208,
            209, 211
Lithium carbonate (Eskalith), for
    aggression, 35

M
Matching Figures Test (MFT), in
    assessment of disruptive behavior
    disorders, 26–27
Medical history, in anxiety disorders, 59
Medication adherence
    contingency contracting for, 212–
        213
    cues and reinforcement for, 212
    follow–up for, 211–212
    parental reinforcement for, 213
    token economies for, 212
Melatonin, for sleep disorders, 113
Methotrexate, for juvenile rheumatoid
    arthritis, 182
Methylphenidate (Ritalin)
    in comorbid conduct disorder and
        attention deficit/hyperactivity
        disorder, 35
    overutilization issue and, 40
    side effects of, 41–42, 43
Metoprolol, for recurrent pain, 195
Milk allergies, in sleep problems, 113
Milk and diary products, constipation from,
    133
Modeling
    filmed
        for procedure–related pain and
            anxiety, 184t, 187–188
        as phobia treatment, 74
MTA Cooperative Group study of stimulant
    medication in attention
    deficit/hyperactivity disorder, 41
Multidimensional Anxiety Scale for
    Children (MASC)
    in anxiety assessment, 61, 62, 63t,
        63–64, 66
    adult agreement with, 64

N
Nail biting, 79, 81

comparison of habit reversal and
negative practice treatment for,
94
prevalence of, 82
Negative practice
comparison of habit reversal with
for nail biting, 94
for trichotillomania, 94–95
long–term follow–up of, 96
Neuroleptics, adjunctive, in chronic pain
management, 182
Nightmare disorder, 101
behavioral strategies for, 120
DSM–IV criteria for, 103
DSM–IV differential criteria for, 104t
Night terrors. See Sleep terror disorder
Nighttime fears, cognitive-behavioral
therapy for, 74
Nonsteroidal antiinflammatory drugs
(NSAIDS)
for cystic fibrosis, 182
for postoperative pain, 181
Nursing Assessment of Pain Intensity
(NAPI), 178

O
ODD. See Oppositional defiant disorder
(ODD)
Operant procedures, for phobias, 74
Opioid drugs
in chronic disease pain, 182
dependence versus addiction and,
183–184
misconceptions and controversies
regarding, 183–184
for postoperative pain, 181
Oppositional behavior, increase in, 45–46
Oppositional defiant disorder (ODD)
behavioral interventions in, 28–29,
28–33
comorbid attention
deficit/hyperactivity disorder and
conduct disorder with, 19–20
defined, 12, 12
DSM–IV criteria for, 12
parent training in, 29–30
pharmacological interventions in, 28
structural family therapy in, 33–34
time–in in, 30, 31
token economy in, 30–33
Oppositional disorders, prevalence of, 18
Oucher Scale, in pain assessment, 173t, 175

Overlearning, in enuresis treatment, 151–152

P
Pain
adult reports of, 177
assessment of, 198
methods for, 168, 169
purpose of, 168
child self–report measures for, 171,
172t–173t, 174–177
in chronic disease states
biofeedback for, 197
cognitive-behavioral therapy for,
196
hypnosis for, 196–197
incidence of, 162–163
intervention studies of, 195–196
types of, 160, 162–163
cognitive-behavioral management of
procedure–related, 184t, 184–190
breathing exercises for, 184–185
distraction for, 185
filmed modeling for, 187–188
hypnosis for, 189–190
imagery for, 185–186
positive reinforcement for, 188
rehearsal/coaching for, 188
relaxation training for, 186–187
cognitive-behavioral therapy for, 198
contributing factors in
child, 164–167
environmental, 167–168
cultural expectations and, 8
definitions of, 159
disease–associated
research needs in, 198–199
experience of
age and, 164–165
coping strategies and, 165–166
gender and, 165
influence of previous experience,
167
temperament and, 166–167
inadequate treatment of
incidence of, 163
reasons for, 164
nociception in, 159
pain diaries for, 173t, 177
pain interviews for
for acute pain, 169–170
for chronic/recurrent pain, 170–171
conduct of, 171

patient–controlled analgesia for, 198
pharmacologic management of,
180–183
in procedure–related (acute) pain,
180–181
in recurrent and disease–state pain,
181–182
physiological measures of, 179–180
pictorial scales for, 174–177
postoperative
pharmacologic management of, 181
procedure–related
combination cognitive-behavioral
and pharmacological
management of, 189–190
recurrent
abdominal, 190, 192, 193t
cognitive-behavioral therapy for,
191–192
headache, 190–191
in recurrent medical conditions
biofeedback training for, 192–193
combination treatments in,
194–195
undertreatment of, 198
Pain diary, 177–178
limitations of, 177
in pain assessment, 173t
Pain disorder
DSM–III–R and DSM–IV and, 160
DSM–IV criteria for, 161
versus somatization disorder, 160, 161
Pain experiences, prevalence of, 160, 162
Parent education
in encopresis, 136
for prevention of sleep problems,
113–114
Parenting groups
for children with conduct disorder,
38–39
for prevention of conduct problems, 39
Parent involvement
in habit reversal training, 93
Parent management training (PMT). See
also Parent training
comparison with problem–solving
skills training, 37
in conduct disorder
effectiveness of, 37–38
procedures in, 36–37
Parents
and child's response to pain, 167–168

Conners Parent Rating Scale, 24, 25, 25t
pain report of, 177, 179
psychopathology of
child anxiety and, 57
Parent training. See also Parent
management training (PMT)
and child pain, 199
with cognitive behavioral therapy,
72–73
comparison with child therapy
for children with conduct disorder,
38–39
maintenance of effects of, 46–47
in oppositional defiant disorder, 29–30
effectiveness of, 29
stepwise approach to, 29–30
time–in for, 30
time–out for, 30
token economy in, 30–33
Parent training programs
for attention deficit/hyperactivity
disorder, 44
Patient–controlled analgesia (PCA)
for acute pain, 181
for chronic disease pain, 181
for pain, 198
Pediatric Pain Questionnaire (PPQ), 171
Peer interventions, adherence and, 219–
220
Peer pressure, adherence and, 218–219
to medical regimen and, 203
Phobia(s)
cognitive-behavioral therapy for,
73–75
school, 74
comparison of cognitive behavioral
and with educational-
supportive therapy, 74, 75
social. See Social phobia
specific (simple). See Specific phobia
Physicians
primary care, referrals from, 10
training and urine–alarm training, 154,
155
Pimozide, haloperidol versus, for Tourette's
syndrome, 87
Poker chip tool, in pain assessment, 172t,
174
Positive reinforcement, for
procedure–related pain and anxiety,
184t, 188
Positive restructuring, as coping strategy, 166

Problem–solving skills, parental, 46
Problem–solving skills training (PSST)
    for conduct disorder, 36
    with parent management training
        for oppositional and aggressive
            youths, 48
Problem–solving skills training with
    practice (PSST–P)
    for conduct disorder, 36
    effectiveness of, 37–38
Progressive muscle relaxation. *See*
    Relaxation training
Psychiatric illness, medical adherence in,
    217
Psychologists
    medication recommendations of, 42
    relationship with physicians, 10
Psychotropic medications
    increased usage of, 40
    use in children, 35–36

R
Recurrent abdominal pain (RAP)
    cognitive-behavioral therapy for, 192,
        193t
        group, 192, 193t
    defined, 190
Referrals, from primary care physicians,
    10
Rehearsal/coaching, for procedure–related
    pain and anxiety, 184t, 188
Reinforced practice, for phobias, 74
Reinforcement, for medication adherence,
    212
Relaxation training
    for disease–related pain, 196
    for headache, 191–192
    for pain in recurrent medical
        conditions, 191
    for procedure–related pain and anxiety,
        184t, 186–187
    for sleep onset problems, 117–119
    for Tourette's syndrome, 94
Research
    in adherence, 205
    in cultural deficiency, lack of, 7
    in disease–related pain, 198–199
    in intervention efficacy, 3–4
    treatment manuals in, 5
Revised Children's Manifest Anxiety Scale
    (RCMAS)
    in anxiety assessment, 61, 62, 62t

Reward system, in simple habit
    intervention, 89
Riley Infant Pain Scale (RIPS), 179
Risperidone
    for aggresison in conduct disorder, 35
    for Tourette's syndrome, 87
Ritalin. *See* Methylphenidate (Ritalin)

S
Scheduled awakenings
    for sleep onset problems, 116
    for sleep terror disorder, 120
    for sleepwalking disorder, 121
School phobia
    cognitive behavioral therapy treatment
        of, 74
        comparison with educational-
            supportive therapy, 74, 75
Screen for Child Anxiety Related
    Emotional Disorders (SCARED),
    62, 63t,
    64
Sedation, for procedure–related pain, 181
Selective serotonin reuptake inhibitors
    (SSRIs)
    for anxiety disorders, 66
Self–control strategies
    in cognitive behavioral therapy group
        treatment, 72
Self–management, parental, 46
Self–management training program, in
    adherence enhancement, 218
Self–report measures
    in anxiety assessment, 61–64, 62t–63t
    for pain, 177–178
Separation anxiety disorder, 49
    comparison of cognitive behavioral
        therapy and wait–list control, 68
    defined, 49, 50
    DSM–IV criteria for, 51–52
    risk factors for, 58
Sickle cell disease
    hypnosis for, 196–197
    opioids for, 182
    pain in, 163
Simple phobia, age and, 56
Simple tics, brief interventions for, 89, 90
Sleep behavior
    assistance with, 100
    cultural diversity and, 8
    night–awakening habits, 100
    normal, 99

requirements for sleep, 100
time to onset in, 99
transitional object and, 100
Sleep diary, 107–108, 109
Sleep intake form, 107, 108
Sleep–onset delays, 100, 105
Sleep onset (primary insomnia). *See also*
    Insomnia, primary
    bedtime routines for, 116–117
    electronic equipment for, 120
    graduated extinction for, 115–116
    ignoring, 114–115
    relaxation for, 117–119
    scheduled awakenings for, 116
    treatment of and daytime behavior,
        117, 118
    white noise for, 119
Sleep problem(s)
    in adolescents, 105
    bedtime resistance, 100
    behavioral assessment of, 106–109
        parent interviews in, 107
        sleep diary in, 107–108, 109
        sleep intake form in, 107, 108
    behavioral interventions for, 113–121
    causes and correlates of, 105
    daytime behavior problems and, 106
    dietary treatments for, 113
    DSM–IV criteria for, 102, 103
    medical assessment of, 106
    medical treatment for, 110–112
    night awakenings, 100
    parental presence and involvement in,
        105
    persistence of, 100–101, 121
    prevalence of, 104–105
    prevention of, 109–110, 111
    primary hypersomnia, 101, 102
    primary insomnia, 101, 102
    sleep–onset and, 100
Sleep terror disorder, 101, 103
    DSM–IV criteria for, 103
    DSM–IV differential criteria for,
        104t
    medical treatments for, 112–113
    reinforcement, desensitization,
        attention reduction for, 120
    scheduled awakenings for, 120
Sleep walking disorder, 101–102, 103
    DSM–IV criteria for, 103
    DSM–IV differential criteria for, 104t
    scheduled awakenings for, 121

Social phobia
    defined, 50
    DSM–IV criteria for, 52–53
Social stigma, negative impact on
    adherence, 219
Somatization disorder, 160
    DSM–IV criteria for, 161–162
Specific phobia
    behavioral interventions for, 73–75
    defined, 50
    DSM–IV criteria for, 52–53
Stanford Hypnotic Clinical Scale for
    Children, 190
State-Trait Anxiety Inventory for Children
    (STAI–C), 61, 63t, 64
Stereotypic movement disorders, 79–80, 81.
    See also Habit disorders
    differential diagnosis of, 83t
Stimulant medications
    in comorbid attention
        deficit/hyperactivity disorder and
        oppositional defiant disorder, 28
    increased usage of, 40
    in oppositional defiant disorder, 28
Stranger anxiety, 49
Stress/anxiety reduction, in habit reversal
    training, 93
Structural family therapy
    comparison with psychodynamic
        therapy, 34
    for oppositional defiant disorder, 33–34
        comparison with other therapies,
            33–34
        effectiveness of, 34
Systematic desensitization, for phobias, 74

T
Temperament, pain experience and,
    166–167
Temper tantrums, prevalence of, 18
Thermal biofeedback, for headache,
    193–194
Thumb sucking
    brief intervention for, 89, 90
    prevalence of, 82
Tics
    behavioral treatments for
        comparison of, 95t
    chronic and transient
        differential diagnosis of, 83, 83t, 84
    DSM–IV criteria for, 80
    defined, 79, 82

differential diagnosis of, 83, 83t, 84
habit reversal procedures for, 93–94
prevalence of, 82
severity rating scales of, 84–85
Time–in
defined, 30
for oppositional defiant disorder, 30, 31
for thumb sucking, 89
Time–out, in oppositional defiant disorder, 30
Tofranil. *See* Imipramine (Tofranil)
Toileting refusal, 124–125
DSM–IV diagnostic criteria for, 132t
Token economies
for adherence to complex regimens, 215–216
in diabetes, Type I, 216
in juvenile rheumatoid arthritis, 215–216
application of, 31–33
for behavior problems at home, 33
defined, 30
Home Chip System for, 33, 223–239
for medication adherence, 212
for oppositional defiant disorder, 30–33
populations served by, 33
for relaxation for sleep problems, 118
Tourette's syndrome
defined, 79, 80
differential diagnosis of, 83t
DSM–IV criteria for, 80
habit reversal in, 92
pharmacological intervention in, 86–87
relaxation training in, 94
tic severity in
scales for, 85
Tourette's Syndrome Clinical Global Impression Scale, 85
Tourette's Syndrome Severity Scale, 85
Treatment manuals
concerns regarding, 5–6
graduate student need for, 6
individual needs and, 6
use in research, 5
Treatments
efficacy research in, 3–4
empirically supported
advantages of, 4–5
comoribidity *versus* single diagnoses and, 6
movement for, 4

Trichotillomania (hair pulling), 81
clomipramine for, 88
cognitive–behavioral therapy for, 95–96
comparison of fluoxetine and placebo for, 87
differential diagnosis of, 83t
group habit reversal training for, 94
habit reversal procedures for, 92
hypnotherapy for, 95–96
negative practice treatment of, 94–95
prevalence of, 82
Tricyclic antidepressants
for anxiety disorders, 66
for comorbid attention deficit/hyperactivity disorder-oppositional defiant disorder, 28
for oppositional defiant disorder, 28
Trimeprazine tartrate, for sleep problems, 112

U
Urine–alarm training. *See also* Dry–bed training
bed–wetting alarms for
availability/cost of, 154, 155
for enuresis, 151, 154, 155t, 157
implementation of, 152
physician training in, 152–153

V
Valium. *See* Diazepam (Valium)
Videotaping, of habit disorders and tics, 84
Visual Analog Scale (VAS), in pain assessment, 172t, 175–177
Vitiello, B., *12*

W
White noise, for infant sleep, 119–120

X
Xanax. *See* Alprazolam (Xanax)

Y
Yale-Brown Obsessive Compulsive Scale (Y–BOCS), for tic severity rating, 85
Yale Global Tic Severity Scale (YGTSS), 85

ABOUT THE AUTHORS

Edward R. Christophersen, PhD, is professor of pediatrics at the University of Missouri at Kansas City School of Medicine and a staff psychologist at Children's Mercy Hospital in Kansas City. He received his PhD in developmental and child psychology from the University of Kansas in 1970 and held faculty appointments in pediatrics at the University of Kansas Medical Center and at the Department of Psychology and the Department of Human Development in Lawrence.

In 1984, Dr. Christophersen was elected Fellow of the Society of Clinical Psychology (Division 12) of the American Psychological Association. In 1997, he was board certified in clinical psychology by the American Board of Professional Psychology. In 1998, he was elected Honorary Fellow of the American Academy of Pediatrics for his unique and substantial contributions to child health.

Dr. Christophersen established a distinguished research and clinical program in behavioral pediatrics at the University of Kansas Medical Center, Department of Pediatrics, which he moved to the Children's Mercy Hospital in 1988. His research and clinical findings have been published in more than 150 journal articles, edited books, book chapters, and conference proceedings. He has popularized treatments that work with children in more than 300 television and radio interviews and more than 180 print interviews. He has served as a reviewer or technical advisor on many federal grant study sections and task forces, including the U.S. Preventive Services Task Force, Bright Futures (American Academy of Pediatrics), and the *Diagnostic and Statistical Manual of Mental Disorders*. He has offered more than 300 continuing education workshops and symposia at national and regional meetings for both clinical psychologists and pediatricians.

Susan L. Mortweet, PhD, is an assistant professor of pediatrics at the University of Missouri at Kansas City School of Medicine and a staff psychologist at Children's Mercy Hospital in Kansas City. She received her PhD in developmental and child psychology from the University of Kansas in 1996. Currently, Dr. Mortweet serves the Section of Developmental and Behavioral Sciences and the Section of Endocrinology at Children's Mercy Hospital. She provides the primary psychological care for children with diabetes and other endocrine disorders. Dr. Mortweet is also an active researcher in the area of diabetes education. Her publications have been in the areas of cultural diversity in the education system and effective teaching strategies for children with mild mental retardation.